9.30.77

THE CONCISE
ENCYCLOPEDIA
OF
PSYCHOLOGY
AND
PSYCHIATRY

THE CONCISE
ENCYCLOPEDIA
OF
PSYCHOLOGY
AND
PSYCHIATRY

Edited by Alice Small

FRANKLIN WATTS
NEW YORK | LONDON | 1977

Library of Congress Cataloging in Publication Data

Main entry under title:

The Concise encyclopedia of psychology and psychiatry.

Includes index.
SUMMARY: An encyclopedia of terminology, organizations, and individuals in the fields of psychology and psychiatry.
1. Psychology—Dictionaries, Juvenile. 2. Psychiatry—Dictionaries, Juvenile. [1. Psychology—Dictionaries. 2. Psychiatry—Dictionaries] I. Small, Alice Louise.
BF31.C68   150′.3   77–71180
ISBN 0–531–01332–4

Library of Congress Catalog Card Number: 77-71180

INTRODUCTION

Psychologists study how humans and animals behave as individuals and in groups. They are concerned with both mental illness and mental health. They examine physiology, emotions, intelligence, and to some extent moral and philosophical questions. The results of their efforts are having a greater impact on our lives than ever before, especially with regard to education, business, community, and personal relations.

The Concise Encyclopedia of Psychology and Psychiatry is designed to clarify the terminology, and describe the issues and current state of the field. Important people and their contributions are included, along with descriptions of such organizations as Alcoholics Anonymous, the American Psychological Association, and the World Federation for Mental Health. Sections discussing the brain, nervous system and sensations add to the reader's understanding of the physiology involved in psychology and psychiatry. Current problems such as drug addiction and juvenile delinquency are also covered in depth. Career and guidance counseling have been included. The remainder of the book outlines aspects of psychology such as abnormal, clinical, developmental, and experimental; kinds of behavior patterns such as autosuggestion and repression; and mental disorders such as autism and pathological lying.

Each major article is cross-referenced for easy research. Diagrams and an index will also assist the reader, along with the many references to articles and books for further reading.

THE CONCISE
ENCYCLOPEDIA
OF
PSYCHOLOGY
AND
PSYCHIATRY

A

ABRAHAM, KARL (1877–1925), German psychiatrist and pioneer in the development of psychoanalysis. A close associate of Sigmund Freud, he introduced psychoanalysis into Germany, analyzing patients and students (including numerous subsequently prominent practitioners). His activities made Berlin an international psychoanalytic center. Abraham's investigations dealt with the development of the libido (the primitive drives of psychoanalytic theory), the hostility of women to men, the roots of manic-depressive conditions, and other psychiatric problems.

ADLER [äd'lər], **ALFRED** (1870–1937), Viennese psychoanalyst and early associate of Freud. Adler became dissatisfied with Freud's emphasis on sexual maladjustment as the basis for neurosis. He developed the doctrine that all neuroses could be understood as an attempt to free oneself from a feeling of inferiority in order to gain a feeling of superiority. From this emerged the concepts of inferiority and superiority complexes and the school of individual psychology. Adler left Freud's group and later held the chair of medical psychology, at the Long Island University School of Medicine.

ADOLESCENCE is the period of life from the beginning of puberty to the attainment of adulthood. Popularly, this is often spoken of as the teen-age period, but strictly adolescence includes a greater length of time than is contained in the teen years. Although there are many individual differences, for girls adolescence begins at about age 12 and ends at about age 21; for boys the age range is from about 13 to about 22.

Adolescence is a period of intellectual as well as physical development. The child who has been somewhat indifferent to intellectual pursuits may show a distinct improvement as he gains experience and knowledge in many areas and as he realizes that he is preparing to enter the adult social and vocational world.

It is somewhat difficult to define intellectual ability but, in general, it involves the ability to learn, to profit from experience and deal with new situations quickly and successfully, to handle effectively those problems of life requiring abstract thinking. During the 20th century, psychologists have striven to develop tests that will measure intellectual ability. Popularly, but inaccurately, such tests are often spoken of as "I.Q. tests." Although the tests do not give perfect measures of intellectual ability, they are very helpful for practical purposes.

Tests of intellectual ability indicate that individuals ordinarily achieve their maximum scores during the late teen years or early twenties. That is, learning ability is potentially as great as it will be during the adult years of

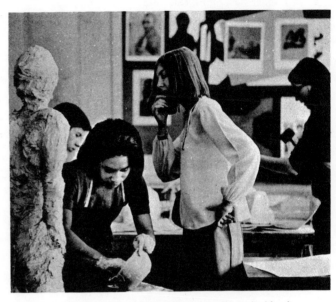

Apart from the family, school is the main focal point in the life of the teen-ager. (HAMMID—RAPHO GUILLUMETTE)

life, and adolescence can be a period of high achievement in education. Fortunately, high schools and colleges are developing special programs designed to challenge adolescent capacities, especially the capacities of individuals of superior intellectual ability.

A question often heard is: "Are girls smarter than boys?" The consensus of psychologists is that there are no true sex differences in general intellectual ability, although analyses of test scores often show that girls tend to excel in verbal items and boys tend to excel in mathematics and science. When adolescents and young adults are given equal opportunities, and when there is sufficient motivation, there seem to be no significant sex differences in either test scores or the ability to achieve success in life.

Problems of Maturing

Intelligence tests do not give the only measure of an individual's intellectual growth and development. The adolescent shows that he is achieving intellectual maturity when he can take personal responsibility, when he can think objectively and fairly about himself, when he can make up his mind without being too dependent upon the opinions of others, and when he can maintain an interest in social problems.

As the individual grows and matures, his values change. When asked to denote their life values by naming the person or persons they wish most to be like, small children

1

usually name one or both of their parents. By middle childhood and early adolescence the ideal person is usually considered to be some glamorous athlete or romantic actor. By late adolescence the ideal is likely to be a real or imagined young adult who is a composite of many desirable characteristics. Young teachers, clergymen, and youth-group leaders probably influence adolescents as much through their presence and behavior as they do through their formal teachings.

College training can contribute a great deal to the adolescent's growth of values, but colleges differ in the extent to which they touch their students' standards of behavior. On the whole, college graduates tend to be more concerned with status, achievement, and prestige than are those who have not attended college. They tend to feel more self-important, are more conservative, but are, at least on the surface, less prejudiced than individuals without college training.

Adolescence is often spoken of as a period of religious awakening. This awakening may be gradual in nature. There is a slow process of change in ideals and religious beliefs as the adolescent adjusts his standards to fit his more mature intellectual ability and personal needs. Although figures differ from one community to another, there is evidence that nearly half of the youth of high school age regularly or usually attend some kind of religious service once a week, girls being more likely to do so than boys. However, about a third of high school youth seldom or never attend religious services. (The remainder of the persons covered in this survey gave vague answers or no answer.)

Feelings of uncertainty, frustration, and conflict lead to a religious awakening in some adolescents. The inability to cope with such feelings causes other adolescents to go in the undesirable direction of delinquency. These youth compensate for their feelings by striking out against society, revolting against adult authority. They are emotionally immature but they try to appear big, tough, and superior. No single factor can be said to be the cause of

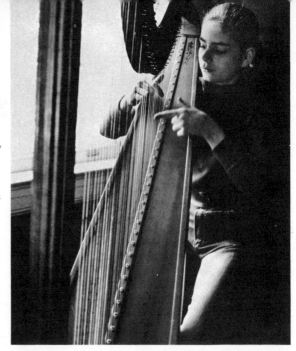

Developing talents help the adolescent acquire a sense of being an individual. (ESTHER BUBLEY)

delinquency, and delinquents come from all kinds of home and community backgrounds. However, various studies have reported characteristics frequently found among delinquents. They frequently come from homes broken by divorce or in which there is little affection and understanding. Their parents have tended to be either too harsh or too lax in disciplinary measures. They often live in rundown areas of cities near business or manufacturing sections. Most delinquents are normal or near-normal in intellectual ability, but they are likely to have unsatisfactory school records. Poverty is not itself a cause of delinquency, but feelings of frustration and inferiority growing out of inadequate income may lead to delinquency.

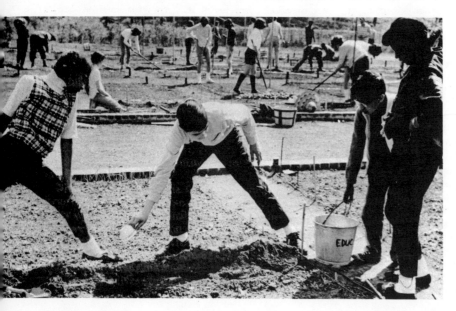

A group of city students at work on an agricultural project. The expanding interests of the adolescent can be channeled into projects that broaden both his education and social relationships. (HAMMID—RAPHO GUILLUMETTE)

Every adolescent encounters frustration; he is made to feel his inadequacies in many situations, and all too often he feels that adult society is threatening him. In order to grow into a truly mature person, the adolescent must develop social maturity. He must master those social techniques that will enable him to get along comfortably with other adults and feel that he is an integral part of a number of social groups. The adolescent must develop emotional maturity. He must learn to restrain explosive behavior such as "flying off the handle" or having adult-size temper tantrums. He must learn to stand on his own feet but without loss of love for his parents. He must leave behind the normal self-love of childhood and attain a love that includes affection for children, friendship with close and casual acquaintances, and a feeling of brotherhood for mankind. He must learn to wait for rewards and satisfactions rather than demanding immediate recognition or pleasure. He must achieve the ability to tolerate, if necessary, personal inconveniences and even discomforts in order to bring happiness to others.

A mature approach to emotional problems is essential. If not controlled, emotional tensions may result in sleep disturbances, chronic fatigue, loss of appetite, digestive disturbances, inability to concentrate, irritability, moodiness, and touchiness (oversensitivity to criticism and reprimands). But while the adolescent must learn to control his emotional behavior, this does not mean that he should try to suppress all such behavior. Adolescence should be a time of enthusiasm, activity, and enjoyment of life. Strong feelings such as fears, angers, and loves can provide useful motivation. Control rather than elimination of emotional behavior is the goal.

Relations With Parents

It is not uncommon for strained relationships to develop between an adolescent and his parents. In his apparent eagerness to achieve adult status, the young person may resent any restrictions placed upon him. Oftentimes he is not willing to admit, even to himself, that he has doubts and fears about taking on adult responsibilities and freedom. The adolescent may say that his parents are over-anxious and overprotective whereas, though not aware of it, he is projecting his own anxiety into them. For their part the parents have for years taken the responsibility of caring for the child and it is difficult for them to shift the responsibility to his shoulders, especially as they realize his lack of experience in dealing with personal and social problems. Furthermore, and again without being aware of it, the parents may try to think of their adolescents as young children because to admit that their children are becoming adult is to admit the unpleasant fact that they themselves are now middle-aged or older. Frank talks between an adolescent and his parents often reveal that the adolescent is basically willing to rely on his parents for protection in many situations. The parents often reveal that they are basically willing to give the adolescent more freedom than he realizes.

Psychologists emphasize the importance of psychological weaning, sometimes referred to as emancipation. This is the process of outgrowing family domination, of working toward the time when the adolescent will establish his own home. Acute nostalgia, or homesickness, is

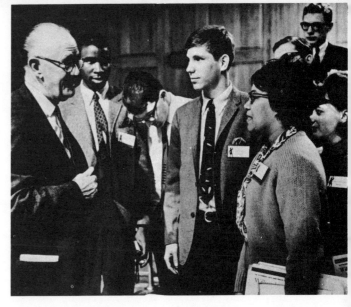

Delegates to a youth congress gain new perspectives as they question a government representative. (AUTHENTICATED NEWS SERVICE)

Team sports use up some of the exuberant energy typical of the teen-ager. (AUTHENTICATED NEWS SERVICE)

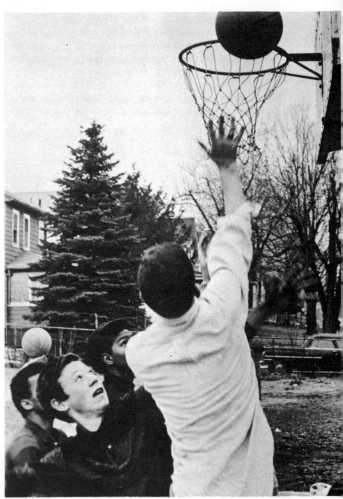

3

one indication of incomplete weaning. Just as the baby, for his own good, must be biologically weaned in infancy, so the adolescent must be psychologically weaned as he approaches adulthood. When the adolescent becomes psychologically weaned he does not cease to love his parents and they do not cease to love him; there is simply a changing and deepening of the relationship.

Parents differ greatly in their attitudes toward control of their adolescent children. Some parents tend to dominate their children by exercising a great deal of authority and by being very strict. Their children tend to grow up to be dependable, honest, good citizens but somewhat submissive, shy, retiring, and docile. Other parents tend to be quite submissive. They give their adolescent children a great deal of freedom and indulge them in many ways. As they grow up, these children tend to be aggressive, independent, and self-confident but somewhat stubborn, antagonistic, and careless. Between these two extremes are the many parents who accept their children for what they are and make child-rearing one of their jobs in life. They exert control, but with sympathy and understanding. They participate in the activities of their children and are interested in their play and work. Studies have indicated that children coming to maturity in such homes tend to be well adjusted, cheerful, and emotionally stable.

Dating and Sex

An area of great concern to young people and their parents involves dating and sex. As to dating, some parents are stricter than others, but the usual pattern in the United States allows considerable freedom to arrange dates and go on dates without chaperons. In other parts of the world, parents regulate the social activities of their children far more strictly.

Nearly half the boys and over half the girls in the United States have had some dates by the time they enter high school. Rather frequent dating has become the rule rather than the exception by the time adolescents are juniors and seniors in high school. High school girls, and especially seniors, date more than do high school boys. They often date with older boys who are out of high school.

Dating serves a number of important functions: it gives valuable experience in learning to adjust to other persons; it develops social poise; it provides opportunities for social life which might not be available otherwise; it tends to build up one's prestige with his peers. Social adjustment in dating is less difficult for those adolescents who from an early age have had frequent and normal social relationships with members of the other sex. Parents, schools, and churches can do much to promote such wholesome relationships.

"Going steady" is a fairly common practice which parents frequently believe to be more serious than is actually the case. Young people often look at the practice as little more than a matter of convenience and an insurance that company will be available for dances and parties. A boy and girl may go steady for only two or three weeks and then change to other partners, although it is true that the relationship may go on for months and lead to thoughts of marriage. The boy and girl going steady are more or less "out of circulation" to other adolescents.

Relationships between boys and girls can involve serious emotional and behavioral problems. Many of the sex problems of adolescents could be lessened if young people were given sufficient and suitable instruction well in advance of the time when sex is an immediate problem for them. Surveys have indicated that for most children the primary source of information about sex is their companions rather than their homes, although other surveys report that adolescents consider the most desirable source of information to be their parents and other adults in the home. Girls are more likely than boys to receive sex instruction in the home. Sex instruction from companions is likely to be incomplete, incorrect, and even sordid.

Education and Career Planning

A major task in the adolescent years is planning for education and a career. In some countries, a person's vocation is determined entirely or largely by the social group into which he is born. In other countries, governmental agencies tend to dictate the kind of work a man or woman will be permitted to do. In those countries in which there is freedom of vocational choice, the adolescent has both the privilege and the responsibility of making a decision concerning his life work and the training that will be needed for it.

Oftentimes the adolescent has not had sufficient experience to enable him to make a wise choice. Fortunately, many high schools have guidance programs. Special courses enable the adolescent to survey the world of work, and various tests are administered to help him assess his interests and abilities. However, no battery of tests can guarantee a wise vocational choice. Individual guidance by well-trained counselors is also needed, and the final choice must be made by the adolescent himself, using all available counsel and information.

Often parents are able to give valuable assistance in career and educational planning, but sometimes parents are unduly swayed by their personal ambitions, rather than by what is best for their children. They may insist that the sons enter the occupational field that has been followed in the family for generations. They may put undue pressure on their children to enter a profession or other line of work which the parents consider to stand high on the social and economic ladder. A father sometimes insists that his son go to the college he attended.

To make a satisfactory vocational choice a person should (1) study his interests, capacities, and abilities; (2) survey the fields of work that are open to him; and (3) select a job that matches his qualifications. He should avoid such common mistakes as picking a field solely because it seems to offer glamour, adventure, or social prestige, rushing into a "job of the future" without careful investigation of the training needed and the actual prospects, or being unduly influenced by a relative or friend.

The choice of a career often controls plans for education. If a technician's job is desired, for example, training may be obtained in a vocational-technical school. Public and private junior and community colleges provide vocational training. There are many possibilities for pre-job and on-the-job training. Information can be obtained from such sources as industries, school guidance offices, colleges, and state employment offices.

For some careers four or more years of college study are

required. Before applying to a college or university the prospective student should make sure that the institution offers all the courses he will need and that it is accredited by educational and professional agencies. It is worth noting that many colleges and universities provide off-campus centers which the student may attend while living at home. They may offer correspondence courses and courses conducted by television.

See also:

AGGRESSION, in psychology, a hostile act, or more generally, a self-assertive action. Aggression can be shown to exist in almost all animal species and may be of two kinds: aggression directed toward animals of a different species (interspecific aggression) and toward animals of the same species (intraspecific aggression). Because of its implications in law and psychiatry, and its relevance to the occurrence of warfare, the latter has been the main subject of recent research. There are two main schools of thought in the research concerning intraspecific aggression. One considers aggression a reaction to stimulation from the external environment. The other holds that aggression is part of the organism's innate drive structure.

Scientists of the first viewpoint have attempted to show that frustration leads to aggression. In man, aggressive tendencies would be kept in check by teaching young children how to inhibit overt expressions of rage. Evidence for this frustration-aggression theory has been obtained in animal experiments. J. P. Scott showed that some animals have to be taught to fight, and that one can diminish the fighting disposition by not exposing the animal to fighting.

Scientists representing the other viewpoint attribute a positive role to aggression. While agreeing that acts of aggression are influenced by learning, they point out that the disposition to fighting and many of the motor patterns used in aggression are innate. Complete adult fighting behavior can be elicited in animals raised in isolation, even at their first exposure to animals of the same species (conspecifics). It has also been shown in many animal species that electrical stimulation of specific parts of the brain elicits complete sequences of aggressive behavior.

Like other instincts, aggression has meaning for the process of evolution. K. Z. Lorenz has reviewed different aspects of aggression for their survival value to the individual, the group, and the species. Obvious roles of aggressive behavior appear in establishing and defending a territory, selection of mates in breeding, defense of the

The attacking and the friendship gestures of a gander differ only in that in the attack (2) he faces the adversary, while he approaches his mate from the side in friendship (6).
(SLIGHTLY CHANGED, WITH PERMISSION FROM K. Z. LORENZ, ON AGGRESSION)

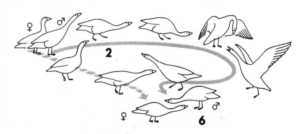

INTRASPECIFIC AGGRESSION				
MANNER OF EXPRESSION	**APPEARANCE AND FORM**		**PURPOSE AND VALUE TO BOTH MEN AND ANIMALS**	
	MAN	ANIMAL	FOR THE INDIVIDUAL	FOR THE GROUP
OVERT AGGRESSION	Fight, Flight		SURVIVAL	
			establishment of territory, selection of mate, etc.	establishment of dominance hierarchy
	INTERGROUP FIGHTING		identification with group	maintenance of group
	War		in modern war, fighting may serve little purpose, since weapons have removed the inhibition man has against killing man, his conspecific	
REDIRECTED AGGRESSION	RITUALIZED BEHAVIOR		DISPLAY OF INTENT	
	greeting rituals	such as a gander running with head and neck held low	upon seeing the display, the other gander may choose flight, rather than engage the initiator (maintenance of territory, dominance hierarchy, etc.)	to the mate, the behavior signifies friendship, communication is served, thereby forging social bonds and other relationships
	DISPLACEMENT BEHAVIOR humor, sport, grooming, etc.		release of tension	intergroup fusion
	Sublimation: hard work, etc.		productivity (creative)	culture and economic welfare
	Suppressed or Repressed: may result in behavior abnormalities, mental illness, suicide		avoidance of useless violence and rage	processes of education and socialization

young, and establishing a dominance hierarchy to facilitate group living. Lorenz emphasizes, however, the function of ritualized fighting. In many animals, acts of friendship and love use the same behavioral units as those which occur in fighting.

Lorenz also points out that aggressive animals in nature, such as wolves, have developed behavior patterns which prevent a fight from getting out of hand by a show of submission from the losing animal. Such a behavior pattern effectively prohibits the winning animal from continuing the fight. In normally peaceful animals, such as doves, no such behavior pattern exists. Once doves start fighting in a place where they cannot avoid each other, such as a cage, they fight to the death. Man has the age-old notion of chivalry and fair play that may inhibit his killing an enemy who has surrendered. In modern war, however, one rarely sees the adversary.

The table attempts to summarize the many forms aggression may take. Most important is the role of redirected aggression and the communicative function of aggression. Displacement occurs when the animal in an aggressive state switches into another activity pattern, such as the cat suddenly interrupting a fight to clean himself, seemingly ignoring his antagonist. Redirected aggression in man may appear in forms described in psychoanalysis, such as defense mechanisms, and sublimation. Although there are indications that animals have a sense of humor and play, it is especially in man that these displacement activities are consciously used to relieve aggressive tendencies. Sports are valuable in reducing intergroup hostility. Long-lasting friendship between individuals, cities, and nations can grow from international sports competitions, such as the Olympic games.

An exposition of the two main theories of aggression appear in *The Natural History of Aggression* by J. D. Carthy and F. J. Ebling (1964). They present the arguments of proponents of the frustration-aggression theory, based mainly on inferences from human behavior and laboratory studies. They also give the viewpoints of students of naturally occurring animal behavior. It is clear that both viewpoints will be needed in a full explanation of aggression, since all behavior has both innate and learned aspects. Since these aspects are not simply separable, in the development of a particular behavior pattern, future studies will have to reconcile both points of view.

Psychology in general, and the understanding of human nature in particular, will benefit from deepened insight into the aggressive drive, analogous to the benefit derived from study of the sex drive, as furthered by psychoanalysis.

See also DOMINANCE HIERARCHY; ETHOLOGY; FRUSTRATION; PSYCHOANALYSIS.

ALCOHOLIC PSYCHOSES, mental disorders resulting from prolonged use of alcohol. Certain individuals are prone to a form of alcoholic psychosis called pathological intoxication. This transitory mental state represents a violent reaction to alcohol, different from ordinary drunkenness. Pathological intoxication may be considered a form of psychomotor epilepsy evoked by the alcohol.

Pathological intoxication occurs only in certain individuals. Prolonged excessive use of alcohol can result

generally in more extended psychotic states. Delirium tremens, a state of weakness, tremors, and impaired interpersonal functioning, is often caused by the sudden withdrawal of alcohol from a habitually heavy drinker. Typical symptoms are terrifying visual hallucinations of small animals or men engaged in odd activities. A patient suffering from the psychosis called acute alcoholic hallucinosis complains of hearing threatening voices, often accusing him of homosexual practices.

Chronic use of alcohol may lead to nutritional and vitamin deficiencies, resulting in psychotic and debilitating states. Alcoholic paranoia is characterized by delusions of jealously and infidelity. Other nutritionally linked alcoholic psychoses are Korsakoff's psychosis, with memory defects, and alcoholic deterioration, in which brain and nerve functions are gradually impaired.
See also ALCOHOLISM; PSYCHOSIS.

ALCOHOLICS ANONYMOUS (A.A.), organization to promote recovery from alcoholism through self-help and the help of former alcoholics. Organized in 1934, Alcoholics Anonymous grew out of the efforts of two men, identified only as Bill W., and Dr. Bob S., to conquer their own drinking problems and to use their experiences for the benefit of others similarly distressed. In 1961 A.A.'s total membership was estimated at 300,000. Within the organization there are autonomous local groups; some hospital and prison groups; internationalists (seamen); and "loners," members not associated with local groups. Alcoholics Anonymous stresses a belief in spiritual values as the way toward cure. The only membership requirement is a desire to stop drinking, and the tradition of anonymity reassures potential members who might fear exposure. National headquarters are in New York City.

ALCOHOLISM, a dependence on alcoholic beverages that causes a deterioration in the physical and mental health of the individual and interferes with his economic and social life. The alcoholic is a compulsive drinker and although he may be aware of the destructive nature of his habit, he is unable to control it.

The addiction to alcohol begins gradually. The earliest sign is the tendency to drink to relieve tension. This is followed by drinking in private, "gulping" drinks, and frequent blackouts. The crucial phase appears when the alcoholic loses control of his drinking and begins to make excuses for his erratic behavior. He becomes aggressive, hoards drinks, neglects eating, and takes regular morning drinks. From this point he may slip into prolonged bouts and is well on the way to developing severer symptoms, such as tremors and impairment of thinking.

Although it was once thought that alcoholism was inherited or in some way caused by physical factors, most present-day psychiatrists emphasize psychological and social factors as causes of the disease. There is some evidence, however, that inherited deficiencies of body chemistry may also be involved.

Alcoholism and Family Life. According to many authorities, alcoholism has its origins in a disturbed family situation in which the mother is typically overprotective and indulgent. As a result the youngster makes excessive demands for emotional contact that are doomed to frustration, especially when he begins to function in the world outside of the home. The pattern persists into adult life. The alcoholic becomes disappointed in and enraged at persons who fail to accede to his demands. He expresses his anger in various ways that leave him with guilt feelings. The guilt leads to depression, and finally relief may be sought through alcohol.

This pattern of childhood experiences applies to other psychiatric disturbances as well and need not lead inevitably to alcoholism. The choice of alcohol as a means of relieving the tensions and frustrations may be influenced by an alcoholic father or by an environment in which social drinking is common. Alcoholism is much less likely to develop in a teetotal culture, such as that of the Quakers.

The Personality of the Alcoholic. The question is often raised whether there may not be certain characteristics that are shared in common by all alcoholics. Most studies have been unsuccessful in disclosing any consistent personality pattern. However, extensive research conducted at the State University of New York College of Medicine has revealed five characteristics that seem to be regularly present in alcoholics:

(1) Schizoid features. Beneath the usual façade of friendliness and sociability there is a deep-seated distrust and an emotional detachment from people. This is found to be associated with a self-centered attitude and immature thinking.

(2) Depression. This may not be apparent as such and may take the form of boredom or loneliness. It may be masked by joviality. Suicidal thoughts are frequent.

(3) Dependency. Like an infant, the alcoholic is demanding; he looks to others to fulfill his needs and feels that he has no control over what happens to him.

(4) Hostility. The alcoholic is frequently aggressive toward parents and others who have frustrated his demands.

(5) Sexual immaturity. Among men there are frequent doubts about one's masculinity. Homosexuality may be a feature.

Physiology and Pathology. Ethyl alcohol, the active ingredient in alcoholic beverages, produces exhilaration in small dosages (blood levels of 100–200 mg./cc.), depression and severe loss of muscular co-ordination with blood levels of 200–300 mg., and, frequently, interference with breathing, and death, if the blood level exceeds 500 mg.

Approximately one-fourth of all alcoholics develop medical problems, such as cirrhosis of the liver, pellagra (a nutritional deficiency), and gastritis. Disorders of the nervous system also are common. Since alcoholics invariably suffer from nutritional deficiencies, because of poor eating habits, there is considerable doubt as to how much of the observed tissue damage can be ascribed to the alcohol itself.

Treatment. Acute intoxication (drunkenness) usually does not require treatment, except when shock develops. In such cases immediate hospital care is necessary. Alcoholism itself presents a far more serious challenge. Three widely differing approaches are worthy of mention:

(1) Antabuse, a drug that makes alcoholic drinking unpleasant, if not impossible; even a small amount of alcohol produces vomiting and palpitations. Antabuse must be taken daily if it is to be effective.

(2) Alcoholics Anonymous, an organization in which former alcoholics actively help those fighting the addiction. They may, for example, intercept a backsliding member who has set off on a tour of the bars.

(3) Psychotherapy, which attempts to help the alcoholic discover the unconscious conflicts that drive him to drinking. This is the only approach that attempts to deal with the actual source of the problem. It may be applied on an individual or a group basis.

Alcoholism as a Social Problem. Estimates indicate that there are more than 4½ million alcoholics in the United States, which thus outranks all other countries by a substantial margin. Eighty-five percent of these are males, though the number of female alcoholics is on the increase. The severe social impact of this affliction results from its crippling effect on family life and upon the economic productivity of the individual.

Alcoholism is also a major problem in some European countries. In recognition of these facts the World Health Organization has set up committees to study the problem and to make recommendations for dealing with it.

See also ALCOHOLICS ANONYMOUS; DELIRIUM TREMENS.

ALLPORT, GORDON WILLARD (1897–1967), American psychologist. As a personality theorist, Allport focused on the uniqueness of the individual and the importance of consciousness. He considered that unconscious factors in the individual's past, as they are elaborated in psychoanalysis, are of great importance primarily in disordered and abnormal behavior. To understand the "functional autonomy" of normal behavior one must look at the individual in an "action setting," away from laboratory or consulting room.

Allport's interest in social conflict led him to his work on *The nature of Prejudice* (1954), a landmark in the development of a comprehensive theory of personality. His theories regarding the development of the ego include the kernel concept of "functional autonomy." This refers to the observable phenomenon that a behavior pattern or activity may become an end in itself. Such a pattern may persist even when there is no further need for it in the life of the individual, acquiring a significance of its own. Many of Allport's ideas have been severly criticized, but his work has had great influence on current psychological thinking.

AMBIVALENCE [ăm-bĭv'ə-ləns], psychiatric term used to describe opposed feelings toward a single person. A common form of ambivalence involves feelings of love and hate toward a member of the family. Hatred toward a parent or other close person is usually intolerable to the conscious mind and is consequently repressed. Frequently this repressed hatred is projected so that the ambivalent person regards himself as the object of hostile feelings held by the other person.

See also PSYCHOANALYSIS; PSYCHOTHERAPY.

AMERICAN PSYCHOLOGICAL ASSOCIATION, INC., major professional organization in the field of psychology in the United States, founded in 1892. It furthers its purpose—"to advance psychology as a science and as a means of promoting human welfare"—by holding annual meetings, publishing 12 journals of psychology, and working toward improved standards for psychological research, training, and service. In an increasing number of states a certificate or license is required for the practice of psychology. Policies for certification are set by the association. The association is a source of information on the profession, on licensing requirements, and on universities having approved graduate courses. A central office is maintained in Washington, D.C.

AMNESIA [ăm-nē'zhə], loss of memory. It may result from disease of, or injury to, the brain (organic amnesia) or may occur as a complication of certain personality disorders (psychogenic amnesia). Organic amnesia may appear during old age, or in cases of alcoholism, concussion, or stroke. In a chronic condition such as cerebral arteriosclerosis, which involves narrowing of the blood vessels of the brain, amnesia develops slowly, and memory of certain recent and remote events may be permanently lost In cases of acute alcoholism and in cases of minor injury to the brain, amnesia is more likely to be temporary. Brain injury may produce distinctive types of amnesia. A boxer may be injured in the early rounds of a bout and continue fighting, unaware of the events following his injury (anterograde amnesia), or he may forget the events that immediately preceded it (retrograde amnesia).

Psychogenic amnesia is most often a symptom of a personality disorder, and appears most frequently in highly emotional persons of a hysterical type (see HYSTERIA). Painful memories may become dissociated, or detached, during periods of great nervous tension. Amnesia of this type, usually limited to specific memories, both appears and vanishes suddenly. In extreme cases the tendency of parts of the personality to become detached from consciousness may be so strong that the individual assumes a second personality: he changes identity and is unable to recall his name, address, family, and all other facts concerning his everyday self.

ANGELL [ān'jəl], **JAMES ROWLAND** (1869–1949), American educator and psychologist. Born in Vermont, the son of James Burrill Angell, he was educated at the University of Michigan, at Harvard, and in Europe. After teaching philosophy at the University of Minnesota he moved in 1894 to the University of Chicago, where he served for many years as professor of psychology and was acting president in 1918–19. One of the founders of the functionalist school of psychology, he was president of the American Psychological Association in 1906. As president of Yale University from 1921 to 1937 he greatly increased the facilities of that institution. His books include *Psychology* (1904) and *American Education* (1937).
See also FUNCTIONAL PSYCHOLOGY.

ANOREXIA NERVOSA [ăn-ə-rĕk'sē-ə nĕr-vō'sə], uncommon neurotic disorder characterized by a persistent lack of appetite associated with disgust for food. It occurs mainly in sensitive, young, unmarried women. Frequently menstruation ceases, and constipation, falling of the hair, vomiting, and extreme emaciation may occur. There is often a previous history of overeating and concern about being overweight. Disturbed mother-daughter relation-

ships and rivalry for parental favor with brothers or sisters are also frequent background factors. Treatment by psychotherapy is indicated.

ANXIETY, in psychiatric usage, an emotional reaction of fear, in which there is usually no clear, visible source of danger. The concept of anxiety forms a central part of psychoanalytic theory. Neurosis is thought to be the outcome of subconscious attempts by the individual to master anxiety. Sigmund Freud specified a number of situations that he regarded as the chief sources of anxiety. These arise in infancy and childhood, and form a basis for anxiety in adult life. An early anxiety-producing situation is the absence of the mother, whose assistance is needed for the satisfaction of the infant's wishes. Others are the possibility of the loss of parental love and the fear of castration. Later, the superego, or conscience, develops, and an anxiety-producing situation arises whenever the conscience threatens to flood the mind with guilt.

According to Freud, anxiety arises when the subconscious perceives the possibility of the emergence of one of these dangers. Thus a child may become anxious as a reaction to an unconscious desire to strike or injure his parents, for this action might result in a loss of parental love. The neuroses develop when defense mechanisms are used to protect the individual from the distressing effects of anxiety. The hostile child may become excessively nice to his parents (reaction formation), or he may say that his brother wants to hit his parents (projection). In adult life, a woman who hates her mother, but who cannot tolerate the possible loss of parental love, may hate instead a second person (displacement). The defense mechanisms constitute the symptoms of neurosis and are effective insofar as the person does not experience anxiety. If the defense mechanisms fail, the anxiety emerges into consciousness and the individual suffers from free-floating anxiety. He becomes depressed, irritable, and unhappy, without knowing why. In its extreme forms this is termed an anxiety reaction and typically affects timid, overconscientious individuals who attempt to live up to severe, self-imposed standards of achievement.

The victim of the anxiety reaction experiences great difficulty in sleeping and may suffer from severe attacks of rapid pulse, sweating, nausea, pain in the chest, and palpitations. Anxiety reactions often develop into phobic reactions in which the anxiety becomes attached to specific objects and situations (see PHOBIA). Tranquilizers are useful in controlling the physical symptoms of the anxiety reaction but psychotherapy is required to treat the deeplying causes.
See also PSYCHOANALYSIS; REPRESSION.

APHASIA [ə-fā'zhə], disturbance of language functions resulting from injury to, or disease of, certain parts of the brain. The nature of the disturbance depends upon the exact region of the brain in which the disease or injury occurs. Three major types of aphasia are:

Expressive Aphasia: Inability to communicate thoughts through speech, writing, or gestures. The individual knows what he wishes to say, but finds difficulty in expressing his ideas.

Receptive Aphasia: Inability to recognize words pronounced by others (word deafness) or written (word blindness), although. these words were familiar prior to the illness.

Amnestic or Nominal Aphasia: Difficulty in finding the right name for a familiar object.

These difficulties sometimes improve without treatment as the brain damage that caused them heals. Other cases require help through remedial training. True aphasia should be distinguished from the language problems that appear in the mentally retarded, and from physical disturbances of the tongue, the larynx, or other parts of the vocal apparatus.

APTITUDE TESTS. In its original meaning, the term "aptitude test" was intended to refer to an instrument measuring some native ability (particularly a capacity to learn in a certain field) existing prior to any environmental influence. Subsequent research has shown clearly that there are few, if any, broad aptitudes, such as clerical aptitude or mechanical aptitude, that are not composed of other elements of ability. Moreover, aptitudes are likely to be greatly modified by experience and training. Possible exceptions may be aptitude in certain areas of music and art as expressed colloquially by such phrases as "a good ear for music." The building stones of native ability seem to be much more specific than was once thought, and they may be combined in any individual in an infinite number of ways.

See also TESTING, PSYCHOLOGICAL AND EDUCATIONAL; VOCATIONAL GUIDANCE.

ARCHETYPE, in Plato's philosophy, the perfect or absolute idea of an object. In the psychology of Carl Jung, the word has a special meaning as part of the collective un conscious.

Jung was impressed by the recurrence of certain characteristic images in dreams, fairy stories, and myths in all cultures, during all periods of history. He explained the universality of these images by postulating that they reveal certain universally inherited structures of mind. We inherit the potential to experience anew the experiences of prior generations. These potentials are given to us in the form of special predispositions. The archetypes are the potential experiences of birth, rebirth, death, power, unity, hero, child, mother, earth, the wise old man, and so on. Works of art, dreams, myths, and rites contain archetypal material. In the signs and symptoms of mental illness, in addition to the symbolization of individual psychologic material, archetypes may figure prominently.

See also SUBCONSCIOUS AND UNCONSCIOUS.

ASSOCIATION OF IDEAS, the basis of a philosophical doctrine concerning the nature of mind. Ideas, which arise primarily through sensory experience, are the irreducible elements of mind, and lawfully developed connections or associations among them account for all mental phenomena. The primary principle of association is *contiguity* (nearness in space or time). Thus, the ideas of "bigness" and "heaviness" seem to go together because they are often given rise to contiguously.

This speculative psychology, which was developed largely by the British Associationists of the 18th and 19th centuries, directly influenced the scientific psychology of the late 19th century. Association Psychology is the name given to the theory that stimuli and responses become associated. Again contiguity, now between stimulus and response, is seen necessary to the formation of associations. This approach supposedly permits indirect study of mental phenomena, while avoiding problems inherent in introspection.

See also FACULTY PSYCHOLOGY; INTROSPECTIVE PSYCHOLOGY; PSYCHOLOGY.

AUTISM [ô′tĭz-əm], the tendency to see the world in terms of one's own needs and wishes. An example of autistic thinking may be seen in the fantasies of children, who populate their world with imaginary creatures and objects. Autism in adults, when carried to extremes, becomes the type familiarly seen in mental illness. The mental patient who thinks he is Napoleon, and expects deference from others, is distorting reality in terms of his own desires. Autism in mental disease is most frequently associated with schizophrenia.

See also SCHIZOPHRENIA.

AUTOSUGGESTION, self-stimulation (such as "talking to oneself," or thinking about particular situations or events). It has the apparent effect of producing behavior changes or experiences for which the normally appropriate physical realities are absent. Autosuggestion can also seem to negate the normal effect of certain physical realities. Thus, for example, preoccupation with the possibility of seasickness may lead to illness regardless of the extent of a boat's motion; or one might in this way "see" ghosts in a cemetery, or "see" an oasis in a barren desert. But also, a soldier might apparently enjoy a tasty meal while dining on field rations, or withstand great pain (apparently "denying" its reality) during field surgery. Autosuggestion may or may not appear intentional.

B

BARBITURATES [băr-bǐch'ə-rǐts, băr-bǐ-tūr'ǐts], group of drugs used principally as sedatives and to induce sleep. The first barbiturate (Veronal, or barbital) was synthesized in 1903. Since then over 2,500 barbiturates have been prepared and clinically studied, and about 50 have been placed on the market.

The barbiturates produce their effects by depressing the activity of the brain and spinal cord. The individual drugs differ in the duration of their action. The effects of the longer-acting drugs, such as phenobarbital, may last for over six hours, while the action of the shorter-acting drugs, such as pentobarbital, may last for less than three hours. Comparatively small doses are used for sedation in cases of anxiety, nervousness, and hyperthyroidism. Larger doses are given to induce sleep. Patients who have difficulty in falling asleep are given short-acting barbiturates, while those who tend to wake repeatedly during the night may be given the longer-acting type. Barbiturates are often given before surgery, and are occasionally used to produce anesthesia. Psychiatrists have employed these drugs to produce a state of deep sedation and relaxation in which a variety of neurotic conditions can be diagnosed and treated (narcoanalysis).

Barbiturates tend to augment the action of certain pain-relieving drugs (analgesics), and are included in some commercial preparations for this purpose.

A serious addiction can develop from the unsupervised use of barbiturates. Acute barbiturate poisoning has occurred accidentally, but has more frequently resulted from attempts at suicide. As a consequence of the potential danger of their use, many states have passed laws forbidding the retail sale of barbiturates without a prescription.

BEDLAM (ST. MARY OF BETHLEHEM HOSPITAL), the first institution for the mentally ill erected in England. Inmates are believed to have been accepted at the end of the 14th century. In the course of time this institution became notorious for its brutality toward the insane. Until around 1770 patients were kept in chains and irons, and visitors were permitted to obtain amusement from their antics. The term "bedlam" subsequently became associated with any scene of general disorder and confusion and as such has become part of the English language.

BED-WETTING or ENURESIS, the involuntary passage of urine during sleep by individuals who are beyond the age when control should have been established. Some children may have voluntary control of urination after 18 months of age, but most achieve full control by the age of 4. Bed-wetting may persist from childhood or follow an interval of successful training. Physical causes are sometimes responsible, but the vast majority of cases result from emotional disturbances. Too early or too vigorous toilet training may produce frustration and guilt, and urination may become the focus of a power struggle between parent and child. Night control is often unsuccessful and the child uses bed-wetting to express his hostility toward his parents.

Enuresis that develops after control has been established is viewed as a return to an earlier mode of dealing with problems. This may be brought on by situations that threaten the security of the child, such as moving to a new home, the birth of a brother or sister, separation from the parents, or efforts to stop thumb-sucking.

Treatment is directed at establishing a secure parent-child relationship in which understanding replaces punishment. Encouraging urination prior to retiring and restricting the consumption of water may help. If bed-wetting persists and is accompanied by other symptoms a psychiatrist should be consulted.

BEERS, CLIFFORD WHITTINGHAM (1876–1943), American humanitarian, founder of the mental hygiene movement. His experiences as a patient in a mental hospital (1900–3) moved him to inform the public about the injustices perpetrated on the mentally ill. His autobiography, *A Mind that Found Itself* (1908), told of his illness and treatment. He founded the first community mental health association, the Connecticut Society for Mental Hygiene, in 1908. He also organized the National Commission for Mental Hygiene (1909), the American Foundation for Mental Hygiene (1928), and the International Foundation for Mental Hygiene (1931).

BEHAVIOR DISORDER. *See* SOCIOPATHIC PERSONALITY.

BEHAVIORISM, the view that the only suitable subject of study for a science of psychology is observable behavior itself. In this view, consciousness, memory, imagery, and the like are unobservable and private, and must be left outside the field of psychology as a natural science.

In its best-known form, as developed by John B. Watson, beginning in 1913, behaviorism was a radical position presented in rebellion against introspective psychology. Behaviorists of that time took classical conditioning as the basic pattern of learning, and considered genetic inheritance relatively unimportant in determining the behavior of an individual. The phenomena under study were not those of consciousness or the mind, but rather those of overt behavior.

Most 20th-century psychological theories (particularly learning theory) reflect the influence of behaviorism both in their emphasis on "responses" as basic data, and in the cautious use by theorists of unobservable factors like drive and habit strength as explanatory devices. Thus neo-behaviorism and behavior theory are common contemporary terms of reference, even though the radical behaviorism of Watson has been essentially rejected. In its place has developed a behaviorism that retains the core of Watson's view (that only observable or objectively measurable phenomena can be granted status in a science), but that is strengthened by the sophistication of positivism and operationism; these provide what was absent in early forms of behaviorism, namely, a useful and meaningful definition of behavior.

See also CONDITIONING; INTROSPECTIVE PSYCHOLOGY; LEARNING; PSYCHOLOGY.

BEKHTEREV [byāκн'tyĭ-ryəf], **VLADIMIR MIKHAILOVICH** (1857–1927), Russian physiologist and neurologist. His work on reflexes was the basis for a theory of all human behavior which he called "reflexology." His system reduced all psychological processes to physiological terms through the use of the conditioned response. This point of view, supported by clinical and experimental research, brought him acknowledgment from American experimental psychologists of the behaviorist school. He founded an institute in St. Petersburg (1907) for psychophysiological research. His books include *General Principles of Human Reflexology* (1904) and *Objective Psychology* (1913).

BENZEDRINE [běn'zə-drēn] **or AMPHETAMINE,** drug with potent stimulatory effects on both the central nervous system and the peripheral (sympathetic) nerve network. Because at one time it was marketed as an ingredient of nasal inhalants, available without prescription, it has been subjected to much abuse by thrill-seekers and drug addicts. Amphetamine and the related compounds dextro amphetamine (Dexedrine) and methamphetamine cause nervousness, alertness, a temporary sensation of elation, and a false sense of increased ability at such tasks as arithmetic, writing, and memorizing. By objective tests, the individual's performance is usually below his best while the drug's influence lasts. Physiologically, it increases pulse rate, blood pressure, and excitability.

It is used by physicians to treat coma resulting from an overdose of sedatives and in certain forms of epilepsy (narcolepsy). Amphetamine is also used to decrease appetite in weight-reduction programs. Appetite loss probably results from dulling the sense of taste and smell and by central brain action. Continued use of the drug may cause true addiction. A few doses can produce feelings of fatigue without the ability to sleep. After frequent repeated doses, severe weight loss, irritability, agitation, tremors, and hallucinations often occur.

Amphetamine addiction is a serious illness. Withdrawal of the drug has severe effects on the brain, cardiovascular system, and peripheral nerves. Its continued use must be considered as serious as narcotic addiction.

BERGSON [běrg-sôN', Angl. bûrg'sən], **HENRI LOUIS** (1859–1941), French philosopher. Born in Paris, he studied at the École Normale Supérieure from 1878 to 1881, then taught school for a time. His doctoral thesis appeared in 1889, translated as *Time and Free Will* (1910).

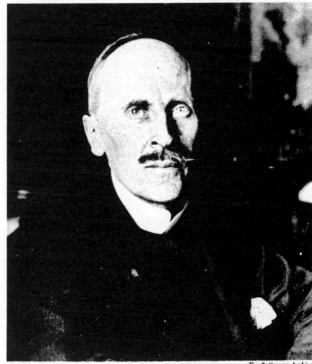

The Bettmann Archive

Henri Bergson, French philosopher who won the Nobel Prize in 1928.

In 1900 he became professor of philosophy at the Collège de France, and received the Nobel Prize for literature in 1928.

In his philosophy Bergson shows pairs of contrasting principles at work, corresponding roughly to static matter and mobile life, and examines the mental operations (intelligence and intuition, respectively) which give access to these. In *Time and Free Will* he demonstrates the inadequacy of psychologies which seek single units of experience (for instance, "sensations"). He regards experience as indivisible and organically meaningful. His thought is thus comparable to Gestalt psychology and phenomenology. In *Matter and Memory*, 1896 (trans., 1911) he contrasts "habit-memory," which is mechanical and practical, with "pure" memory, which provides the sense of personal identity. *Laughter*, 1900 (trans., 1911), explains laughter as a social corrective to absent-mindedness. *Creative Evolution*, 1907 (trans., 1911) contrasts the roles of instinct and intelligence, and in *The Two Sources of Morality and Religion*, 1932 (trans., 1935), the "closed" source is law and precept, the "open" source inspiration from example.

BINET [bē-nā'], **ALFRED** (1857–1911), French psychologist, author of the first standard measure of intelligence. His work embraced personality study, research with gifted and mentally deficient children, and investigation of the reasoning and thinking processes of children and adults. In 1905 the French government asked him to devise a method of detecting children incapable of school learning. Collaborating with Théodore Simon, he produced the Binet-Simon Test of Intelligence, which consisted of tests arranged in age levels from three to twelve. A score called "mental age" was earned according to how many test levels a child passed. A revision of this test, the Stanford Revision of the Binet-Simon Scale, achieved wide use in the United States.

See also INTELLIGENCE; INTELLIGENCE QUOTIENT; INTELLIGENCE TEST; TESTING, PSYCHOLOGICAL AND EDUCATIONAL.

BINGHAM, WALTER VAN DYKE (1880–1952), American psychologist. He taught at Columbia and Dartmouth, organized the Institute of Applied Psychology at Carnegie Institute of Technology, and served as its director (1915–24). A pioneer in personnel psychology, he worked on the classification and use of army personnel during World Wars I and II. His publications include *How to Interview* (with B. V. Moore, 1931) and *Aptitudes and Aptitude Testing* (1937).

BLEULER [bloi'lər], **EUGEN** (1856–1939), Swiss psychiatrist. As head of the Burghölzli clinic and professor at Zurich, he pioneered in the development of psychoanalysis and occupational therapy and in the scientific study of alcoholism. He introduced the term "schizophrenia" into psychiatry and did extensive studies of this illness.

BODY TYPES, categories of human physique based on major anatomical characteristics, and usually developed within theories relating body structure to personality. Relationships between body type and certain personality characteristics may reflect common underlying causal factors; for example, the thyroid gland can affect physique and temperament. It is important to note that certain personality characteristics might include behavior—such as overeating—that would in turn affect physique, and that certain physiques may lead to the success of certain ways of behaving.

Most research on relationships between body build and personality has focused on the theories of a German, Ernst Kretschmer, and an American, W. H. Sheldon. The latter developed three descriptive categories for body build: endomorph, ectomorph, and mesomorph. The endomorph, to give an approximate description, is round and soft, with prominent abdomen, short limbs, small hands and feet, and smooth skin. The ectomorph is thin and long-limbed, with narrow shoulders, long neck, slight muscular development, and thin skin. The mesomorph has strong skeletal structure, well-developed musculature, and thick skin. These descriptions are of extremes which are rarely found; the body builds of most individuals are mixtures of components. A person's physique can be rated to show how much he tends to resemble one of the three categories. Sheldon reported relationships between patterns of body build and patterns of temperament. Persons who rated high in endomorphy tended to rate high in viscerotonia—a term covering such traits as relaxation in posture, preference for physical comfort, sociability, complacency, and tolerance. Persons who tended toward ectomorphy were found to tend toward cerebrotonia—a temperament marked by restraint in posture, secretiveness, desire for privacy, inhibitions, and preference for intellectual activity. Persons who rated high in meso-morphy tended, according to Sheldon, toward somatotonia—a personality description including such traits as boldness, aggressiveness, and liking for exercise, adventure, and risk.

Evidence has been found for the relationships between body build and personality described by Sheldon. The nature and extent of the relationships, however, have not been precisely determined.

BORING [bô'ring], **EDWIN GARRIGUES** (1886–1968), American psychologist. He studied at Cornell and later taught at Clark University. He directed the Harvard psychological laboratory from 1924 to 1949, was made professor in 1928, and emeritus professor in 1957. Among his works are *A History of Experimental Psychology* (1929), *Sensation and Perception in the History of Experimental Psychology* (1942), and *Psychologist at Large* (1961).

BRAID, JAMES (1795–1860), Scottish physician famous for his studies of hypnotism. In 1841 he began to investigate mesmerism, as it was then called, became convinced of its validity, and named it neuro-hypnotism, later shortened to hypnotism.

BRAIN [brān]. The brain of almost every animal is a piece of its living tissue near the front or head end of its body and is usually collected into a compact mass, although occasionally it is found distributed as a chain of small masses. Generally whitish in color, the brain is invariably connected by many strands (nerves) with the sense organs and with the muscles of the body. When cut across, the exposed surface of the brain often shows a mixture of patches of gray and white tissue.

Under the microscope brain tissue at first seems little differentiated, but after treatment with various selective stains it shows an extremely rich structure. Scattered throughout the gray patches are great numbers of nerve cells (in the human brain about 10 billion) each branching out into many ramifying threads, the dendrons and the axons. The branches seem to be intermingled in a network of bewildering complexity. Some of the nerve cells have one especially long and thick branch, the axon, which may travel quite a distance (many feet in the larger animals) before ending either at another nerve cell or at a muscle. The brain thus forms an extremely rich network between the sense organs and the muscles.

All nerve cells are extremely sensitive, and share one kind of special behavior: when a nerve cell is disturbed by an appropriate stimulus, it "fires" by producing an electric wave (the nervous impulse), which then travels over all of its branches. This may be likened to a flame traveling over a network of trails of gunpowder, the flame at each point igniting the next. The impulses are usually set up by the activities of the world around (light, sound, heat, touch) which impinge on the sense organs, since the sense organs contain nerve cells in which the impulses originate. These impulses are conducted over various parts of the nervous network, cell firing off cell in the process. If the stimulation leads to action, the final impulses arrive at the muscles, which they cause to contract.

Chemically, the substance of the brain is mostly protein, like the rest of the body, but with an unusually large amount of special fatty substances (lecithin, for example) which act to insulate one nerve from another, stopping any single impulse from spreading over the whole brain.

The energy for these nervous activities comes largely from the burning of glucose (a simple sugar) by oxygen. The physical and chemical processes used by the brain in the course of its work do not differ in any essential way from those used by other tissues of the body.

Brain Function

The description just given does not suggest what is the main function of the brain and of what use it is to the organism. To answer this, one must go back to the basic facts of evolution. The rough-and-tumble of existence and natural selection (a mechanism of evolution whereby those organisms and particular qualities of an organism, best adapted for survival, are selected and perpetuated), ensure that forms will develop that are extremely resistant to the destructive forces around them. This earth, after about 5 billion years, has produced its well-adapted forms. Among these are the higher animal organisms, such as the mammals, whose power of resistance can be properly appreciated only when we remember that they have survived the ice ages and are, in fact, older than the Alps. In general, the forms produced by evolution tend to achieve their resistance in one of two ways: by developing simple physical hardness (as the tortoise protects itself by an inert but almost unbreakable shell) or by developing complex mobility (as a fly avoids being caught or as a fencer avoids being wounded). The development of complex mobility is the function of the brain: to produce the right action at the right time, so that the threats from the world around will cause no serious harm to the organism. All of the brain's functions can thus be seen as a complex form of homeostasis, or maintenance of internal balance by an organism. This word ("homeostasis") was coined by physiologist Walter Cannon, in 1929, to represent the fact that the body's internal mechanisms, especially the autonomic (involuntary or vegetative) nervous system, always react to disturbance so that the effects of the disturbance are eventually neutralized. The same neutralization, however, is just as essential in the wide-ranging activities of the free living animal. The threat of drying up, for example, leads the organism to drink water, to search for water, or (in man) to build pipelines to bring water. In all cases the end is the same: the brain's activity is so related to the threatening disturbance that the disturbance hardly hurts the organism at all. The organism survives, and the brain, which has read the threat and produced an appropriate action, proves its value to the organism.

When the threat is simple (such as that of drying up) and the cure simple (such as "go toward the smell of water and then drink") a simple brain is adequate. But evolution has shown that there is advantage in being able to deal with more complex threats. "Complex" means here that the threat has many components and what the best reply to each component is depends on the direction of the other components. Thus "red" coming to the eye may at one time be a light at a traffic crossing, at another time part of a meal with red meat and white potatoes, and at a third time a poisonous red berry in green foliage. What the reaction should be to "red" depends, therefore,

on what other stimuli are coming in from other sense organs. It becomes necessary for the brain to receive information from many different sources at once, and to act, using the muscles, in a way depending on complex comparisons between the various partial pieces of information. From this arises the necessity for the brain itself: a central station operating so that the pattern of action sent to all the muscles can depend on an interweaving of what information has come from all the sense organs.

Not only may the correct response to a stimulus depend on what is happening at other places being stimulated, it may also depend on what has happened to the organism in the past. The more highly evolved brains have developed methods by which what happened in the past is preserved in some physical trace, ready to exert its effect on a later process. When this happens, the psychologist says that the organism is showing the effects of memory. Although there is as yet very little known about what form these traces take, there can be little doubt that they are in the form of some physical, that is material, change, possibly in molecular structures in the brain. Discovery of their nature is one of the outstanding problems of brain function awaiting solution.

When a threat recurs there is a clear advantage, once a suitable form of response has been found, in retaining the form of the response so that it can be reproduced at once on future occasions. Living organisms do show this retention. How it is done depends markedly on the duration between the first presentation of a threat and the last. Sometimes the duration is very great, such as the threat of winter's cold, which has recurred annually for millions of years. When the recurrence is over many generations, natural selection tends to develop a uniform reaction which is inherited and transmitted by the genes, so that the young animal produces the correct response on its first encounter. Such a response is called a reflex. The brain of the higher organism contains many such reflexes, each an appropriate reaction to some threat.

Other threats, however, while recurring over a period of time, do not last long enough for natural selection to be able to develop the appropriate response. It is then advantageous if the individual can find a response and retain it over his own lifetime. The higher organisms have all developed special mechanisms by which the individual can find and retain, for his own lifetime, any response that is adaptive for him individually. The mechanisms responsible are those of "learning." The general mechanism is provided by heredity, but the details come from the world around. Thus, it is a characteristic of the species that the kitten can learn, but the details of what the kitten learns—of how to catch mice and of how mice behave—come ultimately from the mice themselves.

To summarize, then, the brain may be characterized biologically as that part of the organism which protects it by receiving information in complex patterns and by recoding these patterns into suitable patterns of action that show in the muscles. Its purpose is to keep constant those variables on which the organism's life depends. It recodes the patterns in the right way, rather than in a random or chaotic way, either because evolution has formed the right nervous mechanisms in it (for those disturbances that recur over the centuries), or because evolution has formed in it the neuronic mechanisms for learning, and actual experience has provided the brain with the details.

Artificial Brains

The whole subject of "brain in general," however, cannot be adequately understood today unless one also considers the artificial, man-made forms of the brain; for the development of the modern, general-purpose electronic computer has thrown a flood of light on what is implied by "brainlike activity."

The point is that the general-purpose computer is a completely willing slave. It will carry out any process that it is told to do, but it must be told what to do in terms that do not require previous knowledge or explanation. The terms must also be totally devoid of ambiguity. Thus the command "be clever" is useless; one must decide what "being clever" means; one must break the instruction down to commands of the most basic and practical type. The attempt to define what one really means by a machine "being clever" has forced much intensive thinking. As a result, we now have an understanding of what is meant by brainlike activity that far surpasses what was known in, say, 1935.

Feedback. One of the discoveries made was the importance, in brainlike activity, of "feedback." Feedback is said to be present if two systems, A and B, are so acting that A has an action on B, and B at the same time has an action on A, so that the chain of cause and effect goes back and forth between the two. A simple example is provided by the heater of a room and the controlling thermostat: the thermostat controls the heater, and the heater acts, through the air of the room, on the thermostat. Another example occurs when one holds a telescope to look at a distant object: movements of one's hands shift the position of the image in the field of vision; but at the same time (if one wishes to keep the image central) the movement of the image causes one to make readjusting movements with one's hands. A continuous double action is produced: the movements of the hands affect what is seen, and what is seen determines the movements made by the hands. There is feedback between position of image and movement of hands.

The recognition of the importance of feedback, and its practical use in such "clever" devices as the automatic pilot and the self-aiming antiaircraft gun, made obsolete the dogma that no machine could correct its own errors. The automatic pilot does this incessantly. Some physiologists had earlier attempted to use the concept of feedback to describe biological phenomena, but the concept is a difficult one that needs a properly developed logic and mathematics if arguments about it are not to break down in confusion. About 1935 certain engineering problems made it necessary to develop an adequate mathematical description of feedback. Today the understanding derived from those early (and subsequent) investigations is of the greatest assistance in making clear what is meant by brainlike activity.

Information Theory. A second development that has thrown a great light on brain function is that of information theory. During World War II, two noted American mathematicians, Claude Shannon and Norbert Wiener, found that "information" could be measured. (In this special sense, information corresponds to the freedom of choice that one has in selecting, from all the possibilities, a message for transmission.) Today there exists an extensive body of knowledge about how information can be received, transformed, lost, recovered, and stored. This knowledge is relevant to brainlike behavior, for we now realize that many of the brain processes that once seemed most mysterious are in fact just those processes that are today well understood in information theory. It is, for instance, an expression of a deep and exact truth to say that the fundamental homeostatic processes in the brain are identical with those that remove noise from a communication system.

Briefly, just as noise is that which tends to corrupt a telephone message and drive it away from its proper form, similarly, when the disturbances of the world threaten to drive a living organism away from its own proper form, brain activity helps to oppose the threats so that the form is maintained. What is important about this identification is that it makes us aware that both natural and artificial (mechanical) brains have a fundamental limitation: any system that is to achieve appropriate selection (to a degree better than chance) can do so only as a consequence of information received.

Information theory has made us realize that all the "remarkable" properties of the brain fall into one of two categories. First, there are processes that were considered unique simply because the living brain was the only known example of a system both highly dynamic (active) and really complicated. The other processes are those that show evidence of intense selection, and they are the ones usually thought of as being peculiarly brainlike. Selection was shown dramatically, in 1846, when J. C. Adams and U. J. Leverrier said to their fellow astronomer, J. C. Galle, "Aim your telescope at the point P in the sky and you will there see a new planet." Here, out of all the points in the sky they selected the particular one, and the planet Neptune was discovered. But selection is also shown just as clearly (though less dramatically) when a person leaves home and, after traveling for hundreds of miles, eventually returns to exactly the same house. Again, the ordinary intelligence test shows in detail how a good score is inseparably connected with the ability to select a small set of (correct) answers from the great range of what is possible.

When a brain, either natural or artificial, is regarded from this point of view, its selective power is limited by the amount of information that has come to it previously. Here one may easily make a gross error by overestimating the amount of information that must be given ("programmed" into) a computer before it can solve a problem, or by underestimating the amount of information held by the brain of the higher organism after it has been shaped by two billion years of evolution (together with all the experiences of youth, and perhaps by the training of school). When the magnitude of the difference between these two quantities of information (programmed and previously stored) is appreciated, we see that as far as the biological activities of the higher organisms are concerned (those, for example, by which they get their food and avoid their enemies), what goes on in the living brain is not essentially different from what goes on in the artificial brainlike mechanisms that can be made today. It can be said that the brain is understood, in the sense that any of its functions can be reproduced mechanically, its function of being "intelligent" not excepted.

The Brain of Man

What of the brain of man—does it show uniqueness? So far as its physical, chemical, and anatomical (in a word, material) properties are concerned, it shows nothing unique. So far as its behavior is concerned, everything that is demonstrable can be paralleled by the behavior of a machine, provided the latter is given as much information as is used by the human being when he produces his behavior. In everything that is demonstrable, the brain, man's included, shows no unfathomable mystery, only great complexity.

At the same time, it would be wrong to conclude that no mystery remains, for not all brain function is demonstrable. The inner awareness that we all possess (when awake) cannot be demonstrated but is nonetheless real. The particular shade of color I see when I look at fresh grass is known to me directly, but is not communicable from me to another. I can communicate to another person the wavelength of its light or point to a certain insect and say that its color is about the same, but I cannot communicate any vision of the color itself, although it is very real to me. Of this awareness, modern science knows nothing. It is outside science's terms of reference.

The modern science of the brain, which has removed almost all "mechanical" mystery from it, has at the same time thrown into sharp relief a deeper mystery. And we are reminded that science does not destroy mysteries; it relates them, and shows the various small mysteries to be facets of one single mystery.
See also Nervous System.

BRAINWASHING. *See* Psychological Warfare.

BRENTANO, FRANZ CLEMENS (1838–1917), Austrian philosopher and psychologist. Ordained a Roman Catholic priest in 1864, Brentano left the priesthood and the Catholic Church in 1873, but remained a theist and taught that the soul is a spiritual entity capable of interaction with the body. Teaching at Würzburg, Germany, and later at Vienna, he made important contributions to almost every branch of philosophy, but is best known for his view that "intentional inexistence"—reference to something beyond itself—is peculiar to what is psychological. This view led to Meinong's "theory of objects" and to Husserl's "phenomenology." Brentano's theory of language, according to which only concrete individual things can be referred to, influenced later positivistic and analytic philosophy. His writings include *Origin of the Knowledge of Right and Wrong* (Eng. trans., 1902).

BREUER [broi'ər], **JOSEF** (1842–1925), Austrian physician, noted for his collaboration with Sigmund Freud during the early days of psychoanalysis. Breuer hypnotized a young woman suffering from hysteria, who then recalled her feelings while nursing her sick father; her symptoms thereupon disappeared. Breuer named this reliving of an earlier experience "catharsis"—a term still used by psychoanalysts. With Freud he wrote *Studies in Hysteria*, a book based on this and other cases. Among Breuer's other discoveries was that of the function of the semicircular canals of the ear in maintaining body balance.

BRILL, ABRAHAM ARDEN (1874–1948), American psychiatrist who helped bring Freudian psychology to the attention of the English-speaking world through his translations of Freud's works. Born in Austria, Brill graduated from Columbia University in 1903 and studied with Freud and others in Europe. He later became head of the psychiatric clinic at Columbia University and taught there and at New York University. An advocate of psychoanalysis, Brill fought against strong opposition for its acceptance by the medical profession and the public. He was a founder and president of the New York Psychoanalytic Society and the American Psychoanalytic Association.

C

CABANIS [kȧ-bȧ-nēs'], **PIERRE JEAN GEORGES** (1757–1808), French physician and philosopher who attempted to understand the relation between mind and body. Considered the father of physiological psychology, he advanced the ideas that the entire body contributed to the activity of the mind and that the brain was the organ of consciousness. During the French Revolution, with which he sympathized, he became the friend and physician of the statesman Honoré de Mirabeau. After Mirabeau's death Cabanis was accused of having poisoned him; in refutation of this charge he published *Journal de la Maladie et la Mort de Honoré de Mirabeau* (1791).

CATALEPSY [kăt'ə-lĕp-sē], a state of muscular rigidity and fixation of posture associated with a lack of response to stimulation, often extending to a complete loss of contact with the world. Cataleptic states are seen most frequently in catatonic schizophrenia; a waxy flexibility (cerea flexibilitas) develops in which the patient tends to remain in whatever posture he is placed for long periods of time. Local catalepsies of the eyelids and limbs can be induced during hypnosis.
See also SCHIZOPHRENIA.

CATATONIA [kăt-ə-tō'nē-ə], an abnormal type of behavior seen in some persons suffering from schizophrenia. The catatonic person is usually in a trancelike stupor, but may occasionally be violent and dangerous. Typically, the catatonic is mute and motionless. He may spend the entire day standing in one position or sitting on the edge of the table. Although the patient seems unaware of the world about him he may actually be alert and thinking actively.
See also SCHIZOPHRENIA.

CATTELL [kə-tĕl'], **JAMES McKEEN** (1860–1944), American psychologist. His early research dealt with reaction time, span of attention, and other perceptual areas. After holding the first professorship in psychology at the University of Pennsylvania (1888–91), he taught at Columbia until 1917. In 1921 he founded the Psychological Corporation, organized to apply psychological methods to practical problems. He edited the *Psychological Review, Scientific Monthly, Science,* and *American Men of Science.*

CHARACTER, that aspect of personality associated with the maintenance of moral and ethical principles. The statement that a person has "good character" implies that he can be depended upon to do the right, decent thing. Also, "good character" often implies perseverance, determination.

Psychologists do not agree as to whether character should be considered a unitary aspect of personality, or as a cluster of specific habits, some, all, or none of which may be displayed by a given person. Common usage, and often experience, favor the first meaning. Thus, for example, if a person is a frequent churchgoer, he is expected to be honest in his dealings with other people. Some psychological research, however, suggests that people who are honest in some situations may not be so in all situations and that only specific habits or ways of behaving in particular situations are learned. That is, a person may be honest in his dealings with other individuals and yet be dishonest in computing his income tax.

Character is often used synonymously with conscience, but some writings imply that character is determined by conscience.
See also CONSCIENCE.

CHILD CARE. *See* CHILD DEVELOPMENT.

CHILD DEVELOPMENT is the growth of children in all aspects—physical, psychological, and social—from birth to maturity. The period of development is ordinarily divided into a preadolescent and an adolescent phase, marked off by the onset of puberty. Adolescence is treated in a separate article, and the present discussion deals only with changes during the years before puberty.

At birth, an infant can eat, eliminate, cry, and sleep—but he can do little else. A child of three is fairly agile, shows a considerable amount of self-control, and has developed to a respectable degree the ability to talk and to understand, which makes him uniquely human. By the time he is 12 he is capable of athletic accomplishments requiring intricate physical co-ordination, and his intellectual and other capacities are more like those of an adult than of an infant. Attitudes, desires, and beliefs that will affect him all the rest of his life have already been formed. These changes, and the principles that govern them, are of interest to parents, teachers, psychologists, pediatricians, and other professional and nonprofessional groups. Understanding children and the way they grow is important in its own right, but the study of child development is also significant for understanding the behavior of adults, whose characteristics are largely formed in childhood.

The Normal Course of Development

A great deal of research has been aimed toward charting the normal course of human growth. Children are observed at different ages, changes in behavior are noted, and when enough research has been done, it is possible to describe the typical characteristics of new-born infants, two-year-olds, or children of any other age. In reading such accounts, including those to follow, it is important to keep in mind that they represent averages and nothing more. Descriptions of typical behavior help people know what to expect of children in a general way, and they are

STAGES OF DEVELOPMENT

No child exactly fits any arbitrary pattern of physical and social growth, but children pass through stages of maturing and learning. The photographs here show typical behavior through 5 stages described in the article.

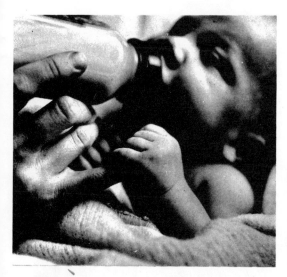

FIRST STAGE: The infant, helpless except for his reflex actions. (ESTHER BUBLEY)

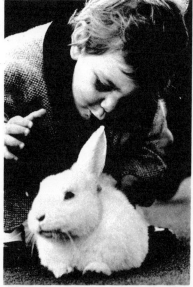

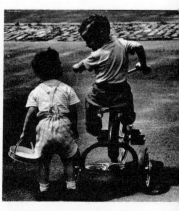

SECOND STAGE: The crawling-walking period (6 mos.—1½).
(TED SPIEGEL—RAPHO GUILLUMETTE)

THIRD STAGE: The more sociable toddler (1½—2½). (ESTHER BUBLEY)

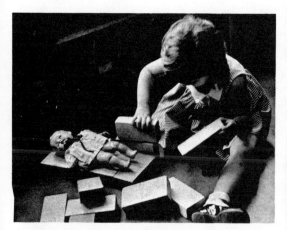

FOURTH STAGE: The preschool years (2½—5), marked by increasing dexterity, imagination, and independence. (KEN HEYMAN)

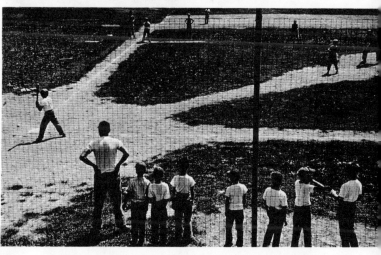

FIFTH STAGE: The early school years (6—12), during which ideas multiply, physical skills are developed, and interests outside the home increase. (KEN HEYMAN)

essential for determination of lawful behavior sequences, but this does not mean that every child must conform precisely to the behavior pattern of other children his age.

Behavior of the Newborn. All the basic sensory capacities of man are present when an infant is born, but these function in a rather poorly organized way. The newborn infant (neonate) can see, hear, taste, smell, and respond to touch, but he has little ability to arrange sensations into coherent patterns and to attach meaning to the things that happen around him. He must learn before he can tell what

an event signifies. The subjective experience of the neonate cannot be known directly, but a classic statement from William James' *Principles of Psychology* is probably very close to the truth: "The baby, assailed by eyes, ears, nose, skin, and entrails at once, feels it all as one great blooming, buzzing confusion."

He is capable of a considerable variety of reflex actions. If the palms of his hands are touched, the fingers will close in a surprisingly strong grasp. If he is held with his feet just touching a surface he will make prancing movements with his legs that are not unlike the movements involved in walking later on. If his cheek is touched when he is hungry he will turn his head, and if a nipple is present his lips will close about it and he will begin to suck. He may choke and sputter a bit at first, but he will soon be able to manage the rather complex cycle of acts required to suck, swallow, and breathe in a smoothly co-ordinated way. And, as any parent knows, he can cry. The average newborn infant cries 113 minutes per 24-hour day, though babies differ widely in this respect as in others. Some cry less than an hour a day; others cry more than four hours out of the 24.

Conditioned responses can be established at this time. If a signal, such as a buzzer, is repeatedly followed by presentation of a bottle from which the infant takes food, he will soon begin to make sucking movements with his mouth whenever he hears the buzzer, even though he is not given any milk. In a primitive way, he has learned to expect the bottle to appear after the buzzer sounds, and this is just one experimental example of an important kind of learning that continues to take place from birth on. The conditioned responses, however, are difficult to establish and do not last very long. There is no reason to suppose that learning just after birth has any extraordinary effect on later behavior, and there is evidence to suggest that most of the learning of specific responses that takes place at this time is very feeble indeed. Certain early deprivations, including severe denial of maternal attention, can have harmful and probably permanent effects on intelligence, personality, and social behavior; but these effects evidently appear only if the damaging conditions are extreme and endure into infancy and early childhood.

The First 18 Months. Perhaps the most striking changes that occur during the first year and a half of life are those having to do with the ability to move about and inspect the world. From a squirming infant the child is transformed into an active, self-directed person, poking, searching, exploring, "into everything." After one month the infant can lift his chin, before another month has passed he can lift his chest from a supporting surface and assume the pose so popular in photographs of nude babies. By the age of four months he can sit if someone supports his back, and two or three months later he can sit alone. In still another month he can stand with help, and at nine months he can pull himself to a standing position by the bars of a playpen. In his crib he may have been rocking back and forth on hands and knees and occasionally flopping forward. These movements are integrated, usually at about ten months, into actual creeping. By 11 months he can walk if someone holds onto his upraised hands, and shortly thereafter, near his first birthday or a little later, he takes his first steps alone. Nobody has to teach him to do this, and the common phrase "learning to walk" is a rather misleading term for what actually goes on. The nervous system matures, the ankles straighten, the muscles grow and become better co-ordinated. These changes come to pass no matter what parents may do, though opportunity and encouragement have an influence on the child's rate of progress.

The ability to manipulate objects develops in much the same way. The earliest attempts to grasp things are jerky, lurching movements not only of the arms, but of the shoulders and trunk as well. The hands are ordinarily fisted at birth but tend to remain open after the infant is around 16 weeks old. He is then able to manage a crude palming of objects, but the thumb and fingers are basically nonfunctional. At six months a baby can not only grasp an object, but he can voluntarily let it go; this reflects his growing control over movements that before were little more than automatic reflexes. By the time he is a year old his actions have been refined to the point where he can rather daintily pick up a pellet with his thumb and forefinger.

If at the same time he has become able to walk, he will begin to explore the world about him with tireless energy and curiosity. He looks at, listens to, feels, shakes, bangs, lifts, pokes into, pulls at, and chews everything he can. As far as possible, dangerous and breakable objects should be kept out of his reach at this time. Parents can teach him to avoid unmovable dangerous objects, such as electric outlets, by saying "No," and following with a slap on the hand or elsewhere; but household life is simplest if the number of forbidden objects and situations are reduced to a minumum.

All the while the infant's motor skills are growing, his awareness of the world, and especially of other people, develops at a prodigious rate. At one month he begins a wavering, cross-eyed inspection of the faces hovering above him. These faces often smile at him, and at six or seven weeks of age he rather crookedly smiles back. Up to the age of six months he may smile at any face that appears, but after a half year he becomes more discriminating, and the face of a stranger often brings forth a howl of distress. If an infant is exposed to various other people during this time, and if the other people are reasonably calm and composed, the fears will generally subside. By one year most babies are quite sociable with adults, playing peek-a-boo and pat-a-cake until the patience of

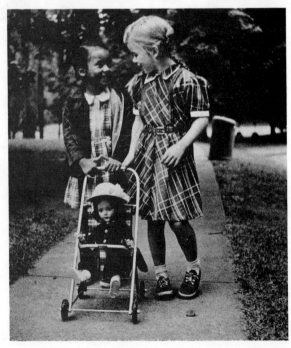

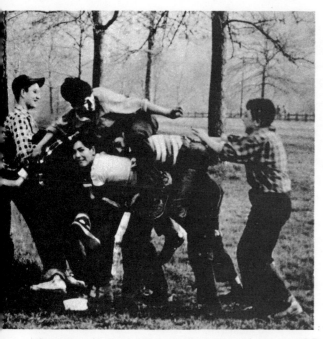

dramatic play can often be seen in a two-year-old. Instead of biting or banging a toy telephone, he pretends he is talking to someone. He may put a doll to bed; he may solemnly inform his mother that he is going to work and then say "Bye-bye" as he leaves the kitchen. The scenes he enacts are simple and quickly performed. They will later be elaborated, improvised, organized, and other children will be involved in "playing house" or "cowboys and Indians," but even the earliest ventures at dramatic play involve important advances in maturation and learning. To "pretend" usually requires taking the role of another person, and out of this experience grows the capacity for looking at things from different vantage points. The child begins to be able to perceive himself from the point of view of other people, and this is a crucial factor in the development of a sense of personal identity.

The sense of autonomy grows. More and more, the child comes to think of himself as a distinct human being, with desires, capacities, and limitations of his own. His desires are urgent, his capacities are only partly developed, his limitations are many, and he is often in trouble. This stage of development has been called the "Terrible Two's"—and for excellent reason. Temper tantrums are at their peak, especially before meals and at bedtime, and children in Western society usually go through a period of negativism when they are about two and a half, countering practically any suggestion parents might make with a vigorous "No!" Punishment of these tendencies seldom has any beneficial effect, except possibly to offer the parent some release; and it is generally agreed that if parents can firmly continue to put the child into bed or do whatever else is necessary without becoming unnecessarily involved in a battle of wills, the tantrums and unrealistic objections of the child will gradually diminish. He will learn that there are better ways to satisfy his needs.

There are other difficulties during this year. Sooner or later children have to be toilet trained, and if this is badly done certain problems may arise. Bowel training can often be established when a child is about a year and a half old —whenever he can signal that he "has to go." Muscle control for bladder training is not generally achieved until the child is two or older, and it is still another year before most children can stay dry at night. Alertness and patient effort are required to get a child trained. Attempting training too early or punishing failure too severely may attach more emotional importance to elimination than this simple body function deserves.

During this time children are strong in motility but weak in judgment. As they test the limits of the world, certain restrictions have to be set on their behavior. Discipline is probably necessary to their own security and is surely essential to the comfort of others around them. The beginnings of self-control can be seen in a two-year-old as he says "Hot!" and stays away from a stove, or pats the head of a baby sister very gently as his parents have taught him to do. But such control, and the eventual emergence of a conscience, comes slowly. Meanwhile, controls must be imposed by parents and others outside.

The Preschool Years (2½ to 5). Rapid changes in behavior continue during the next three years. At two the child uses a kiddy-car with vigor and determination but little ability to control his direction, at three he can pedal

the older person has been exhausted. The one-year-old also shows a strong interest in others his own age. He may babble enthusiastically when he sees another baby and perhaps hand him a toy, though he will usually want this returned along with anything else that captures his interest. His sense of the difference between his own and others' possessions is largely unformed, and while he may play contentedly alongside another child for rather long periods of time, cries of outrage will occasionally arise from the playpen as toys are snatched back and forth.

For all these difficulties, the child has changed tremendously in the first year and a half. Never again will so much progress be made in so short a time. He can walk and he can, probably, talk a little. His language development has advanced to the point where a few of his needs can be communicated and some of the desires of others can be understood. In a poorly differentiated way he is aware of himself as distinct from other people, and he is on his way to becoming an autonomous, but socially conscious, person.

The Toddler (Age 1½ to 2½). A child between the ages of one and a half and two and a half does not toddle for long. He much prefers to run, and as soon as his muscular co-ordination and balance permit, that is what he will do. Walking is much too slow. He loves wheeled vehicles and drags or pushes them through the house with no concern whatever for the condition of walls and furniture. He prefers activities calling for use of large muscles—bouncing on a bed until he is taken off, climbing on a chair and getting down again—though he is also capable of such small-muscle accomplishments as the construction of a sizable block tower. His attention span is short and he is easily distracted.

In his play, he is more sociable than before, taking evident pleasure in the company of another child, but he seldom works co-operatively with his playmate in any joint endeavor. That will come later. The beginning of

THE GROWTH OF UNDERSTANDING

Children's growth in skills and deepening understanding of the world about them are reflected in their drawings. There is great variation owing to individual personality, but development occurs in discernible stages. Scribbles are replaced by object symbols, which are refined as awareness of details increases.

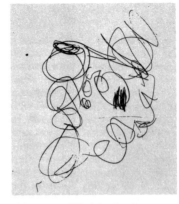

Elaborate scribble (preschool).

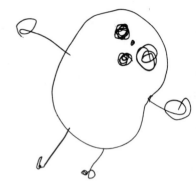

Rudimentary human object (3—5 years).

a tricycle, and by the time he is five he may be riding a bicycle with only a little wobbling. Two-year-olds are continually falling down, three-year-olds are much more surefooted, four-year-olds can skip, though somewhat clumsily. At five, the highly complex co-ordinations required for skipping have matured. From banging kettles and scattering blocks, the child progresses to the point where he can play with rather complicated mechanical toys; and at five he may be using his father's tools to build boats and airplanes. Crude as these may seem, he is very proud of his creations and will play with his own airplane or some other barely identifiable thing for hours, leaving its expensive manufactured counterpart in the box.

The ability to think, to form concepts, and to solve problems by using ideas instead of acts develops along with other skills. If a pair of two-year olds get into a dispute over a doll, they will tug at it until one wins and the other cries. Three-year-olds are more willing to share, and if arguments arise, these are often settled by appeals to a nearby adult. By five, fewer of the arguments are over things. They often deal with such social concerns as fairness and rules for play ("I shot you and you won't stay dead!"). Some arguments between five-year-olds may be directly concerned with the validity of ideas ("There is *too* an Easter bunny!"), and the difficulties are commonly dealt with on a verbal plane. This is not to say that physical assaults abruptly cease, only that the ability to use ideas has developed enough to permit many problems to be solved by words rather than blows. Number concepts expand. Three-year-olds have little sense of number, but four-year-olds can distinguish between one thing, two, and lots of things. At five, most children can count ten objects, know their age, and can manage some simple addition. Changes in the ability to think and plan are manifest in the drawings children make. The beginnings of representative drawing typically appear around three, but a child of that age often draws first and decides afterwards what he has made. At five he can draw a recognizable man, and it is clear as he works that he is setting out to portray something he has previously thought about. He is executing a plan.

The ability to think and imagine has in it obvious potential for dealing with human and physical problems. Now the child can wait a while for something he wants and fill in the delay with reasonably clear ideas about what is going to happen later on. Not only can he antici-

pate the future, he can also mull over the past and, in some measure, profit from his experience. But like so many of man's abilities, imagination can lead to trouble. Two-year-olds are more afraid of the novel and sudden than anything else. They are terrified by loud noises and strange situations. These fears have greatly diminished by five, and children of that age tend instead to fear imaginary objects or vague threats of danger. They are worried about ghosts and animals in the bedroom; they anxiously wonder what it is like to die. With further maturation, the fearful child will be more able to distinguish fantasy from reality, but now he has difficulty keeping them apart. If his fears are excessive, professional help may have to be obtained at a child guidance clinic or similar facility, but many irrational fears are "outgrown" as fact and fancy become distinct, and spooks and goblins are put in their place.

With the growth of ability to imagine how he looks to others, the child develops a new social awareness. At two he wants his way, at three he mainly wants to please, at four he wants to be noticed. He shows off, he plays the clown, he indulges in childish word-play. He calls a playmate a silly name and is convulsed with laughter at his own wit. Sibling rivalry is most severe if a new baby arrives when the older child is around three or four years of age. He is old enough then to have some awareness of his position in the family, he wants attention very badly, and the newcomer may constitute a real threat to his security. Bringing the older child into preparations for the arrival of the brother or sister, and helping him feel that the baby is his too, can help somewhat. But it is dangerously easy to overdo the preparation in a gushy sentimental way, and no parent should be surprised if, in spite of his efforts, the older child starts to suck his thumb again or tries to hurt the baby. There is no substitute for seeing to it that the older child actually does not lose his place in the family, though his role must change; that he still gets the attention he needs, though he may not be able to have all the attention he wants; and that his basic security is truly unimpaired.

In any case, the preschool child is beginning to sever some of the ties with his parents and is no longer as completely dependent on them as is the toddler. Other people —playmates, perhaps a kindergarten teacher—assume progressively greater importance in his life. With his new sense of who he is, and the growing awareness of what he can do, the five-year-old may be arrogant and domineering at times; but in playing with other children he generally works with them rather than against them, and he is rarely content just to play beside them in the parallel activity of his earlier years. Roles are exaggerated in his dramatic play, and adults have been known to receive some sobering insights into their own characteristics as they listen to five-year-old "parents" arguing with each other and screeching at the children.

There are problems during the preschool years, as at any other age, but children of three, four, and five are more delightful than otherwise. They are not nearly such a care as they were before. They do not have to be watched all the time, though they still need some supervision. In general they like to conform, can be surprisingly dependable, are fairly sure of themselves, and normally tend to trust other people. By this time, they have a tolerably clear idea of who they are and where they stand in the world. Some basic character structures have been established, and though changes will continue throughout life, the distinct core of personality is already formed.

The Early School Years (6 to 12). Between the ages of six and 12, children slow down a bit in their growth. The rapid physical changes of the earlier years have levelled off somewhat, and the growth spurt of adolescence has not yet begun. Still, motor skills continue to improve as the muscles of the body come under increasingly refined control. At six, children are inclined to wriggle and sprawl, especially at table, and their abundant energy is worked off elsewhere in rather aimless running, jumping, and chasing. A six-year-old can care for himself in a reasonably thorough way, but there are flaws in his competence. He can bathe himself, but he usually needs some encouragement to wash his ears and neck; he can dress himself, but his sweater may be put on backwards. At nine, all these actions are more nearly automatic, and the small muscle movements involved are far better co-ordinated. New abilities are expressed through a growing interest in activities requiring fine dexterity, such as playing marbles and catching a ball. By 12, boys particularly are concerned with attaining excellence in performing certain physical feats. They may spend hours learning to juggle or making jump shots in basketball. The sudden growth of adolescence may later introduce the appearance of gangling

awkwardness; but even before puberty, motor skills of a highly refined sort can be quite fully developed, and feats that would defy an adult can often be performed with consummate grace by a 12-year-old.

Ideas multiply and are more and more clearly differentiated during the school years. Children then are greedily concerned with finding out about the world they live in, with what is and what is not, with ideas of the most far-reaching kind. Their information comes from every possible source: personal observation, teachers, books, parents, and more and more from other children. It is the task of each generation of second graders to tell the less sophisticated beginners about Santa Claus. Facts and myths about sex and reproduction are spread among the children—with typical confusion over the difference between birth and elimination. After six, memories are fairly continuous, rather than isolated and episodic. With more coherent awareness of the past comes a constantly improving ability to plan ahead. Elementary school children become progressively more able to think in abstract terms. Six-year-olds are inclined to think in a concrete or purely functional way. A chair is to sit on; milk is to drink. At that time, they are mostly concerned with the differentiation of ideas, and are able to recognize differences between objects in a fairly clear way. By the time they are eight, they can note and verbalize similarities between such objects as wood and glass, and at 12 they are capable of defining such abstract terms as loyalty and courage.

In school, in their games, and in the other activities that children carry on together, they truly become members of society at large—the society outside the home. Aside from the information and attitudes they incorporate at school, this is probably the most important thing that happens to them during the school years. At six, most children are still somewhat babyish and like to be held now and then. They typically think their parents know everything that matters. At nine, they are somewhat embarrassed by displays of affection, and they are likely to recognize their parents' limitations. Other adults, and particularly their own age group, "the gang," have assumed greater importance as sources of essential knowledge. At 12, most children are ostentatiously disdainful of childish ways and may scorn their parents in a fierce effort to be independent. In the search for autonomy, they may ex-

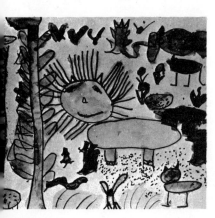

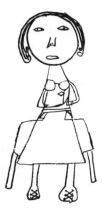

Objects become more coherent (early school).

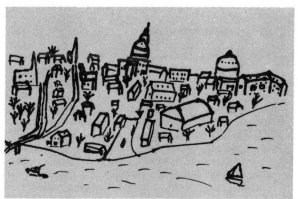

Studio for Young Artists, Annapolis
The child develops a better understanding of the world around him.

change dependence on parents for the tyranny of other children, who decide what will be worn, what will be done, which children will be outcasts and which heroes. But growing away from the family and forming intimate attachments to other children constitute an important, perhaps a necessary, step on the road to self-direction and personal integrity.

Some of the most dangerous threats of this time lie in the standards of conduct maintained by the groups with which the child becomes affiliated. If the group happens to be a delinquent gang, where acceptance and status can only be gained by stealing, fighting, and defying adult authority, the new member is likely to adopt those standards as his own. It is difficult for adults to remember the desperation of a child's need to be accepted by other children, but parents should be aware that children will sometimes do outrageous things to gain that acceptance. Here, as throughout childhood, some restraints may be necessary. Children of 12 are not ready for complete self-determination, and cries of "All the other kids are doing it" sometimes have to be met with every bit of conviction the parents can muster. Still, children have to be given some freedom to make their own decisions—even wrong decisions—if they are ever to learn to get along on their own. This is the eternal dilemma of growing up. Every child must learn to satisfy his needs and become an individual within the limits set by his society. Every parent must restrict his child yet still let him go—and to do this the parent must use all the good judgment, love, and common sense at his command.

Principles of Development

Observations of behavior during childhood have led to the formulation of certain principles that summarize the general character of growth, suggest causes that determine change, and carry some implications for putting knowledge about child development to use in rearing and educating children.

Differentiation and Integration. The direction of behavior change is, first, from mass activity to specific activity. Specific functions are then integrated into larger behavior patterns. The earliest attempts to throw a ball, for example, involve movements of the entire body. The child thrusts energetically with both arms, his face is contorted with effort, he may jump clear of the ground, though this movement is irrelevant to propelling the ball. Later, only the muscles needed for throwing are used, superfluous movements have dropped out, and the action is performed much more smoothly and effectively than before. At the same time the child may have been learning to swing a bat with his arms and shoulders, instead of moving trunk and limbs stiffly together in a cumbersome effort to hit the ball. Still later these two specific skills are integrated with others, such as running and catching, in the complex activity of playing ball.

Not only motor behavior but also perceptual tendencies and ideas change in accordance with principles of differentiation and integration. Out of the "blooming, buzzing confusion" of infancy, shapes, colors, sounds, images, ideas, and meanings are distinguished one from another. Horses and cows look much alike to a two-year-old; later he can tell them apart. When he is older still he can connect his ideas of these and other things, of himself and other people, into a coherent frame of reference for his own role in the world.

Maturation and Learning. Two processes are involved in all behavior change: physical maturation of the muscles, neural tracts, glands, and other body structures; and the learning of information and skills through experience. In any given accomplishment both processes are inextricably involved. If a child obtains a score of 130 on an intelligence test, he does so because his brain has matured to a certain level and because he has had certain opportunities and experiences in his life. One process or the other, however, may be predominant in determining behavior change. If most children walk at a given age despite severe environmental restriction and lack of experience, it is reasonable to attribute this change principally to maturation. If a child in a wretched home environment develops emotional conflicts and an inclination to avoid other people, one may legitimately assume that learning has been primarily involved.

Developmental Readiness. It is inefficient and sometimes harmful to begin training in any activity before children have matured enough to respond to the experience. It is senseless to try to teach a baby to walk when he is six months old. Insisting on performance of which a child is maturationally incapable can only lead to distress and disappointment on the part of everyone involved. On the other hand, the principle of developmental readiness offers no excuse for parental negligence, as in the case of a rude and insolent nine-year-old whose parents explained that he was not yet ready to learn manners. Nor does it exclude the problems that arise when educational measures are delayed too long. The principle amounts merely to a statement that changes in behavior are most efficiently and painlessly fostered if training procedures are paced to coincide with periods of optimal developmental readiness. As such, the principle is very important for parents, educators, and others to comprehend, but it is difficult to apply. Judicious pacing, to challenge a child without placing impossible demands upon him, requires a good deal of knowledge about the norms of child development and a fine sensitivity to the differences in capability that individual children show.

See also:

CHILD GUIDANCE CLINIC, a psychiatric agency designed to diagnose and treat personality and behavioral problems of children. The first demonstration clinic was established as the result of a survey, conducted in 1915 by the National Committee for Mental Hygiene, which revealed the existence of extensive behavior problems and lack of treatment facilities in the public schools. Under the joint sponsorship of the Commonwealth Fund and the National Committee for Mental Hygiene, a five-year demonstration program of clinics was instituted in 1922.

The standard child guidance clinic is staffed by a psychiatrist who acts as director and child therapist; a psychiatric social worker whose scope of investigation and treatment extends from the child to the family, the school, and the other recreational and institutional agencies affecting the child's behavior; and a clinical psychologist who provides diagnostic testing. The clinics function in relation to courts, public and private social welfare agencies, and schools. Only a very small percentage, however, operate on a full-time basis.

CHILD PSYCHOLOGY. *See* CHILD DEVELOPMENT.

CHILDREN, CARE OF. *See* CHILD DEVELOPMENT.

CLAIRVOYANCE [klâr-voi'əns], perception of a thing or event by some means other than the recognized sense organs. Clairvoyance and telepathy are forms of extrasensory perception. *See* PARAPSYCHOLOGY.

CLARK, KENNETH BANCROFT (1914–   ), American Negro educator and psychologist. He was born in the Panama Canal Zone and became a U.S. citizen in 1931. Clark was educated at Howard University and Columbia University. He has been a university teacher and an administrator of programs to aid the underprivileged. Clark has written a number of books on the psychological effects of prejudice on Negroes. His work, *Desegregation: An Appraisal of the Evidence*, played an important part in the historic *Brown v. Board of Education of Topeka* (1954) Supreme Court decision on school desegregation.

CLIQUE [klēk], a small group of persons who meet frequently and whose relationship is close and confiding. The group is informal and usually without rules, officers, stated purposes, or name. Cliques are often formed in a larger organization among persons who feel different from and uncomfortable with the others. In a study of a business firm, it was found that those employees who had grievances against the company most often formed cliques. They had no group plan of action, but found relief and support in commenting sarcastically about superiors or about the plans of the organization. A study of life in a small town showed cliques arising to help the members' efforts in social climbing.

The term usually has a negative connotation. Those in a clique often appear exclusive and unwilling to associate with outsiders. Members are perceived as planning activities intended to benefit insiders, to the detriment of excluded persons. Members of a clique are often intolerant of those in another clique, and thus the unity of the larger group of which the cliques are a part is weakened. A strong clique, however, can strengthen a larger organization by supporting its goals. New members are accepted with difficulty and the loss of a few old members may destroy the group; thus cliques are usually relatively short-lived.

COCAINE [kō-kān'], an organic nitrogen-containing chemical obtained from the leaves of certain South American trees. For centuries leaves containing this substance have been chewed by South American Indians to increase endurance by stimulating the brain. Sir Arthur Conan-Doyle represented his famous fictional detective Sherlock Holmes as taking cocaine for the same purpose. Cocaine is addictive and its use is subject to narcotics regulations. The drug was once extensively used to produce limited, or local, anesthesia, but it has been largely replaced by less toxic compounds.

COMBAT FATIGUE, also known as combat neurosis, combat exhaustion, or shell shock, is a form of nervous breakdown that appears under the stress of battle. Although common misconception has it that it is usually the passive, timid, and emotionally immature personality who succumbs, even normally strong personalities may also collapse under the strain of prolonged combat.

The breakdown is ordinarily preceded by certain danger signals, such as a lack of appetite, insomnia, irritability, and a lack of interest in maintaining one's equipment. If, at this point, the soldier is not given an opportunity for rest and recuperation, he is likely to "freeze" in the next combat situation, developing amnesia, extreme anxiety, sweating, and palpitations. In severe cases, he may pass into a stupor in which he loses contact with reality or he may impulsively flee from the battlefield.

A chronic form of combat neurosis develops gradually over a period of time and is characterized by a limited emotional response and a reliving of combat experiences in the form of nightmares, anxiety, and convulsions.

Most cases of combat fatigue respond quickly to rest and relaxation.

COMMUNITY PSYCHIATRY, branch of psychiatry dealing with the prevention and treatment of mental disorders outside a hospital. It might also be termed preventive psychiatry, or more positively, community mental health service. The idea was first described in 1963 by President John F. Kennedy in his special message on Mental Illness and Mental Retardation. It was the first official pronouncement by a head of government that prevention, treatment, and rehabilitation of the mentally ill and mentally retarded are a community responsibility, not a private problem of patients, their families, and doctors.

State and local governments have provided facilities for the treatment and care of psychiatric patients for a long time. But these have not been comprehensive efforts integrating the services of hospitals, clinics, and private practitioners, and the resources of the public at large. Such an organized program would provide a framework within which medical doctors, psychologists, and auxiliary health workers could focus on the prevention of mental and emotional disorders.

The need to go beyond individual personality factors in the study of mental illness became apparent after World War I. Conditions of daily living, and social problems as factors in emotional health, received attention initially in the child guidance movements.

Approach. There are four phases in the community mental health approach. First, there are attempts to control the incidence of mental disorder. These include such preventive measures as child guidance, maternity clinics, and vocational and marriage counseling. Second, there is the attempt to reduce the duration of private treatment, or of hospitalization, when the latter becomes necessary.

Here the accent is placed on the doctor-patient relationship and professional care. The community is becoming more involved in this phase through community mental health centers, and welfare and Medicare programs. The third phase seeks to minimize disruption of family and community life by reducing the stigma attached to psychiatric treatment and hospitalization. Last is the attempt to aid the patient in his return to a life within the community. This is the area of family and job counseling, and follow-up services, such as aftercare clinics or patient clubs.

The extent of federal support for such a program in the United States is shown in the development of one service entering all phases of community psychiatry—the community mental health center. By mid-1967, $130,000,000 of federal funds had been spent on 256 centers that serve 41,000,000 people in practically all parts of the country. Plans call for 2,000 such centers by 1975. In view of the program's rapid expansion, there are urgent manpower needs, but a practical basis for true community psychiatry has been established.

See also MENTAL HEALTH; PSYCHIATRY.

COMPENSATION, one of several so-called defense mechanisms, is defined by behavior that is aimed (usually) at indirect or partial achievement of a goal when direct achievement is frustrated or leads to anxiety. For example, the boy who is unable to make the school basketball team may achieve partial satisfaction from being official scorekeeper. Much of the play and fantasy of children and daydreaming by adults may be considered compensatory in nature, when goals that are unattainable in reality are achieved in imagination. In addition, behavior designed to correct or "make up for" a real or imagined deficiency may be considered compensatory. The deaf person who learns to read lips and the blind person who learns to depend on other senses for knowledge of the environment provide examples of constructive compensatory behavior.

Some forms of compensation are less constructive, and may be indicative of major adjustment difficulties. Examples might be the father whose feelings of inferiority (imaginary or real) are compensated for by harsh disciplining of his children or the unmarried woman who spends her life "babying" cats and dogs instead of caring for children.

See also MENTAL HEALTH.

COMPARATIVE PSYCHOLOGY. *See* PSYCHOLOGY: *Comparative Psychology.*

CONDITIONING, psychological term referring to two methods for changing an organism's behavior in a relatively permanent fashion. The term "conditioned reflex," or "conditioned response," came into use as a result of experiments by Russian physiologists, notably I. P. Pavlov. In a famous study, Pavlov fed meat powder to a hungry dog. Eating the meat was accompanied by a flow of saliva. Before the dog was given meat, a bell was rung. After the bell-meat-salivation combination had been repeated a few times, the bell alone caused saliva to flow.

Respondent Conditioning. This "classical" or "Pavlovian" conditioning is now often referred to as respondent

conditioning. It is a method for causing responses of the glands or the smooth muscles (also called involuntary muscles—for example, muscles of the blood vessels) to be brought on by stimuli that would not ordinarily have any effect. This method begins with an innate or unconditioned reflex. In the case of Pavlov's dog, the action of salivation in response to meat in the mouth was an unconditioned reflex. If a stimulus such as a bell, which initially has no effect upon salivation, is presented together with the unconditioned stimulus (meat) for a series of trials, the neutral stimulus (bell) acquires the power to elicit the response (salivation). In this way a new, or conditioned, reflex is formed consisting of a conditioned stimulus (bell) leading to a conditioned response (salivation).

The conditioned reflex depends upon the unconditioned reflex for its strength, for if the meat in the above example is omitted for a series of trials, the conditioned reflex disappears (extinguishes). The unconditioned stimulus is therefore said to reinforce the conditioned reflex. The term "conditioning" is derived from the observation that the new reflex is conditional upon the occurrence of the reinforcement.

Operant Conditioning, also called instrumental conditioning, is a method of training responses of the striated muscles (also called voluntary or skeletal muscles—muscles of the arms and legs, for example). If a response or movement of the organism is followed by a reinforcement (or reward), the tendency to make that response increases. Thus if a small pellet of food is delivered each time a rat presses a lever, the frequency of lever-pressing increases. This is often called the law of effect since the probability of the response depends upon the effect which the response produces. As in the case of respondent conditioning, omission of the reinforcement weakens or extinguishes the response.

These two types of conditioning are considered to be basic to an understanding of learning, and most learning theorists attempt to derive details of the learning process from the laws of conditioning.

See also LEARNING; REFLEX.

CONFORMITY, the acceptance of and adherence to rules defining how members of a human group ought to think, feel, and act in social situations. It is commonly construed to involve motivation and choice in several forms rather than to derive from habit. It may remain a private subjective attitude of acceptance, unspoken and acted upon. It may be apparent, expressed, or communicated as a public avowal of socially sanctioned and doctrinally shared sentiments, beliefs, ideas, values, and standards. Or it may be openly and observably expressed as behavior or action in accordance with the rules, irrespective of the person's covert attitudes or overt professed beliefs. Conformity requires not only that the individual comply with the relevant rules governing his own action but also that he assume responsibility for applying rewards or penalties to others as they adhere to or deviate from accepted regulations. Research indicates that conformity in one form, type, or institutional area is not necessarily linked with that in another.

Personality, culture, and social structure are all considered to be important in engendering and maintaining conformity as a universal feature of social order. To be relatively predictable, conformity must be grounded in the needs of the personality during childhood. If the rules have been appropriately incorporated in the self, the individual will not experience conformity as an unavoidable response to external coercion. He will, instead, be motivated because compliance is emotionally gratifying, instrumentally effective in attaining his goals, and morally satisfying to his conscience. Since socialization also tends to instill a desire for social approval, the positive or negative responses from others, which the individual can anticipate in his imagination, act as additional incentives to conformity.

The character of the culture is another important consideration. Possible conflicts of rules may be prevented by specifying their application to different times, places, or groups. In instances in which such separation is impossible, conflict can be minimized by a socially sanctioned hierarchy of values which will stipulate an order of precedence or priority of rules. An official or unofficial ideology, with its systematic justification of the social status quo, also contributes culturally to conformity.

The social structure of the society and its constituent groups comprise a third source of conformity. Widespread dissemination of a sense of loyalty, common social interaction, observability of behavior, integration of subgroups, explicitness of informal or formal sanctions buttressed by immediacy and certainty of their imposition by members of the group are important in conformity. The vigilance of vested interests, groups enjoying special but legitimized advantages from present social arrangements, may also be consequential.

In addition to studying conformity as a universal social phenomenon, social scientists and others in the United States have been preoccupied with the distinctive features of the problem in American society. The traditional values of individualism and freedom have been subjected to strains from such internal developments as accentuated urbanization, centralized formal organization, expanded mass communications, and emergent mass society, which have been aggravated externally by the rise of successful, aggressive, highly centralized foreign social systems.
See also CULTURE; PSYCHOLOGY: *Psychology of Personality.*

CONSCIENCE [kŏn'shəns], the internal sense of right and wrong with respect to moral or ethical conduct. It is revealed both in self-control (resistance to temptation) and in self-censure (guilt). To many psychologists conscience is not a specific faculty but is a designation for various learned ways of guiding, or reacting to, one's own ethical behavior.
See also SUPEREGO.

CONSCIOUSNESS, like "experience" and "awareness," is a word which cannot be adequately defined in terms of more elementary concepts. In daily language consciousness is used to denote those kinds of experiences which almost anyone can privately verify. Public knowledge about consciousness can only be inferred from behavior. When an organism is able to react to its environment and to take past events and future possibilities

into account, it fulfills a necessary condition for being considered "conscious." It is generally considered that consciousness is a characteristic found in the animal kingdom, and that it coincides with a functional state in which instincts, or drives, are carried out to the advantage of the organism.

The following examples outline the progressive increase of consciousness in the animal kingdom. By attributing a subjective life to an animal we are employing *empathy,* which becomes quite speculative for animals low on the evolutionary scale. The drives of insects, for example, appear to have no overall goals, such as avoiding pain or finding pleasure. Action follows immediately upon stimulus, or impulse, even if this leads to the destruction of the organism. The attraction to light will lure a moth to a flame where, not feeling pain, the moth will burn. There cannot be consciousness in such an action. Behavior at this level consists of reflex, tropism, and instinctual action.

In vertebrates the beginnings of sensory awareness are apparent. Sensory experience becomes indirect because of the possibility of perceiving space and time. This results in virtual imagination and striving for overall goals, rather than merely carrying out individual instincts. Starlings with the "cat-danger" figure held in memory will postpone the pleasure of eating insects on a freshly mown lawn when a cat is present, thus avoiding danger. They may mob the animal and by acting as a group chase him away, thereby consciously removing danger. In man, awareness of the impressions made upon one's senses and awareness of one's actions is constantly present, except during periods of sleep and central nervous system malfunction.

Another meaning of consciousness is the awareness of one's awareness, of one existence and mental states. This is a reflexive state in which indirect experience can be related to something else. One might say, "I experience that my head aches." In this sense consciousness can be perfected only through that extension of the human brain known as language. Only language gives man the ability to objectify the experiences of pleasure and pain of which he is aware. Through mental acts, he may suppress his experience, and thought can then be his guide to action. Man has thereby surpassed the animal stage of evolution in which experiences themselves can be determinants of action. This in turn is an improvement upon the lower animals, whose instinctual drives determine all action.
See also SUBCONSCIOUS AND UNCONSCIOUS.

COUÉ [koō-ā'], **ÉMILE** (1857–1926), French psychotherapist whose formula "Every day in every way I am becoming better and better" is now proverbial. Born in Troyes, France, he was educated as a chemist and served as such in his home town. He studied hypnosis and suggestion with the physician Hippolyte Bernheim and later developed his own method of psychotherapy. In 1910 he established a free clinic in Nancy where he applied his new method. He taught individuals how to use autosuggestion to heal themselves.

CRIMINOLOGY [krĭm-ə-nŏl'ə-jē], the study of the development of criminal behavior, the organization of criminal activities, and the methods of dealing with the criminal—his apprehension, trial, and subsequent treatment. It investigates the causes of crime, seeking through comparative studies to separate general widely applicable principles from fortuitous or accidental circumstances.

The systematic study of criminal behavior was undertaken only 80 or 90 years ago when speculations about the nature and causes of crime began to be replaced by the accumulation of information based upon systematic investigation of social phenomena. The sociologist has a definite contribution to make to criminological research by his persistent search for the uniformities in the social behavior related to criminal acts. Ideally, he sets aside considerations of vengeance, justice, and moral condemnation and studies crime as a social and socio-psychological phenomenon. He seeks to establish and test various hypotheses regarding criminal behavior in order ultimately to develop techniques for controlling crime.

History. Scientific investigation in criminology began with Adolphe Quételet (1796–1874), the Belgian statistician who applied the term "social physics" to his work. Quételet charted the environment of crime and related his findings to social conditions in diverse urban areas and national regions. The most influential early work was done by three Italian investigators, Cesare Lombroso (1836–1909), Raffaele Garofalo (1852–1934), and Enrico Ferri (1856–1929). Lombroso, with his student Ferri, attempted to correlate criminal behavior with bodily form and work out a theory of the biological origin of crime, according to which criminals were an atavistic type of human being, that is, a reversion to an earlier stage in human evolution. According to this view criminals constitute a distinct biological type and can be identified by such characteristics as small capacity of the skull, fusion of the skull bones instead of the normal sutures, retreating forehead, protruding jaws, and low sensitivity to pain. According to Lombroso, these marks did not cause crime, but they were the symptoms of the degeneracy and reversion to a primitive stage of development which predisposed the individual to criminal behavior. Lombroso later rejected his theory and introduced socio-psychological factors into the etiology of crime. Although Lombroso's findings were discredited, his approach, which emphasized the study of the criminal to explain crime, was followed by later criminologists.

Enrico Ferri made original contributions, both in the study of crime as an individual fact, by his researches on prisoners, and in the study of crime as a social fact, by using French criminal statistics. He tried to reconcile the social elements in the genesis of criminal behavior with the physical and anthropological ideas of Lombroso, and his *Sociologica Criminale* (1884) stimulated the study of crime by sociologists. Garofalo, another of Lombroso's students, also incorporated social factors into his interpretations of the causes of criminal behavior. The early combination of sociology and the study of criminal behavior culminated in America in the publication of Maurice Parmelee's textbook, *Criminology*, in 1918.

With the decline in the acceptance of Lombroso's theories there appeared numerous attempts to explain criminal behavior as the result of inherited mental defects, particularly, feeble-mindedness. Studies subsequently undertaken largely discredited this theory when it was found that criminals were not necessarily persons of low intelligence. Various attempts have been made to relate neuroses, psychoses, and psychopathic states to criminal activity. Claims were made that one or another type of mental illness or emotional disturbance underlay criminal behavior. Such explanations are questioned, though psychiatrists and psychoanalysts have made basic contributions to the study of criminal behavior.

Modern Views. In the second decade of this century the "multiple-factor" approach was developed. It recognized the complex conditions under which specific instances of criminal behavior may develop. Modern criminology recognizes a distinction between systematic crime and occasional or erratic crime. Systematic crime involves a complex network of social relationships, including a division of labor, special training, group morale, and specific relationships with the police, courts, and politicians. Systematic crime is thus distinguished from individual isolated instances of criminal acts by people who are otherwise not closely connected with the criminal system. The predominant contemporary view is that criminal behavior results from a process essentially indistinguishable from that involved in behavior in general. Criminal behavior, like other behavior, is one result of a learning process; in this case, the learning of antisocial behavior from others. Criminality is thus acquired by the individual from his environment, if it is conducive to such behavior. A definite contribution by American sociologists has been the theory that criminal behavior results from cultural conflict and the weakening of the force of the mores upon members of society, the resulting social disorganization being characterized by confusion, uncertainty, or ambivalence regarding contradictory moral and ethical standards. Coupled with materialistic values, these conditions drive individuals, particularly those who are emotionally unstable, to fulfill their desires by antisocial or criminal behavior.

At the same time, most criminologists do not limit their explanation to environmental factors, but maintain that the personality of the individual plays a role; it is in the interaction of personality and environment or in the impact of environment upon personality that explanations must be sought. This approach is thus a kind of synthesis of the contributions of sociologists, psychiatrists, and psychoanalysts, the main difference being one of emphasis.

Another view of the nature of crime is found in the work of E. H. Sutherland, whose theory of white-collar crime maintains that the total picture of the contemporary criminal is incomplete and incorrect, since it is based on data concerning individuals in prison and omits the many businessmen, industrial leaders, and professional people who are rarely imprisoned. Thus, theories which relate crime primarily to the lower classes, to poverty, to low intelligence, or to psychopathic states, are erroneous, and remedies which consider only these factors are bound to fail.

In Europe the tradition has been to restrict criminology to the status of an offshoot of legal science, while in the United States the field has been characterized by numerous empirical studies relating to contemporary aspects of crime and by the publication of general textbooks containing recapitulations and reformulations of research and theory.

The main difficulty has been, and continues to be, the difficulty of establishing a satisfactory definition of the word "crime." In common usage the term designates not only acts which deviate from the imperatives of various ethical systems but also numerous other acts which appear to some persons, or by some standards, to represent merely improper behavior. Thus the inexactness of the definition of the word "crime" and the inability to characterize homogeneous units of behavior remain formidable handicaps to the development of comprehensive interpretations of criminal behavior.

See also JUVENILE DELINQUENCY.

CRITICAL REALISM, name loosely applied to the philosophical theories of perception which, like those of René Descartes (1596–1650) and John Locke (1632–1704), in contrast to naïve realism, affirm the irreducible dualism of the perceived object and the sensory datum through which the object is known. Sometimes it is applied more specifically to the views of a group of 20th-century American philosophers, including George Santayana, who maintained that sensory data are essences and not existents.

CROWD BEHAVIOR, actions among the members of a large gathering of persons within sight or sound of one another. These actions are made possible by certain characteristics of a crowd, such as the temporary duration of the gathering; the lack of officers, rules, division of labor, or other qualities of an organization; and the anonymity of the members.

Members of a crowd are ordinarily indifferent to one another, but any event which appeals to their emotions at once generates interaction and ready contagion of feelings among them. Each person's impulses are strengthened by his observation that others are reacting in a way similar to his own, and the characteristics of the crowd provide almost no restraints on impulsive behavior. The result is that members engage in uninhibited behavior they would ordinarily never reveal in public.

Crowd behavior in reaction to fear, anger, or hate can be uncontrolled and dangerous. The behavior of a crowd may also be a source of enthusiasm for useful purposes in political rallies, religious festivals, and community celebrations. The irrational aspects of crowd behavior are reduced when the crowd is broken into small groups, when a new focus of attention is provided, or when the members are reminded of their places and positions in the community.

CULTURE AND PERSONALITY. People who have grown up under different cultural conditions reveal, as groups, substantially different response tendencies or social personalities. Cultural anthropologists carry out culture and personality studies in order to identify differences in social personality and to learn the cultural conditions that bring them into being.

In America Margaret Mead pioneered in the study of culture and personality with the investigation reported in what has since become an anthropological classic, *Coming of Age in Samoa* (1928). The problem on which she reported was adolescence, a stage of human growth in all societies. Some psychologists used to believe that the teen-age years inevitably brought stormy adjustment problems. Biological changes occurring at this time acted directly on other aspects of personality, they theorized, and caused unrest. Mead doubted this theory and went to a relatively simple, uniform society, Samoa, to test it. She found that, unlike American and European girls, Samoan girls experienced no upheaval in personality when they reached adolescence. Their smooth transition from childhood to adulthood she attributed to specific conditions that distinguished Samoan culture. Growing up in Samoa was easy because Samoan life demanded few strong choices from a teen-ager. In contrast to a girl growing up in the United States, the Samoan girl escaped having to decide between conflicting standards of morality and differing religious denominations. She had not, during her earlier years, become utterly dependent on a few relatives whose strong influence could now arrest spontaneous growth and development. In short, Mead discovered that culture rather than biology produced the adolescent storm and stress observed in America and Europe.

Early in the 1930's another American anthropologist, Edward Sapir, began to call for a new approach in studying culture. He urged anthropologists to examine culture from the viewpoint of persons whom it directly involved. Then Ruth Benedict achieved renown with *Patterns of Culture* (1934), in which she deals with cultures as though they express their carriers' personalities. She contrasts the Indians living on the Great Plains west of the Mississippi River with the village, or Pueblo, Indians inhabiting the American Southwest. Judging from Plains Indian culture, as it existed prior to the white man's westward expansion, the Plains Indian disdained the commonplace and delighted in skirting the edges of excess. He loved and sought risks in warfare, and in ceremonies he heroically practiced self-torture or released unbridled grief for the sake of supernatural aid. (The use of peyote to induce unusual psychological states is a recent example of his bent for going to extremes.) The Pueblo Indians, on the other hand, distrusted excess. They preferred restraint and kept to the middle of the road. Occasionally they found it necessary to go to battle, but warriors did not seek out a fight. In their rain ceremonies the Pueblo people practiced repetitive dancing and chanting but avoided spectacular eruptions of emotion and heroic displays of individual initiative. Plains and Pueblo Indian cultures each reflected a unique social personality. Actually, Ruth Benedict's *Patterns of Culture* was not based on psychological studies of the individuals she described. She drew her conclusions about personality mainly from culture as others had described it. Subsequent culture and personality research, however, nearly always sought information about social personality through the intimate study of living persons with whom the researcher himself lived. Practical problems connected with World War II did much to stimulate culture and personality studies. The war turned anthropologists' attention from personality in small, isolated societies to the national characters of Englishmen, Russians, Germans, and Japanese. Due to the war subjects for such research often had to be found and interviewed at some distance from their homelands.

Are there really social personalities? Perhaps we mislead ourselves in believing that differences in dress, food, language, and nationality are accompanied by more deeply embedded psychological differences. The Rorschach test, which requires a subject to tell what he sees in each of 10 amorphous ink blots, has been used to answer this question. The test assumes that everyone will find the blots equally ambiguous, regardless of his culture, and that a person will react to the blots in a way that expresses his customary personality. Rorschach records from different societies indeed reveal fairly consistent differences from one people to another. This indicates that people who have been reared in the same culture do possess generally similar response tendencies that lie below the surface of their actions. In some respects every individual is, of course, unique in his psychological makeup. But he shares some attributes of personality with people who have been reared as he has. Within the same society, further distinctions in personality coincide with status. Middle-class Americans in a small American city exhibit personality traits that a lower-class neighborhood would find hard to understand. Today many American Indian tribes are split into factions, each possessing some unique personality characteristics. There are tribesmen nostalgically rooted in the vanished past and others who are deeply anxious over whether to adopt the white man's ways. Still others have fully adopted many values and a large part of the psychological outlook of their non Indian contemporaries.

Similar experiences that affect most or all of the individuals born into a specific society shape social personality. Experiences peculiar only to a specific status give rise to those variations in the over-all social personality called status personality, for example, a middle-class personality. The lifelong process which engenders social personality is called socialization. Some socialization is quite direct and deliberate. Parents and teachers hold out explicit expectations and inducements that shape the growing child's unfolding response patterns. Americans learn to be competitive in part through such direct teaching. But the deeper areas of personality often depend more on how than on what a child is taught. They also depend on conditions and circumstances that accompany growing up. The Samoan girl's easy transition to adulthood had not been taught to her deliberately but stemmed from the casual atmosphere which characterized nearly all of Samoan life and in which she had been reared. The less deliberate side of socialization includes the impression that history leaves on society. Those decades when millions of European immigrants landed in America, eager to make their fortunes, shaped American attitudes toward class. The idea of a future unlimited was then welded into the American dream. An American regards class as measuring how far he has come; he is not frozen in his class for life. This idea is still being perpetuated by each generation of parents and teachers.

Culture and personality research also inquires how cultural conditions relate to mental health and illness. For example, the content of a psychotic's delusions varies from one culture to another, and even alters as culture changes. Invention of the radio gave the paranoid, suffering from delusions of persecution, a basis to fear that he was being influenced against his will through wireless. People's confidence in mental health programs and their willingness to trust a psychiatrist also depend on culture. Due partly to their lack of mental health knowledge, people of lower socio-economic status in the United States who are undergoing psychiatric treatment tend to suffer from more severe mental illness than citizens of a higher social class. Many cultures possess their own psychotherapy which periodically comes into operation to relieve tension or anxiety and provide reassurance.

Like anthropology in general, culture and personality study teaches that cultural conditions do much to shape individual behavior. Aggression, adolescent turmoil, cutthroat competition, and high rates of mental illness are far from inevitable. They are encouraged by certain cultural arrangements rather than others. Because culture is man-made it can be brought under man's control. One big problem is how to effect such control. Another is how to do so without sacrificing democratic and other values.

D

DEFENSE MECHANISM, a psychic device for guarding the self against such instinctive but unpleasant feelings as guilt and anxiety. The attempt is unconscious and often directed toward the maintenance of self-esteem. The theory of defense mechanisms is one of the cornerstones of psychoanalysis, which probes the workings of the personality. Sigmund Freud used "defense" to refer to the efforts of an individual to protect himself against various instinctual demands continuing throughout life, as well as the general conflicts arising during childhood from cultural-social conventions. If the personality handles these individual and general demands successfully, they cease to be disturbing. However, an unsuccessful defense necessitates a repetition or perpetuation of the defense reactions. A person plagued by fear of being left alone in a house may adopt the defense mechanism of checking to make certain that the house is indeed empty. If his fear persists, the defense mechanism may become compulsive, and he will resort to needless checking and rechecking.

The best known defense mechanism is "repression," that is, the unconscious dismissal of an idea, emotion, or thought from awareness.
See also ANXIETY; NEUROSIS; PSYCHOANALYSIS.

DÉJÀ VU [*dā-zhà vü'*] (Fr. "already seen"), the illusion of having previously experienced that which is currently taking place—as the feeling of familiarity with a city to which one has never been before. The phenomenon is usually explained by the subconscious association of certain aspects of the new situation with previous events which have been forgotten. *Déjà vu* may occur in normal persons, as well as in those suffering from nervous disorders, such as hysteria and epilepsy.
See also PARAPSYCHOLOGY.

DELINQUENCY. *See* JUVENILE DELINQUENCY.

DELIRIUM [*dĭ-lĭr'ē-əm*]. Once a synonym for insanity, the term now describes a form of mental disturbance characterized by varying degrees of bewilderment, restlessness, confusion, hallucinations, and illusions. The symptoms fluctuate in intensity and may be more marked at night than during the day. There is always an alteration in the state of consciousness, ranging from mild confusion to deep stupor. The patient is usually incoherent and may suffer from delusions of persecution. Delirium is most commonly associated with high fever and infectious diseases and with diseases that seriously impair bodily functions. It is sometimes seen in extremely agitated mental patients. Treatment is directed at the underlying cause; sedatives are given to relieve the symptoms.

DELIRIUM TREMENS [*trē'mənz*], a serious mental disturbance that usually develops in chronic alcoholics during, or following, a drinking bout. The delirium appears suddenly, often with frightening visual hallucinations, such as grotesque animals, which leave the patient in panic. All intellectual functions are affected, resulting in confusion concerning time, place, and identity. A characteristic tremor appears in the muscles of the face, tongue, and fingers. The victim is feverish and loses body water. The condition usually passes in a few days, but it may be fatal. If heavy drinking is continued the disturbance recurs, possibly resulting in a fully developed psychosis.
See also ALCOHOLISM.

DEMENTIA [*dĭ-měn'shə*], a deterioration of intellectual faculties resulting from brain damage produced by disease, injury, or changes accompanying old age. The afflicted person suffers from a loss of memory, restriction of interests, difficulty in grasping and retaining new ideas, and confusion as to his identity and whereabouts.
See also SENILITY.

DEPRESSION, in psychiatric usage, describes a feeling of despondency which may range from simple unhappiness to complete despair. It may be seen as a common reaction to misfortune, in association with physical illness, or bodily changes, or as part of a fully-developed psychotic condition.

Depression following the death of a close friend or relative normally disappears with time. Distressing personal relationships or occupational problems often cause a severe depression, which may include loss of appetite, loss of interest in usual activities, and insomnia. In some cases, physical and mental activity is impaired and the individual may contemplate suicide. In children and adolescents depression may arise as a reaction to an intolerable family situation. It is frequently seen in children living in institutions, and in those separated from their parents.

Change-of-life in both men and women may bring on depression as a reaction to the prospect of vanishing youth. In older persons failing health, the death of close friends and relatives, and financial dependence on their children may bring on depression. Physical illness is a common cause of depression, especially among active persons who cannot tolerate limitations of activity—as, for example, in the case of an energetic businessman who becomes partially disabled following a heart attack.

Depression is a characteristic feature of a mental disorder called manic-depressive psychosis. In this condition the individual alternates between moods of great elation (mania) and profound depression. In general, depression which does not arise from an obvious cause, such as death of a loved one, and which persists for more than a few days, should be referred for psychiatric care.

DEWEY, JOHN (1859–1952), American philosopher and

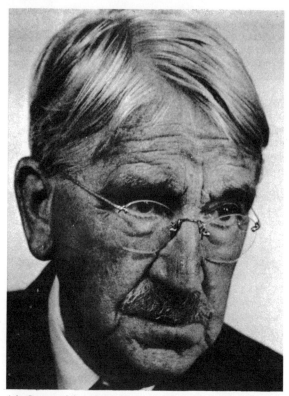

John Dewey, philosopher and leader in education. (COLUMBIA UNIVERSITY)

educator. A professor of philosophy at various universities, he taught at Columbia from 1905 until his retirement in 1929.

In philosophy he was an advocate of a form of pragmatism to which he gave the name "Instrumentalism." The area of philosophy with which Dewey was most concerned was ethics. He believed that success in formulating an adequate ethical code would only come about when men came to base their value systems on human experience in the natural world. Dewey's ethical views are discussed chiefly in *Human Nature and Conduct* (1922) and *The Quest for Certainty* (1929).

In educational theory he was one of the founders of progressive education. While at the University of Chicago from 1894 to 1905, Dewey established an experimental school to develop his theories of education. His educational philosophy is expressed in *The School and Society* (1900) and *Democracy and Education* (1916). Both of these were translated into a dozen foreign languages and had wide influence.

From the time Dewey came to teach at Columbia until his death, he had an international reputation, being invited to China, Japan, Turkey, Mexico, and the Soviet Union as an educational consultant. He was also in the forefront of many social movements in the United States, including woman suffrage.

See also FUNCTIONAL PSYCHOLOGY.

DISCIPLINE IN HOME AND SCHOOL. All societies have standards of conduct that must be met by their members.

Any effort by authorities to encourage conformity to those standards can be regarded as a disciplinary measure. When someone says that a child "needs a little discipline," he often means that the child should be punished. But discipline has a positive as well as a negative aspect; it involves not only the prohibition of unacceptable behavior but also the encouragement of behavior which meets approved standards.

The goals of discipline go beyond mere obedience, at least in democratic societies. As long as parents and teachers are bigger and more powerful than children, obedience is relatively easy to obtain. The major goal of discipline in a democracy is self-control on the part of the governed, and this goal is more difficult to reach.

Numerous investigations are in general agreement on the following principles. Reasonable limits on child behavior are necessary for the good of others and contribute to the well-being of the child himself. Too many restraints confuse children and produce the impression that the world is an excessively forbidding place. A limited number of restraints, stated with the greatest possible clarity and coupled with an effort to channel behavior into areas of freedom, foster feelings of stability and security at a time when self-control is poorly developed.

Approval for "right" behavior has more predictably beneficial effects than punishment for "wrong" behavior. Punishment does not directly reduce the tendency to perform a forbidden act. It creates a drive, fear, and once fear is instilled forbidden behavior may be avoided, at least as long as the punisher is present. Severe punishment is often proposed as a corrective or preventive measure in the control of delinquency, but the results of research suggest that severe punishment is an ineffective way of controlling behavior. The parents of delinquents have been found to be much more prone than the parents of nondelinquents to use physical punishment in disciplining children. In a study comparing children from strict and permissive homes, those from permissive homes were more self-reliant, persistent, imaginative, spontaneous, and above all more cooperative and better adjusted socially than those from strict homes. In another study, harsh discipline by teachers led to an increase in misbehavior on the part of children who had watched the punishment being meted out to others. Severe punishment may control behavior in the situation where it is imposed, but it is likely to arouse hostility along with fear, and this can have enduring and damaging effects.

Lax and neglectful treatment, letting children do as they please, can also be damaging. Firmness and consistency are needed in the application of controls. But these are best internalized by children, so that they can control themselves, if the limits are set in an atmosphere of love and understanding.

See also ADOLESCENCE; CHILD DEVELOPMENT.

DISEASE, PSYCHOSOMATIC AND MENTAL

Psychosomatic Diseases. In recent years it has been realized that many bodily ailments, such as peptic ulcer, high blood pressure, and asthma, may be caused or influenced by emotional disorders. A dramatic example of the ability of the mind to interfere with bodily function appears in hysteria, which may cause blindness or paralysis in the absence of any organic injury or disease. The number of diseases placed within the psychosomatic group is steadily expanding.

Mental Disease. The two broad classifications of mental disease are the psychoses and the neuroses. The psychotic individual is usually regarded as having lost contact with reality. The neurotic is aware of reality, but is the victim of powerful unconscious drives which distort his behavior. Little is known of the causes of mental diseases and a long-standing controversy in the field concerns the extent to which these diseases are of physical or mental origin.

In conclusion, it is frequently not possible to place a disease within a single classification. For example, since some metabolic diseases are inherited they could be grouped in the hereditary category. The causes of other diseases, such as rheumatoid arthritis, are not completely understood, making categorization even more difficult. One can expect that, as the knowledge of diseases and their causes becomes more extensive, the classification of diseases will change considerably.

DISSOCIATION, in psychology, the breakdown of a complex conscious mental process into simpler components, which continue to function autonomously but which can only become conscious singly. After a severe accident, a person may enter a dreamlike state in which he perceives everything around him but in which everything seems unreal. In this state, his perception has become dissociated from his emotions, and only the former remains conscious. Similar cleavages in the psyche may also occur during illness with high fever, and in hypnosis, or trance.

Most often, dissociation is seen in emotional disorders where the splitting off of parts of consciousness may lead to a dual personality. In such cases the patient may be in a so-called fugue state, during which his awareness is narrowed and his memory impaired. The patient may lead a totally different life, and if he regains knowledge of his former life, he may forget everything he experienced during the fugue. Stevenson's *Dr. Jekyll and Mr. Hyde* is an example of alternating fugue states, resulting in a multiple personality.

DOMINANCE HIERARCHY, a concept in animal behavior that refers to the tendency of group-living animals to arrange themselves into a rank order. By knowing their status in the order and accepting this organization, animals minimize aggression. Group life with very little conflict is thereby made possible.

T. Schjelderup-Ebbe made the fundamental observation that the members of a bird flock recognize each other as individuals. In a small group of hens, which have been living together without crowding, there is very little aggressive behavior. If a competitive situation is set up by providing a little pile of grain, the so-called alpha animal will come to the food and start to peck. Should another animal try to peck some of the grain, the alpha individual will threaten and eventually chase it away. If the alpha hen is removed, another hen immediately takes her place and, apparently by common consent, is allowed to dominate the source of food in the same manner. Schjelderup-

Ebbe has shown that the group consists of individuals who form a hierarchy of procedure—in this case for who gets a chance to feed first. Such procedure in competition is called behavioral dominance, and it has been shown to play a role in various degrees and forms in all social behavior of animals. In chickens the hierarchy is clear-cut and linear; alpha pecks all other hens, beta pecks all hens except alpha, and so on. In other animal species the organization may be more subtle and may vary for different situations.

It is important to realize the interaction between dominance and aggression on the one hand, and dominance and territoriality on the other hand. Dominance behavior has a role in minimizing aggression, thereby preventing the waste of energy which would occur if the strongest animal at all times had to secure his part of the spoils by actually fighting off all the others. However, a subordinate individual animal sometimes needs freedom from the restraints of those higher on the totem pole, such as during reproduction. Nature has allowed for this by providing him with the urge to occupy and defend a territory. In cats, for example, the tomcats show a definite rank order for acquiring mates in the mating season, but even a low-ranked tomcat is respected by the dominants on his home ground.
See also AGGRESSION.

DREAMS, a series of images, thoughts, or emotions occurring in the mind during sleep or daydreaming. Dreams have aroused interest and reverence since the beginnings of mankind—examples of prophetic dreams and dream explanations are found throughout the Bible. In many primitive societies the dream state is considered a sojourn of the soul outside the body during sleep.

For the individual, fantasy and dreams may be considered irrational symbolic ways of dealing with reality, comparable to the use of myth and legend by societies. Sigmund Freud published *The Interpretation of Dreams* in 1900. This study of the nature of dreams shows them to be expressions of unconscious processes, such as suppressed wishes or unresolved problems.

According to Freud, the confused, illogical, and contradictory features of the dream represent the attempt of a censoring mechanism to disguise and symbolize the unconscious contents, thus allowing sleep to continue. Without this censoring mechanism, controversial thoughts and ideas might wake the dreamer, since direct confrontation with unconscious material cannot normally be tolerated and must be suppressed in the waking state. The loss of contact with reality, as experienced in the dream, resembles that occurring in psychosis, but the sane person realizes that he is dreaming, whereas the insane accepts his hallucinations as real.

Certain other aspects of the dream were elaborated by Carl Jung. These include the role of archetypes and problem-solving mechanisms, as well as the occurrence of compensatory and prospective dreams.

Dream research has acquired a physiological aspect through the discovery of periods of Rapid Eye Movement (REM) during sleep. It is during REM periods that occur the vividly detailed, unrealistic, and "hallucinatory" dreams remembered after awakening. Although rapid eye

DRUG ADDICTION

movements are the most obvious indicator of such REM periods during sleep, other changes have also been documented, such as changes in the brain-wave patterns and increases in respiratory and cardiovascular activity.

Four to five REM periods normally occur each night, lasting approximately 20 min. each. These REM periods are separated by Non Rapid Eye Movement (NREM) periods, lasting approximately 90 min. NREM periods produce realistic, though vague, dreams, which are difficult to recall upon awakening. Deprivation of REM sleep, by awakening the subject every time he shows signs of REM, leads to increasingly disturbed mental life. The significance of this observation for determining the causes of mental disease is under extensive study.
See also SLEEP.

DRUG ADDICTION, a term used in drug abuse discussions, is frequently confused with psychological dependence (or habituation) and physical dependence. These expressions are often erroneously interchanged, causing semantic confusion. The World Health Organization (WHO) has recommended that these terms be replaced by a single generic expression, "drug dependence," which is itself qualified by designating the particular drug under discussion—for example, "drug dependence of the barbiturate type." Common usage and many laws employ all of these terms and they should be understood in the following context:

Psychological dependence is a state of drug abuse which exists when the user feels that the effects of the drug are necessary to maintain a sense of well-being. There is an emotional or mental adaptation to the effects of the drug, since continued usage appears to satisfy some emotional or personality needs of the individual. The user may experience a degree of psychological involvement ranging from desire to craving to compulsion. An accepted synonym for this particular state is habituation.

Physical dependence is a physiological adaptation in which the drug is required to prevent the onset of a withdrawal or an abstinence syndrome. Abstinence syndromes vary depending upon the particular drug dependency. When a heroin addict is intoxicated, he is sedated, but in withdrawal, a state of excitation predominates. The intoxicated amphetamine user is agitated and excitable, but in withdrawal, a state of depression and exhaustion prevails, and the individual often lapses into deep sleep for long periods. It is probable that physical dependence occurs, at least to a certain degree, after a single dose of an opiate or barbiturate. The aftereffect of this initial drug experience may be a slight aggravation of the underlying anxieties which led to the use of the drug originally and the beginning of the withdrawal phase. The cycle of chronic and repetitive use may thus have been triggered in the susceptible user. The absence of physical dependence, such as noted with most hallucinogens or psychedelics, for example, LSD, does not prove that such drugs are innocuous.

The exact cause or mechanism of the abstinence syndrome is unknown. The reaction to the sudden deprivation of a drug which causes physical dependence depends, to a large degree, upon the dosage level and frequency of use of the particular drug. The withdrawal symptoms disap-

pear as the body readjusts over a period of time or if the drug is reintroduced.

Tolerance is a potentially serious medical and pharmacological problem, in which increasing quantities of the drug must be taken in order to obtain the same effect. This becomes especially dangerous when dealing with narcotics, amphetamines, and the sedative-hypnotic group of drugs, such as the barbiturates and alcohol. The various effects of a particular drug are not necessarily affected by this phenomenon at the same rate. For example, insomnia persists in the amphetamine user as do the constricted pupils of the opiate user, regardless of changes in dosage or frequency of administration. Tolerance is most often associated with drugs causing physical dependence.

Addiction is properly defined as a state of periodic or chronic intoxication produced by the repeated consumption of a drug. Associated with this state is a compulsive and overwhelming involvement on the part of the addict with the procurement and use of the drug. Addiction to the specific drug involves psychological dependence, tolerance, and usually, physical dependence. Physical dependence may be present without "addiction," in this generally accepted sense, as evidenced by the newborn child of a heroin addict. Clearly, there is no psychological involvement on the part of the infant.

Types of Addiction

In general, the commonly abused drugs fit into four major categories: *narcotics, central nervous system stimulants, psychedelics,* and the *sedative-hypnotic group.* In a broad sense "drug abuse" is defined as the self-administration of a drug in a manner that deviates from approved social patterns. In reality, this may involve any drug, but we are here referring to the abuse of drugs that are taken for the purpose of producing changes in mood and behavior, and which are obtained illicitly (not forgetting the other major problem of legal drug abuse). Implicit in this concept is the consideration that society's acceptance of various drugs changes from time to time and from culture to culture—for example, the practice of opium smoking was accepted in China until quite recently.

Narcotics. This group includes opiates derived from the opium poppy, such as morphine, or chemically related derivatives, such as heroin or methadone. They are best characterized as effective analgesics (actually, there is an altered reaction to pain, since the pain itself may be perceived), and profound central nervous system depressants. The frequently described euphoria associated with narcotics may be due to the relief of pain, tension, and anxiety in those with low thresholds. The terms "addiction" and "addict" most commonly refer to the problem of opiate dependence, which is now considered a medical illness rather than a form of criminality. Criminal activity results from the need to obtain a supply of the drug rather than from the effects of the drug itself.

The majority of the effects of opiate addiction, excluding so-called overdose and respiratory depression, are not directly related to the drug action. Most complications or untoward medical effects such as serum hepatitis, skin infections, blood poisoning, anemia, tetanus, and malnutrition are related to the manner in which the illicit drug is used and the kind of life the addict lives.

Recognition of the chronic narcotic addict by means of his pin-point pupils and scars or pigmentation over the veins is usually not difficult. The major medical problems due to the action of the opiates are related to overdosage and to abstinence symptoms. The nonfatal overdose can be diagnosed promptly in the suspected user if widespread fluid accumulation in the lungs is accompanied by stupor, small pupils, and either a normal or slowed breathing rate. The overdose produces profound central nervous system depression, including respiratory center depression, leading to the paradox of fluid accumulation in the lungs without the usual increase in rate of respiration. Since the effects are reversible, the use of specific antinarcotic chemicals and prompt supportive treatment, including positive pressure oxygen and maintenance of the blood pressure, may be life-saving.

In the United States most of the illicit narcotics use involves heroin, the most potent of the opiates. If the narcotic addict cannot obtain his drug, he displays the abstinence syndrome. The intensity of withdrawal increases with the degree of physical dependence, symptoms usually starting 8 to 12 hours after the last "fix" and peaking at 36 to 72 hours. Symptoms include any or all of the following: nervousness, anxiety, sleeplessness, yawning, tearing, profuse perspiration, muscle cramps and twitching, vomiting and diarrhea, rapid heart beat and breathing rate. Administering methadone, itself a synthetic narcotic, or certain tranquilizers for three to five days eases the withdrawal symptoms, and there is no objection to the use of sedatives.

Whereas the initial medical withdrawal from narcotics is relatively easy, the prospects for long-term success are not good. In addition to the effects of tolerance and overwhelming drug dependence, the high percentage of failure of rehabilitation efforts may result from the considerable reinforcement of the habit due to the following factors: (1) heroin suppresses all disturbing sources of the user's anxiety (those related to pain, sexuality, and expressions of aggression)—a total satiation of drive; (2) acceptance into the fraternity of other addicts; and (3) conditioning, an eventual state whereby even after long-term withdrawal, there is an intense craving for the drug in situations where the drug is known to be available. Occasionally, an addict's mere presence in a familiar neighborhood has been said to precipitate a modified abstinence syndrome.

Concerning long-term therapy, it is generally agreed that there is no universally acceptable program nor any single effective method for the rehabilitation of all narcotic addicts. Arrest and incarceration have taken addicts "off the street" but have not acted as deterrents to increased drug addiction. The United States Public Health Service hospitals at Lexington, Ky., and Fort Worth, Tex., established for the treatment of narcotic addicts, likewise have a high readmission rate. Self-help communities run by ex-addicts and following the Synanon-Daytop model have been developed while the chemotherapeutic approach, most notably using methadone in high doses to block the euphoric effects of heroin, is being expanded.

Central Nervous System Stimulants. The abuse of amphetamines, the major representative of this category, is a major health hazard due to the rapid increase in their use and the drugs' inherent biological dangers. The amphetamines are powerful central nervous system stimulants and with moderate dosages, an increase in work performance, alertness, agitation, sleeplessness, diminished fatigue, and loss of appetite are usually observed. With chronic and increasing use, the following adverse effects often occur: irritability, insomnia, aggression, bizarre and sometimes inappropriate repetitive actions, and, eventually, panic, confusion, and paranoid psychosis. Other medical problems include effects related to unsterile intravenous usage, as noted with heroin addiction. The use of the stimulant to augment energy and produce euphoria is often intermittently counteracted by the use of barbiturates to allay agitation and insomnia—the "yo-yo" phenomenon or the "ups and downs" syndrome. There is a rapid onset of tolerance and considerable psychological dependence on the part of the user.

Although a characteristic withdrawal syndrome does not develop when amphetamines are suddenly stopped (thus there is no true physical dependence) there is a reaction phase of exhaustion, sleep, and depression (the "crash"). Because of the sometimes overwhelming psychological dependence they produce, amphetamines are considered addicting. In some areas, young persons are told that heroin eases the crash, and the increasing use of heroin in the schools and suburbs may, in part, reflect and parallel the "speed," or amphetamine, epidemic. In addition, in order to augment the opiate euphoria, intravenous amphetamines are now frequently being used together, with heroin substituting for the older cocaine-heroin combination (colloquially known as the "speedball").

Psychedelics. Because of its potency and widespread availability, LSD is by far the most important hallucinogen, Marihuana, the object of a greater notoriety, is a minor medical or pharmacological drug. The psychedelics are potentially capable of producing psychological dependence in the user, but there is no evidence that they cause physical dependence or addiction. LSD, and probably the other psychedelics, act almost entirely on the higher central nervous system centers. Apparently they permit a bombardment of sensory stimuli, which are unaffected by the usual selective filtering-out processes that function in the brain. A short-lived tolerance occurs with LSD whereby a loss of hallucinogenic effect is noted after a few doses are taken within a short period. After a few days, the psychedelic effects are again evident. A cross-tolerance to other psychedelics such as mescaline also occurs.

Sedative-Hypnotic Group. The model is the barbiturates, the "downs" or "goof-balls," but the group includes among others, alcohol. Each has a potential for abuse, and chronic use results in tolerance and psychological and physical dependence. Taken in combination, there may be a greater reaction than when each is used alone, and each, especially on withdrawal, can cause convulsions, coma, and death.

The initial feeling of tranquility, elation, and well-being, which low doses of barbiturates provide, soon gives way in the chronic, excessive user to irritability, impairment of mental ability, reduced motor co-ordination, confusion, lack of concern, time distortion, inappropriate mood shifts, and general emotional instability. He simultaneously experiences a decreased inhibition of basic drives with the resultant exaggeration of basic conflicts. This state differs from that of the opiate addict, who usually experiences a total satiation of drives.

Despite tolerance, the lethal dose for the addict does not differ greatly from that for the non-addict. The innocent cocktail party thus may prove lethal for the barbiturate addict. Withdrawal from barbiturate addiction is serious, often deadly, clearly more difficult to handle than heroin withdrawal, and should be treated only in a general hospital setting. The withdrawal mimics the delirium tremens of alcohol, and similar brain-wave abnormalities are noted. This is really a "general depressant withdrawal" syndrome.

Symptoms of withdrawal, resembling those of intoxication and starting in about 12 hours, include restlessness, anxiety, fine tremors, abdominal cramps, nausea and vomiting, and low standing blood pressure. After 24 hours, coarse tremors and hyperactive reflexes begin and the addict literally pleads for the drug. Convulsions and coma follow within a few days if therapy is not initiated. Actually, withdrawal should be a gradual, tapering process, lasting several weeks.

See also BARBITURATES; DRUGS; HEROIN; LSD; MARIHUANA; NARCOTICS; NARCOTICS TRAFFIC; OPIUM; PSYCHOPHARMACOLOGY.

DRUGS, substances used in the treatment of disease. Drug therapy is one of the oldest forms of medical treatment. The Ebers Papyrus, an ancient Egyptian medical treatise, contains recipes and prescriptions for the treatment of diseases of the eyes, skin, and internal organs. In China and India "herbals," or collections of herb remedies, were compiled hundreds of years before the birth of Christ. Primitive tribes used quinine for malaria, ipecac for dysentery, and rauwolfia for a host of ailments.

Until the 20th century drugs were obtained primarily from plants. Beginning about 1900 drugs from animal sources became available. These included the hormones, such as epinephrine (adrenalin), insulin, and the male and female sex hormones. The development of organic chemistry made possible the synthesis of pure compounds to replace the crude mixtures prepared by brewing or steeping plants.

Many drugs can now be synthesized more cheaply than they can be isolated from plants and animals. In some cases new and better compounds can be synthesized.

Types of Drugs

While there is no completely satisfactory or logical method of classifying drugs, most can be grouped on the basis of their general effects on the body, or by their medical use.

Drugs used to combat infections and infestations caused by bacteria, viruses, protozoa, or worms, are known as "antiparasitic" drugs. The antibiotics are included in this group.

Drugs Which Depress the Central Nervous System. A large category includes those drugs which depress the activity of the brain and spinal cord. Some of these drugs produce a loss of sensation and consciousness and are used for general anesthesia (ether). The narcotics (opium, morphine) are important pain-relievers. Sedatives and hypnotics produce calm and sleep, respectively. The most important sedatives are the barbiturates, which are found in many sleeping potions. The "anticonvulsants" reduce or prevent the epileptic seizures seen in epilepsy. Aspirin and related compounds are termed "antipyretic analgesics," because they have the dual action of relieving pain and reducing fever. A comparatively new group of drugs are the tranquilizers, which calm anxiety and dull emotional responses without producing drowsiness.

Drugs Which Act upon the Automatic (Autonomic) Nervous System. A large group of drugs act on certain portions of the nervous system (the autonomic nervous system) that control automatic, involuntary functions such as the rate of heartbeat, blood pressure, intestinal movements, and the size of the pupils. These autonomic drugs include epinephrine, a substance normally present in the body, which helps to prepare the body for muscular exertion by increasing the blood pressure and heart rates and by stimulating the release of sugar into the blood stream. Other autonomic drugs, such as methacholine, lower the blood pressure and stimulate the movement of the digestive tract and the flow of digestive juices.

Other classifications of drugs include those which help prevent clotting of the blood (anticoagulants) and those which stimulate kidney action (diuretics). The term "digitalis" describes a group of drugs obtained from digitalis and related species. These drugs strengthen the force of the heartbeat and are useful in treating certain types of heart disease. Hormones, such as insulin and thyroxin, may be used as drugs to meet the deficiencies which may arise from the malfunctioning of the pancreas and thyroid glands. Cortisone and hydrocortisone are hormones which are used to treat a large number of diseases involving inflammatory responses.

The Administration of Drugs

The method of giving a drug is often determined by the manner in which the body acts upon it. Many commonly used substances are readily absorbed from the stomach or intestine, and so can be taken by mouth. Examples of such drugs are aspirin, the sulfonamides, and the barbiturates. Certain drugs, however, cannot be readily absorbed from the gastrointestinal tract and so must be injected under the skin, or into muscles or veins. The hormone insulin must be injected, since it is not absorbed well from the gastrointestinal tract and it is destroyed by digestive enzymes.

Disposition in the Body. After entering the body, some drugs remain in the blood stream. Others may leave the circulatory system to penetrate the tissue fluids. Still others may gain access to particular regions, such as the brain or eye. The action of the drug will be influenced by its ability to penetrate to the target area and the manner in which the body acts upon it. The chemical activity of the body may rapidly change the drug to an inactive form. Also of importance is the rate at which the substance is removed from the body. In the case of potentially harmful drugs their rapid removal from the body may make possible their use.

Drug Action. Knowledge of the exact mechanism by which drugs produce their effects is as yet quite hazy. While it is known, for example, that when insulin is given to the diabetic the blood sugar will be lowered, the manner in which insulin achieves this effect is not clear. Similarly the ability of ether to produce stimulation in small doses and loss of sensation and consciousness and ultimately death, with increasing dosages, is familiar but poorly understood. The question remains as to exactly what changes ether causes in the cells of the brain and spinal cord.

Drug Toxicity. Since drugs are by definition chemicals that alter body function, it is clear that excess doses of any drug may produce harmful effects. The difference between the dose of a drug producing a desired effect (the therapeutic dose), and that producing a toxic effect (toxic dose), is sometimes referred to as the margin of safety.

This margin varies, both for different drugs and for different individuals given the same drug. In some cases the margin is so narrow that undesired actions ("side effects") will appear. In addition to toxicity there is the possibility of an allergic sensitivity even to small doses of the substance which are quite harmless for the nonallergic subject. A well-known example is penicillin, which is normally not toxic for man at the doses needed to kill susceptible bacteria. In rare cases, however, a patient may experience a violent allergic reaction even to minute doses of penicillin.

E

EBBINGHAUS [ĕb′ĭng-hous], **HERMANN** (1850–1909), German experimental psychologist. His studies included color vision and techniques of measuring intelligence in children. He is most famous for his pioneering experiments with memory and the time factor in retention. Of his books the most important was *Memory: a Contribution to Experimental Psychology* (1913).

EGO [ē′gō]. According to psychoanalytic theory, the ego is the part of the mind which deals with the real world. The infant's mind consists of the id, which is the seat of primitive desires. When the id faces the real world part of it becomes differentiated into the ego, which has the task of satisfying the id within the limitations imposed by society. The id, for example, may demand immediate satisfactions of sexual desires: the ego, recognizing the impossibility of such satisfactions, must transform the id desires into socially acceptable conduct. Later the rules of social behavior may be incorporated into the ego, forming a new structure, the superego, or conscience. The mature ego is thus charged with the responsibility of serving at least three taskmasters: the id, the superego, and the real world.

EMOTION usually refers to mental states or processes accompanied by marked bodily reactions, which occur in anticipation or realization of frustration or satisfaction of needs. Such states also are termed "affects," since they typically are accompanied by feelings of pleasantness or unpleasantness. They were called "passions" by early Greek writers. In Latin, emotion originally meant an inner turbulence, as in a storm cloud, which discharged its forces outward. Today, the Latin terminology is accepted. Emotion, for man, connotes an inner turbulence with outward expression.

The earliest writings concerning emotion probably are in the Sanskrit literature. The Vedas (3000–1500 B.C.) and the Upanishads (800–500 B.C.) contain descriptions of pleasure, pain, and sexual enjoyment. Theories about the emotions can be found in the works of the Greek philosophers. Aristotle provided the first extensive classification of "the passions," using words that most of us continue to employ. Other Greek writers held that the passions originated in the body; they were affairs of the heart, the bowels, or the womb. The Greek Stoics decried any lack of control over the passions. To them, passion in any form was bad since it interfered with reason, which was good. The influence of such thought is still with us. One point of view in psychology today is that emotion is disruptive: it interferes with proficient thought or motor performance and should be controlled, although a few "beneficent" emotions are acknowledged.

By the 18th century man had become convinced that the brain was important in behavior, and the supposedly subservient body was largely forgotten. The passions, now called emotions, were considered mental experiences; bodily changes were secondary. In the hands of the mentalistic philosophers of the 18th and 19th centuries emotion became a "thing of the mind." Only the French psychophysiologists, from Descartes on, gave credence to possible physiological bases of the emotions.

Theories. At this time all theories of emotion take one of three forms. Theory I may be stated as follows: emotion is an indivisible mind-body reaction. Many authors disagree, and their proposals take two general forms. Theory II, the most frequently encountered, may be stated thus: emotion is a mental event which depends upon other bodily events. Less prevalent is Theory III: emotion is a bodily event which may produce mental events.

In the first half of the 20th century the second theory was dominant. It was stated most explicitly by William James in 1884: ". . . bodily changes follow directly the perception of the exciting fact, and . . . our feeling of the same changes as they occur is the emotion." For James, emotion was a mental event (feeling) dependent upon physiological events.

In 1885 Carl Lange, a Danish physiologist, published a similar but slightly different point of view. He held that changes in the circulatory system were the essentials of emotion; mental events were secondary. Perhaps because of translation difficulties, James later stated that Lange had published a view similar to his own, and many writers have erroneously referred to the "James-Lange theory of emotion." Actually, Lange's view is a circumscribed class III theory. For Lange, emotion was a bodily event which might or might not produce mental events.

The next major theory to appear was that of Walter Cannon. His physiological experiments had suggested that peripheral bodily events were unimportant in emotion but that integrated patterns of emotional behavior disappeared after destruction of the central portion of the brain (the diencephalon, which includes the thalamus and the hypothalamus). He concluded that emotion resulted from activation of these brain structures. He still believed, however, that emotion was a mental event and, like others today, ascribed most mental events to the outermost layers of the brain (the cortex). His conclusions constitute, therefore, another class II theory.

In 1927, and in 1948, international symposia were held in the United States on "Feeling and Emotion." To date none of the views presented, other than Cannon's, has had marked influence. One deserves special mention, however, since it introduced a new element—the concept that emotion is a continuous process, with ups and downs. This view, presented by an American psychologist, Knight Dunlap, in 1928, was not developed further. Basically a class III theory, it claims that emotion is the dynamic background of all behavior—it is the continuous flux and counterflux of internal bodily responses.

An extension of this view, and of Lange's, has been presented by the present writer. He subscribes to a class III theory and defines emotion as activity of the autonomic nervous system (that automatic portion of the nervous system which controls the basic functions of life such as circulation, heat control, digestion, and elimination). Since this activity is continuous in life, emotion is held to be continuous. Thus, instead of speaking of the presence or absence of emotion, one would speak of the kind of change that has occurred. In this definition the influence of skeletal muscles and endocrine (ductless) glands is minimized but not excluded. Emotional change is seen as a series of complex bodily responses which give rise to a series of different feelings, but which also may be observed in animals or in a human who cannot report his feelings. Feeling and emotion are thus conceived as separate but related phenomena.

Such a point of view questions all present classifications of the emotions. It would hold that extensive knowledge is needed of the possible changes in autonomic response patterns before classification of emotional change is possible. Meanwhile some calculated guesses may be made.

Of particular interest in this respect are attempts to classify emotional behavior in human infants. John B. Watson believed there were three primary emotions which he first called X, Y, Z. He later named them fear (elicited by loud noise or loss of support), anger (elicited by interference with activity), and lust or love (elicited by mild tactual stimulation of erogenous zones). He believed that all emotional life developed from these three behavior patterns.

Watson's views were much criticized, and the explanation advanced by K. M. B. Bridges became popular. She claimed that the primary infant emotion was excitement and that all other emotional responses became differentiated from this one response.

Behavior Patterns. The view of the present writer is that Watson's approach was appropriate but that he should have extended and modified it. He describes eight behavior patterns in infants or young children that may be regarded as distinct emotional changes:

(1) Startle, to sudden intense stimulation;
(2) Struggle, to interference with movement;
(3) Muscular arrest-tumescence, to sustained gentle stimulation of the skin;
(4) Exaggerated withdrawal, to sudden pain-producing stimuli;
(5) General activity, to sustained unpleasant internal sensations;
(6) Quiescence, to relief from unpleasant stimulation;
(7) Spitting-mouth aversion, to unpleasant tastes;
(8) Exhaustion-whimpering, to persisting and unrelieved unpleasant stimulation.

These eight patterns of behavior are believed to occur without learning and to form the bases from which develop the emotional behaviors we recognize as (1) fear, (2) anger, (3) sexual excitement, (4) pain, (5) excitement,

(6) pleasure of relief, (7) disgust or revulsion, (8) disappointment or grief.

If these patterns of behavior are discrete in human infants they should be relatively discrete in adults. These views are now being tested. Few decisive experiments have been conducted, but Nina Bull has demonstrated differences in muscular attitude among some of these commonly accepted emotions, and many experimenters are attempting to determine precise differences in autonomic and endocrine responses to stressful situations.

EMPATHY [ĕm'pə-thē], in aesthetics "feeling" or "projecting" oneself into or identifying oneself with an artistic work, object, or natural process. For example, a thin column supporting a heavy capital might arouse in an observer a feeling of straining to hold up the weight. This use of the term "empathy" is sometimes extended to cover such things as the involuntary movements spectators make while watching an athlete strain to reach his goal.

Empathy also means intellectually understanding another person's emotions without necessarily experiencing these emotions at the same time. It may be considered primarily a form of intellectual identification and is distinguished from sympathy, which implies a more intense sharing of emotions. This does not mean that affective or emotional identification is entirely excluded. A person understands and "feels" himself into the mood or attitude of another, without specifically and intensely having the same emotional experience. Thus a psychotherapist can understand a patient's anguished tears, yet not shed a tear himself. It is also possible to have empathy with a group or cause as well as with a person, object, or process. A neutral observer can appreciate and understand the attitudes or feelings of an oppressed minority group, while neither being part of the group nor aiding its cause.

ESQUIROL [ĕs-kü-ē-rôl'], **JEAN ETIENNE DOMINIQUE** (1772–1840), French physician, called the father of French psychiatry. A student of Pinel, the man who liberated the mentally ill from their chains and other inhuman constraints, Esquirol advanced Pinel's reforms by persuading the French government to build a number of asylums for the mentally ill. He produced one of the earliest treatises on mental illness based upon scientific observation under hospital conditions.

ETHOLOGY, biological study of animal behavior in its natural state. For the ethologist, all animal behavior must be analyzed not only in regard to its cause, but also for its function in furthering survival. The mechanistic views held by science around the turn of the century favored other psychological theories, notably behaviorism, which explains an animal's action on the basis of its response to a stimulus. Experimentalists are looking for "how" the animal behaves, but the ethologist first asks "why." In the last few decades, especially through the work of K. Z. Lorenz and Niko Tinbergen in Europe, the naturalistic observation of behavior has come to supplement the laboratory study of behavior which has burgeoned in the United States.

The ethologist likes to make a dossier of all the animal's behavior, called an ethogram. The units of behavior in this catalogue are subsequently analyzed, especially stereotyped behaviors that could have an instinctive background. In such behavior sequences it is possible to find motor actions that seem automated because they always proceed in the same manner—the so-called fixed action pattern (FAP). They are brought about by a "sign stimulus," or releaser. It is hypothesized that a drive makes the animal look for the specific stimulus situation needed for such actions. The predictable defensive behavior of the male European robin, when it sees another male robin while patrolling its territory, may serve as an example. The releaser for the robin's threatening actions is the orange-colored breast of the intruder, since it has been shown that a stuffed robin without the orange breast is not attacked, and a tuft of orange feathers is attacked by the irate territory-owner.

Another typical animal behavior pattern revealed by ethological studies is imprinting. Imprinting is the rapid establishment of social preferences in the young animal, which will remain in force for life without continuous reinforcement. Lorenz imprinted himself on young geese by being present at their hatching. They followed him as their mother, and when they were mature they even tried to mate with him. This type of instantaneous learning differs both from instinctual activities and from other types of learning, such as conditioning.

By careful description of the objective behavior of organisms, ethologists have revived interest in the instinctual basis of behavior and the processes by which learned and unlearned behavior merge imperceptibly. The study of ethograms provides insight into innate behavior patterns that determine social behavior, such as the phenomenon of imprinting, and the releasers and fixed action patterns which are components of complex behavior. The concept of drive, the purposiveness of many behavioral activities and their meaning for the survival of the species, have become legitimate concerns for the comparative psychologist. Laboratory research based on ethological findings has very much increased. Such research is an important supplement to the experimental findings of studies based on stimulus-response and learning theories which held the dominant position. Consequently, many new insights into the motivational aspects of animal behavior are now available for possible application in testing theories of human behavior, such as the drive theory of psychoanalysis, which hitherto could not be substantiated.

See also AGGRESSION; PSYCHOLOGY; TERRITORIALITY.

EXCEPTIONAL CHILDREN

The term "exceptional children" has been defined by the National Society for the Study of Education as including those children "who deviate from what is supposed to be average in physical, mental, emotional, or social characteristics to such an extent that they require special educational services in order to develop their maximum capacity." The deviation from normal can be toward the higher or lower end of the scale. Hence the category of exceptional children includes the gifted as well as the handicapped. Other terms sometimes used are "atypical" and "deviant." Many sources, including publications of the United Nations Educational, Scientific and Cultural Organization (UNESCO), use "special education" to cover this area of school services.

Classification of Exceptional Children. In the United States, children may be classified as exceptional if they (1) are of high mental ability or are creative or talented, (2) are mentally retarded, (3) are on the border line of mental retardation (slow learners), (4) have visual handicaps, (5) have impaired hearing, (6) have speech problems, (7) have orthopedic handicaps (are crippled), (8) are neurologically damaged, (9) have chronic medical problems, (10) are socially and emotionally maladjusted, (11) have a cultural handicap, and (12) are educationally retarded. Further comment on these categories is given below.

A similar classification of exceptional children has been made in Canada. Under the broad heading of (1) mentally exceptional and emotionally disturbed children are grouped children who are (1a) mentally retarded, (1b) mentally gifted, and (1c) emotionally disturbed. Under (2) physically handicapped children are listed those who are (2a) blind or partially sighted, (2b) deaf or hard of hearing, (2c) speech defective, (2d) "cerebral palsied," (2e) orthopedic, (2f) hospitalized, (2g) tuberculous, in sanitoria, (2h) homebound, (2i) delicate, in open-air schools. Two additional categories are (3) delinquent and (4) orphaned and neglected. England and Wales use similar categories except that there is no special "gifted" clasification. The tendency in other countries is to make less detailed breakdowns. Italy, for example, provides special schools for three groups; mentally abnormal, blind and deaf-mutes, and physically deficient.

Historical Perspective. Special care of exceptional children is a comparatively new idea in history. Early civilizations exposed cripples to die and treated the mentally retarded as possessed of demons or as objects of ridicule. As late as the 19th century it was a common practice for parents to hide away chronically ill, physically handicapped, or retarded children for fear of social disgrace. Many such children were confined in institutions till they died. Some attempts at scientific care and training of the blind and deaf were made in France in the late 18th century. In the United States, Thomas Hopkins Gallaudet opened a pioneer school for the deaf at Hartford, Conn., in 1817. Special training for the mentally retarded was initiated in France and the United States in the 19th century, and around the end of that century signs of progress appeared in a number of fields. Special classes for the mentally retarded were introduced in Providence, R.I., in 1896 and Springfield, Ill., in 1897, and by 1910 more than 200 such classes had been started in the United States. The first Braille class for the blind was organized in Chicago in 1900 (other systems of teaching the blind to read had been used earlier). Programs for the gifted and for children with speech problems, for the socially and emotionally maladjusted, and for the culturally handicapped developed more slowly than programs for children with more obvious special needs. In general, large-scale educational programs for exceptional children were virtually unknown until the 20th century was well under way.

Various factors brought about changes in public attitudes toward atypical children and led to an expansion of programs. The passage of compulsory-education laws in all states by 1918 made the public schools responsible for all children. It soon became clear that children with special problems needed special services. Experience during two world wars led to increased understanding of the needs and the usefulness of handicapped persons. Organizations were formed to promote research and treatment. The growth of cities made it possible to group together enough children with similar problems to make special classes economically feasible. Progress in medicine and psychology led to earlier identification of problems. New techniques and new devices such as improved lenses and hearing aids made treatment and teaching more effective. The number of specialists in all fields increased as training programs in such fields as physiology, social work, psychology, and special education expanded.

Modern Programs in the United States. Programs for exceptional children can be discussed as follows:

(1) The public or private residential, or boarding, institution represents the oldest form of care for exceptional children. Many of these institutions used to be little more than places where children were kept in custody, in crowded conditions and with poor staffs and facilities. Modern institutions—often under such names as "state school," "industrial school," or "parental school"—have in some states improved to the point of having excellent programs, plant, and personnel. The cost for care of blind, deaf, retarded, crippled, or chronically ill children is usually paid by the state government, with parents contributing up to the limit of their ability.

(2) The special school, which serves children from a limited area and is not a full-time residential institution, provides the major portion of the education and training for certain types of exceptional children such as the blind and partially seeing and the deaf and hard of hearing.

(3) The special class, located in a regular school, was developed in an effort to overcome the most serious objections to institutions and special schools, while providing exceptional children with an effective program based upon their educational needs. Special classes have been organized for every type of exceptional child.

(4) In a further attempt to integrate exceptional children into the regular school program, educators introduced the resource room, a room in a regular school that is set aside for special programs conducted by a specially trained teacher, and the itinerant teacher, who travels from school to school to provide special programs and to help the regular class teacher.

One notable trend in programs for exceptional children is an emphasis upon keeping the child at home, in his regular school, and in a regular class if possible. When a child needs placement in a special class, the trend is to integrate this class into the regular school program and to make it as much a part of the regular school as possible. The trend toward special classes rather than special schools obtains in Sweden as well as in the United States. When a child is in need of special school placement, a determined effort is made to keep the contacts with the home as normal as possible and to give these children many of the experiences that the more normal children have. When no other placement is possible, some form of institution is called upon to provide a program for exceptional children. Local school systems are increasing their staffs of professional personnel. States have organized separate divisions of their education departments, sometimes under a director of pupil personnel and special services.

The research being carried on by universities and other agencies can be expected to improve methods of treatment and teaching and to reduce the incidence of some kinds of handicap. At the same time the total number of handicapped children can be expected to increase because of two factors, population growth and the ability to keep alive children whose handicaps would once have been fatal. Although great progress has been made in special education, the problem remains enormous. A conservative estimate for the early 1960's set the number of U.S. children needing special services at about 6,000,000. Only 15% to 20% of these children were actually enrolled in special programs.

Gifted Children

Definition of the Gifted, Talented, or Creative. Like other terms for exceptional children, "gifted" and approximate synonyms for it (talented, creative, genius, superior) are hard to define. In general, children who achieve high scores on tests of mental ability, do outstanding work in school, and show unusual talent or creative ability are considered gifted. A group of gifted children may include those who have a talent for writing, acting, art, or some other form of creative expression; children who are superior in mathematical, scientific, and mechanical work and are interested in investigation or experimentation; children who show leadership ability and are capable of planning and organizing on a high level. In the words of the National Society for the Study of Education, "The talented or gifted child is one who shows consistently remarkable performance in any worth-while line of endeavor." In the United States, gifted children are estimated to make up 2% to 3% of the school-age population.

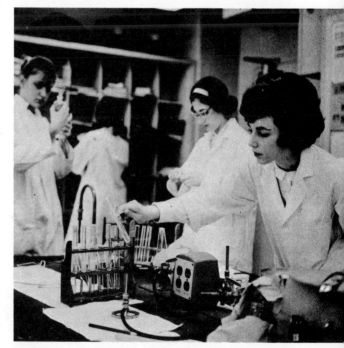

High school students in an advanced chemistry class learning qualitative organic analysis. (JANE LATTA)

As the scope of this definition might suggest, no single method has proved successful for identifying children with superior ability. Evidence ordinarily consists of teachers' judgments, school records, and scores on group achievement tests and on group or individual tests of mental ability. Some experts take an intelligence quotient (IQ) of 120 as the dividing point for special grouping ("normal," or "average," being between 90 and 110). Others would class as gifted those with IQ's of over 135. Aptitude tests are often used as a means of identifying children who are likely to succeed in college.

Tests have undoubted value, but their results must be used with due caution. In the first place, not all children are given the same or comparable tests. In the second place, some kinds of talent may not be revealed by the commonly employed tests of mental ability and achievement. In the third place, test results do not always show an individual's true level of ability. Teachers' judgments have also been found to be an uncertain means of identifying the gifted. Generally, teachers can recognize about half of the exceptionally able children in a classroom.

Programs. Historically, education of the gifted has received less attention than education of the handicapped. Flexible promotion (skipping grades) was tried in the 19th century, but programs for superior students did not become widespread in the United States. After World War II numerous comments on the training of gifted children were published. Some authorities pointed out that while programs were provided for the "average" person, the "superior" person was neglected. The value of superior abilities was given publicity by fears that the Soviet Union was surpassing the United States in training scientists and technicians. Bright children were seen as an important national resource. It was pointed out that a majority of the young people who had a capacity to do college work did not attend college, and that the outstanding students were relatively neglected in the high schools. Reports in the early 1960's gave the number of pupils in special programs for the gifted as less than 25% of the number of pupils in programs for the mentally retarded. Studies of the high schools by James Bryant Conant stressed the need to have academically talented students give more time to mathematics, science, and foreign languages.

Various plans have been used in an effort to provide programs for the gifted in the schools of the nation. One —acceleration, skipping, or flexible promotion—has already been mentioned. Its advantages lie in the fact that the child is challenged to work to the limits of his ability. Several studies have shown that acceleration was not particularly associated with problems in the later life of the gifted. Children who were accelerated were found to be more successful in college than those who had not been in this type of program. An increasing number of colleges are accepting carefully selected superior students for advanced placement. Nevertheless, acceleration has not been popular with many American educators. Although it is agreed that most gifted children succeed in the academic areas and in social and emotional adjustment while participating in this type of program, many children break down emotionally if too severe pressure is placed on them by the school or by parents.

Special classes are another means of providing enriched programs for gifted children. Talented pupils grouped in one class can be given additional work in all subjects. Research projects, individual study in areas of special interest, and pupil-teacher conferences are features of these programs. Foreign language instruction may begin in the elementary grades.

The grouping together of superior students is most common in the high schools. Elective subjects, honors courses, and college preparatory courses have been planned to give educational opportunities to the talented. Less demanding courses are scheduled for pupils who are headed for vocational schools or who, for other reasons, are not likely to enter college.

Some studies of students in special classes indicate that they reach a high level of achievement in scholarship and are characterized by high levels of co-operation, social consciousness, leadership, and responsibility. Objections to special groupings have been made on such grounds as that these classes are undemocratic, cause some students to overwork, and are prohibitively costly. The difficulty of identifying talented students is a problem.

Another means of providing special education for the gifted is termed "enrichment." Students are left in the usual classes, not grouped according to ability. Special studies and activities are offered on an individual basis to students who can benefit from them. Favorable conditions, including small classes and teachers with versatile skills, are needed to make the program succeed.

A number of communities have experimented with providing for the gifted through part-time programs and special rooms. In these programs gifted children are members of regular classes. In the elementary school, schedules are arranged so that children are free for part of the school day. In the junior high school, special project classes or honors classes are used as part of a flexible scheduling arrangement. This program permits these children to be with their regular class for part of the day and yet to have an opportunity to move at their own pace and to explore areas of their own interest. This part-time program has been evolved in an effort to overcome unfavorable criticisms of the other types of programs.

Programs for the Handicapped

Education of Children with Retarded Mental Development. "Mental retardation" as used here includes such designations as feeble-mindedness, mental deficiency, mental handicap, amentia, oligophrenia, and the levels indicated by the terms "idiot," "imbecile," and "moron." The term "mental retardation" has been chosen as the most acceptable by the American Association on Mental Deficiency. Children who are mentally retarded usually have a combination of medical, social, maturational, physiological, and educational problems, rather than a single clinical symptom. Mental retardation is often confused with mental illness. Although mentally retarded children may also be mentally ill and mentally ill children may also be retarded, each category is conceived of as a fairly distinct area of exceptionality. The retarded must be distinguished from those who are classed as socially or emotionally maladjusted (see below). Mental retardation

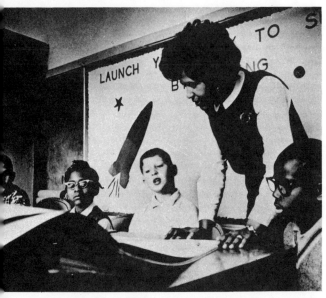

A teacher in a remedial class assists children with various reading problems. (ROBERTS—RAPHO GUILLUMETTE)

has been defined in terms of being below average in one or more of three areas: rate of maturation in early childhood of such skills as crawling, standing, walking, talking, and training in useful habits; learning ability, particularly in school; and social adjustment in the sense of the ability to live independently and earn a living.

For educational purposes mentally retarded children are classified in three groups, usually called educable, trainable, and custodial or severely retarded. At a conservative estimate, 2% of the U.S. school population is mentally retarded. Of this group, 85% is educable, 11.5% trainable, and 3.5% severely retarded. The term "educable mentally retarded" is applied to children of school age who will achieve no more than a maximum of 12 years in mental age at maturity. Characteristic of this group is achievement at no more than 4th or 5th grade in academic ability. However, they are capable of becoming self-sustaining, independent adults who can work in unskilled or semiskilled occupations after they have completed proper training and have been helped in finding a job. Their IQ's generally range from 50 to 75 on an individual test of mental ability.

The term "trainable mentally retarded" is applied to children of school age who will achieve no more than a maximum mental age of seven at maturity, and who for school entrance are able to walk, to have clean bodily habits, to communicate their needs, and who are responsive to simple commands. These children do not usually learn to read or compute to any usable extent, they are limited in their ability to communicate, and they will be semi-dependent or dependent as adults, needing a sheltered environment under close supervision. They often have physical disabilities. Their IQ's generally range from 25 or 30 to 50 on an individual test of mental ability.

The terms "custodial" or "severely retarded" are applied to children who are not eligible for entrance into public school because they require almost total care. Such cases usually require total care for their entire lives. Their IQ's are usually below 25 or 30 on an individual test of mental ability—if it is possible to test them at all.

Modern practice with the educable mentally retarded is to place a child who has been so identified in a special class. A majority of educators working in this field agree that special classes for the educable mentally retarded should be located in a regular school building with classes for normal children. There are a few instances, however, in which these special classes are grouped to form what is in reality a special school. When it is necessary for children to be institutionalized, an educational program is provided in a special school within the institution.

In general, the basic characteristics of the special class are as far as possible those of the regular class. Trainable and educable mentally retarded children are not grouped in the same class. In establishing special classes, major differences among pupils as to age and physical size are avoided. Every effort is made to develop a sequence of four classes so that each child will spend no more than three or four years in any one group.

The curriculum for the educable mentally retarded emphasizes the development of practical and useful knowledge, skills, and attitudes in the areas of citizenship, occupations, communication, arithmetic, health, safety, and recreation. Other areas of training and guidance are socially acceptable behavior, motor co-ordination, self-acceptance and self-confidence, vocational competence, and civic responsibility. A high school program that includes actual job experience is provided in whatever occupations are available. The school co-operates in placing these children in jobs.

Prior to 1950 there were few classes for trainable mentally retarded children in the public schools, but after the middle of the century there was a large increase in the number of these classes throughout the country, despite the fact that some educators question the responsibility of the school for these children. Groups of parents of retarded children have been especially active in this area.

The curriculum for the trainable mentally retarded child emphasizes development of the use of the senses, good health habits, self-care and personal adequacy, motor skills, communication skills, and simple number skills. The lives of these children will usually be circumscribed by the boundaries of the home, school, immediate neighborhood, and the sheltered shop, or, as a last resort, the institution.

Education of Slow Learners. Above the level of the mentally retarded, but below the normal range of ability, are children classed as "slow learners." Such labels as "dull normal," "borderline normal," "borderline retarded," and "limited ability" are sometimes applied to this category. Children whose scores are between 75 and 90 on repeated tests of mental ability are frequently put in this group. Such pupils can achieve some degree of success in school subjects but require more time and greater effort than pupils of higher ability. About 20% of pupils in U.S. schools fall into this classification.

Besides learning at a subnormal rate, slow learners seem to differ from more normal children in ability to think abstractly, to generalize from specifics, to memorize, to think critically, and to work for long periods on school subjects. As a result of inability to be successful in school, slow learners often develop secondary personality problems and sometimes become behavior problems. It has been found that a large number of behavior problems in the school are slow learners for whom no special program has been provided.

The majority of schools attempt to care for the slow learners by nonpromotion, and many leave school as soon as they reach the upper limit of compulsory attendance. Recommendations for effective programs include early identification, smaller classes grouped according to range of ability, the employment of interested and specially trained teachers, and careful guidance.

Education of the Visually Handicapped. The visually handicapped category of exceptional children includes those who are classed as blind and those who are classed as partially sighted, or partially able to see. The partially sighted use sight as their chief means of learning.

A great expansion in facilities and programs for the visually handicapped occurred during the middle decades of the 20th century. In general four types of program for the visually handicapped are in use today: (1) the state residential school; (2) the special class; (3) the integrated or co-operative program; and (4) the itinerant teacher approach. Early identification of children who need care in one of these programs is especially urgent, since corrective work during the early years can ameliorate some visual problems. Despite progress, it is estimated that eight out of nine partially sighted children do not have any type of special educational program.

The program of the residential school is similar to a regular school program. Children are grouped by age and grade and follow the same course of study as do more normal children. A number of special methods and devices are used, of course. Among these are Braille reading and writing, typewriting from the 3d or 4th grade on, "talking books" (recordings of books), and relief maps. Often blind students who are ready for a high school program attend a regular local high school and receive special help.

The placement of blind children in a residential school has aroused controversy among professionals working with this group. Many feel that the specialized problem of the children can best be met by a facility that is specifically geared to meet these needs. Others, however, feel that the regular public school, using a special teacher, can provide the needed help while keeping the child part of his family group. There is general agreement that the partially sighted are best served in regular schools with special services. Efforts have been made to develop educational programs in which the visually handicapped and the sighted could attend school side by side.

A number of large school systems have provided special classes for the partially sighted in regular school buildings. Complete segregation of these children is not considered desirable. On the other hand, the handicapped child must remain in the special class long enough to learn the skills he needs in order to work with the normal class. The partially seeing must not be expected to compete too soon with children having sound vision.

The co-operative plan requires a special teacher for the

visually handicapped and a special room from which their program is planned and directed. Part of each day is spent in regular classrooms. Under what is called the integrated plan for the visually handicapped, these children are enrolled in regular classes. A trained teacher of the blind is available on a full-time basis to assist the regular teachers.

The use of itinerant teachers is another plan to keep the handicapped child in a regular class in his neighborhood school. In this case, the specially trained teacher serves a number of schools, providing individual instruction and special equipment where needed and advising teachers and parents.

Services for the blind are included in the special education programs of most nations. The predominant plan is to put blind children in special schools; Austria, Bulgaria, Finland, Germany, Italy, and the Soviet Union are among the nations reporting special schools, often boarding institutions giving vocational and general training.

Education of Children with Impaired Hearing. Just as there are degrees of visual handicap there are degrees of deafness. From the educator's point of view, the distinction between children with moderate hearing loss and those with profound hearing loss is particularly important. The former can learn speech by ear whereas the latter cannot. Children born deaf present a problem different from that of children who lose their hearing after they have learned speech.

Three out of four children with severe loss of hearing are in residential schools. Because of the relatively low

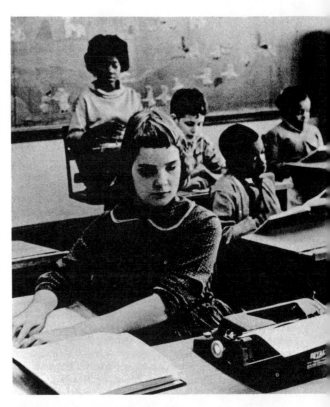

With special help, a blind girl successfully attends class with children having normal vision. (BATTLE CREEK, MICH., ENQUIRER AND NEWS)

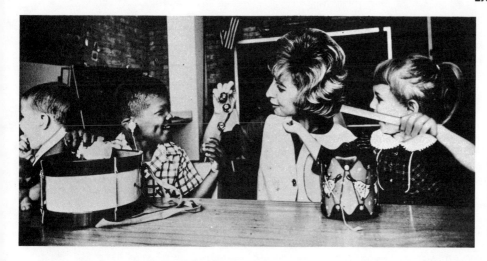

Deaf children of preschool age receive special training in a Houston, Tex., hearing clinic. Such early instruction helps avoid problems that may develop later.
(SPIEGEL—RAPHO GUILLUMTTE)

rate of incidence, it is only in the large metropolitan areas that there are enough children for the formation of day classes and special classes. Lip reading (or in some cases the manual alphabet), speech correction, auditory training, as well as the mastery of school subjects, represent the major areas of work with these children. A precision-built group hearing aid is the most essential piece of equipment for a class of deaf children.

The hard of hearing who are not, educationally, "deaf" are usually placed in special classes or in the regular classes in the public schools. However, some children with moderate hearing losses who have other problems and children with severe hearing losses need placement in a special class. The schoolwork in the special class does not differ materially from the work in the regular classroom. The classroom is usually located in a regular school building, and some general activities are shared with normal children. Every attempt is made to give the hard of hearing children enough background and training so that they may move into a regular school program. When the hard-of-hearing child is in the regular class program, the availability of a trained speech and hearing teacher is essential.

Education of Children Who Have Speech Problems. Objectively, a child may be said to have a speech defect when his speech is such that it presents a problem to him in communicating easily with a normal listener. Subjectively, speech may be said to be defective if the speaker is aware of or fearful about a problem in his speech. Speech defects are frequently divided into four major types: (1) defect in articulation (sound production); (2) defects of phonation (voice production); (3) defects of rhythm (stuttering and cluttering); and (4) language dysfunctions (delayed speech or aphasia).

In current practice, children who are in need of speech help remain in the regular classroom. The speech and hearing teacher works with children who have either speech or hearing problems, dealing with them singly or in groups. Itinerant teachers are usually assigned to cover several schools; they may work with a single child or a group having similar problems.

Generally, state legislation for the physically handicapped provides for educational programs for children with speech handicaps. The number of programs is increasing in the United States. Many other countries use the old category "deaf-mutes" and place children so classified in special institutions.

Education of Children with Orthopedic Handicaps. The term "orthopedic" is used to indicate the purpose of correcting or preventing deformity. Many kinds of handicaps are included in this category, among them being crippling as a result of poliomyelitis, club foot, spinal curvature, tumors, and loss of limbs in accidents. More important than the exact nature of the crippling are such factors as the attitude of the child's family and associates, the reaction of the public, and the personality of the child.

All states now offer aid to crippled children of school age, and a majority of states have provisions for financial aid to public schools that operate programs for the orthopedically handicapped. Many areas still lack effective programs, however.

In general the programs that are provided for orthopedically handicapped children can be classed under five headings: (1) hospital schools; (2) special schools; (3) special classes; (4) home instruction; and (5) services in regular classes. Hospital schools are used to serve children who must remain in the hospital for a considerable length of time. Special techniques are used and teachers are often called upon to make major program adjustments to accommodate medical and hospital treatment. Special schools have been organized in many large cities. These facilities are usually created for children who are in need of special care or treatment that could not be given in a special class. In addition to classrooms, special schools usually have medical and health facilities, therapy rooms, rest areas, and a lunchroom. Some educators feel that such special facilities should be part of a regular school and that children should be returned to the special or regular class as soon as feasible. Special classes are organized to serve children with lesser orthopedic handicaps. These classes are usually located on the street level of a regular school building or are accessible through the use of elevators or ramps. The special classroom may have such equipment as standing tables, special chairs, parallel bars, and reading devices. Physical therapy, where needed, may be provided in the school or children may be transported to another community facility for this service.

Children who must have an extended period of rest, who are not able to travel or move around, or who can work only for a short period of time receive home instruction. The use of school-home telephones appears to have a number of advantages, and the use of educational television programs for these children is being studied.

Education of Children with Neurological Impairments. From a medical point of view, "neurological impairment" refers to damage to the brain or central nervous system. Specific problems may be diagnosed, for example, as epilepsy, cerebral palsy (which is characterized by impaired control of muscles), or aphasia (an impairment of the ability to use or comprehend language).

Since educational programs are designed to attempt to ameliorate symptoms rather than deal with causes of behavior, the types of programs vary with the nature of the particular neurological problem of each child. Children whose major symptom is motor impairment, which is evidenced by difficulty in walking or running or in using their hands, are usually placed in a program for the orthopedically handicapped as cerebral palsied. This program may be located in the hospital, special school, special class, at home, or in the regular class, depending upon the severity of the involvement. Since damage to the brain is not usually limited to a single area, children may have defects in vision, hearing, or speech in addition to motor impairment. Therapy for children who have cerebral palsy is an extremely important aspect of the program. Teaching cerebral-palsied children requires imagination and ingenuity.

Epilepsy manifests itself in seizures. It is not considered crippling from a medical point of view but rather by teachers and parents who come in contact with the child. Except for children with uncontrollable seizures, epileptic children under medical supervision can attend regular classrooms when the teacher and the children understand the problem and accept the child.

Children whose intelligence is affected by neurological impairment and who are mentally retarded are usually placed in a program with other mentally retarded children. Aphasic children are usually enrolled in special classes located in schools for the deaf. There are only a small number of such school programs in the United States.

Education of Children with Chronic Medical Problems. Conditions that may be classed as "chronic medical problems" include rheumatic fever, tuberculosis, nephrosis (kidney disease), hepatitis, allergies, diabetes, cancer, and malnutrition. Epilepsy could be put in this category. Historically, there is little evidence of attempts to provide special programs for children with such problems until modern times.

As with other exceptional children great emphasis has been placed on keeping children with chronic medical problems in the regular classroom. There are, however, instances when special classes, special schools, home instruction, and hospital programs are needed.

The teacher who works in their homes with children who have chronic medical problems needs to have specialized training in working with the handicapped. Most children receive three to five hours of instruction a week utilizing a schedule of two or three sessions of one and a half hours per day rather than several one-hour sessions. The use of closed-circuit television and the home-to-school telephone have broadened the horizons of the home instruction program.

Since the objectives of all the special programs are to enable the child to move as rapidly as possible into the main stream of a regular educational program, the special school or class may provide an intermediary step in this process. There are also some children with chronic medical problems who cannot make the adjustment to the regular classrooms and need the special school or class. Many of these children are placed in classes with children having other handicaps, where special provision to handle their problems may be made. When children with chronic medical problems can be accommodated in the regular classroom, extra care and planning by school personnel such as the school physician and nurse are required. The placement necessitates careful consideration and a sensitive teacher who accepts the child and his limitations and does not isolate the child in the classroom.

Education of Children Who Are Socially and Emotionally Maladjusted. "Social and emotional maladjustment" is manifested in one or more kinds of problem behavior: difficulties in learning that are not explained by any of the handicaps already discussed; poor relations with other children and teachers; "strange" behavior, inappropriate to the circumstances; tendencies to have depressed, unhappy moods; fears, pains, and illness associated with schoolwork. Children who have such problems may become truants or be otherwise delinquent.

Society's first reaction to children who were socially and emotionally maladjusted was to attempt to isolate the offending individuals in order to protect itself. Later it attempted to reform them, and many institutions for reformation were opened in the 19th century. In modern practice children who are socially and emotionally maladjusted are provided services in a number of settings: institutions, hospitals, special schools, special classes, and regular classes. If the problem is not too severe, and the teacher is capable, the child may remain in the regular classroom. The teacher may need assistance from staff psychologists and social workers in order to plan a program for these children. Work with the family may require the co-operation of the school with outside agencies such as a family service or child guidance clinic. The special class for the socially and emotionally handicapped is of help to children who, because of serious and continuous deviations from normal behavior, cannot profit from a program in a regular class. Large cities or a group of small communities may have enough children to form a special school. The problems in these schools may be more difficult than those in a regular school because of the concentration of children who have social-emotional handicaps. Institutions and residential centers have been set up to provide for the socially and emotionally maladjusted on a total basis. A psychiatrically oriented institution can provide well-rounded services for these children.

Education of Children Who Have Cultural Handicaps. Children who have a "cultural handicap" are (1) those who have a cultural background different from that to which they are exposed in school (foreign-born, members

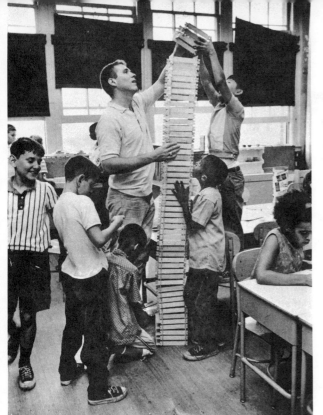

A young teacher working with culturally deprived children in a special summer remedial program.   (LISL STEINER)

Extensive social changes in the United States have brought to schools children who are not prepared for the ordinary program. The increase in the number of working mothers, desegregation of schools, the influx of Puerto Rican children, and the continued arrival of foreign-born children present a challenge for the conscientious teacher. Head Start, a program of pre-school activities intended to provide experience for children with this handicap, has had some success. Much needs to be done, however, to enable culturally handicapped children to begin school on an equal footing with their more culturally acclimated peers.

Education of Children Who Are Educationally Retarded. This category, "educationally retarded," is a broad one. Sometimes children who are not working at the level expected for pupils of their intellectual capacity are called "under-achievers." They are not in the "slow learner" or "mentally retarded" category. Their slow pace may be caused by one or more of the physical, emotional, or cultural handicaps already described or by other factors such as ineffective teaching, poor study habits, poor attendance, frequent transfer from one school to another, poor school facilities, crowded classes, lack of space to study at home, and inappropriate curriculum. Since reading is the tool most used in other subject areas, retardation in reading represents the most serious problem.

With the advent of advanced procedures for testing and appraising pupils, the specific causes of educational retardation have emerged in some school systems. Children whose educational retardation is caused by severe handicap may be helped through special programs. Thus, a child with a reading problem caused by a hearing loss would be given help in the area of speech and hearing improvement as well as remedial work in reading. As communities move toward better curricular practices, smaller classes, and better prepared teachers, the number of children who are educationally retarded is usually reduced.

of minority ethnic groups, and children of migrant workers); (2) those who are culturally deprived because of the lack of exposure to experiences and motivations normally brought to school by other children (children from groups low on the socioeconomic scale).

F

FACULTY PSYCHOLOGY, the point of view that the mind is an aggregate of specific powers, such as memory, will power, judgment, and imagination. Such a view is frequently implied by laymen in their use of these and similar words: "He has imagination but no will power." In scientific psychology such terminology is considered a form of "word magic" which lacks explanatory usefulness. To say that some behavior illustrates a person's good memory does not explain the behavior, but only calls it by a different name and adds nothing to the original observation. Memory does not seem to be a single factor, for while a person may long remember some things he may have considerable difficulty remembering other things.

Phrenology, a pseudoscience that attained popularity in the 19th century, represented the most elaborate form of faculty psychology. Phrenologists made charts of the head showing areas believed to control faculties and traits. Subsequent advances in knowledge about the structure and function of the brain have rendered such theories untenable.

See also PHRENOLOGY.

FIXATION, term used in psychoanalysis to describe an arrest in psychic development at some infantile level. According to Freudian theory, an excessive amount of psychic energy remains attached to some phase of early development, interfering with the normal process of personality growth, and leading to neurosis in adult life. For example, an overly dependent adult is said to be fixated at the oral level, the earliest psychosexual stage, when dependency is normal and at its height. Fixation is distinguished from regression, in which an individual who has progressed beyond a particular stage subsequently returns to it.

See also PSYCHOANALYSIS.

FREE ASSOCIATION, the process in which a patient undergoing psychoanalysis speaks any and all thoughts which come to his mind, without attempting to conceal those which he might feel to be embarrassing or unimportant. The analyst uses this technique to attempt to understand the unconscious drives which underlie the patient's behavior. The process was originated by Sigmund Freud and constituted the basic tool with which he developed his theories of human behavior.

The literary style known as "stream of consciousness" is an attempt to utilize free association for the purposes of artistic creation.

See also FREUD, SIGMUND; PSYCHOANALYSIS.

FREEMAN, WALTER (1895–   ), American neurologist and neurosurgeon best known for his work in introducing prefrontal lobotomy into the United States. In this procedure a portion of the cerebrum is detached from the lower brain to treat certain mental disorders. Freeman's best-known works are *Neuropathology* (1933) and *Psychosurgery* (with J. W. Watts, 1942).

See also LOBOTOMY.

FREE WILL, understood philosophically, is the power of the individual agent to determine his choice (of action or inaction) by and of himself. Free will may also be defined negatively as "uncaused choice," where "uncaused" is understood to mean that no force or power external to the chooser is operative in determining his choice.

The affirmation and denial of free will constitute one of the most important and persistent controversies in the history of Western thought. The issue is important, because metaphysics, theology, ethics, jurisprudence, and psychology all meet here.

The free will question first became important during the early formulation of Christian theology. The doctrine that Christ, the Son of God, came to earth to save man from sin seemed to suggest man's need of external aid; yet sin implied his moral responsibility, hence his freedom. Moreover, divine omnipotence and omniscience appeared incompatible with human freedom of will. St. Augustine (354–430) and John Calvin (1509–64) tried to reconcile these divergent elements by their doctrine of predestination: In Adam the whole human race was (negatively) free to choose good or evil. Adam's choice of evil corrupted all men, rendering them justly subject to eternal damnation. But God's inscrutable act of grace has elected certain souls to the acceptance of the Gospel (positive free will) and the eternal salvation following therefrom.

Since the Renaissance the remarkable progress of the physical and biological sciences has presented the free-will problem in a new light, showing will as only one aspect of the human spirit. Scientific thought, moral decision, and artistic creation all seem to many thinkers essentially meaningless, if viewed scientifically as only a series of causally determined events.

The case for negative freedom of will (freedom from causal determinism) is weak. Many have claimed that without such freedom moral judgments on human decisions would be absurd, since the moral "ought" is incompatible with the scientific "must" and "cannot." The obvious reply is that a decision which does not spring from the agent's own character is not a decision for which he is morally responsible.

A case for positive freedom of will (freedom through causal determinism) is to be found in the pantheism of Benedict Spinoza (1632–77). Here God is the unitary, self-sufficient, self-explanatory Whole of Reality from which all existent details follow with a rigorous necessity, both causal and logical. Determinism pervades the universe; there is no arbitrary freedom of uncaused choice, divine or human. The essential nature of every finite being, including man, is a striving to preserve and increase its power (freedom). Power consists of causes, and a cause is what explains, what necessitates its effect. So to have insight is to have freedom. The more men understand the necessary dependence of all things on God, the more their minds expand toward the mind of God, as they grow in power and freedom. In this process men are united rather than separated, since knowledge (from which power and freedom spring) is a co-operative rather than a competitive good. Free will is the affirmation of a Reality absorbed into one's own mind through the very necessities pervading it.

FREUD [*froid*], **ANNA** (1895–   ), psychoanalyst, the youngest child of Sigmund Freud and the only one to follow in his footsteps. She was educated in the schools of Vienna, her home city. She became her father's secretary and studied psychoanalysis with him. In 1923 she began specializing in the psychoanalysis of children—a specialty neglected since Sigmund Freud's successful analysis of a five-year-old boy in 1908. She accompanied her father to London in 1938 and has lived there since. After serving as co-director of the Hampstead War Nurseries for Homeless Children, she became head of the Hampstead Child-Therapy Clinic where she continued to practice child analysis. *Ego and the Mechanisms of Defense* and other writings have enlarged the horizons of general psychoanalysis.

FREUD, SIGMUND (1856–1939), Austrian physician widely known as the founder of psychoanalysis. Freud entered the medical school of the University of Vienna in 1873 with the intention of preparing himself for a career in science. In medical school he studied with the eminent physiologist Ernst von Brücke, from whom he learned to regard the living person as a dynamic system to which the laws of chemistry and physics apply. During his eight years in medical school and for several years following graduation, Freud engaged in original research on the nervous system. His investigations were well thought of and he was rapidly making a name for himself in science. Anti-Semitism in Austrian universities and the practical necessity of supporting a family, however, led Freud to choose private practice over an academic career.

Because of his scientific interest in the nervous system, Freud specialized in the treatment of nervous disorders. In order to improve his skill as a practitioner he studied in Paris during the winter of 1885–86 with the leading French psychiatrist Jean Charcot, who used hypnosis for the treatment of hysteria.

Freud's work in psychoanalysis grew out of his association with another Viennese physician, Joseph Breuer, who had devised a new method for treating hysterical patients. This method consisted of hypnotizing the patient and having him express the suppressed emotions which were associated with the origin of the hysterical symptoms. Freud and Breuer collaborated on a book, *Studies in Hysteria* (1895), which discussed their use of this method.

Shortly after this work appeared, Freud and Breuer dissolved their association, because Breuer was unwilling to

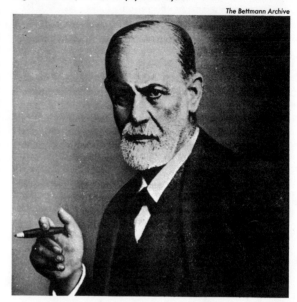

Sigmund Freud, founder of psychoanalysis.

The Bettmann Archive

accept Freud's hypothesis that sexual conflicts were the cause of hysteria. Freud abandoned hypnotism, which had proved inapplicable to many patients, and substituted the method of free association, in which the patient was encouraged to allow his ideas to flow in an unrestricted stream and to speak his thoughts as they came. This method enabled Freud to explore the unconscious mind and to develop a theory of human behavior. The early results of his investigations were set forth in his book *The Interpretation of Dreams* (1900), in which he dealt with the psychological mechanisms underlying dreams.

This book and other writings which appeared during the first decade of the 20th century brought his work to the attention of other psychiatrists. Alfred Adler of Vienna and Carl Jung of Zurich joined with Freud and helped to promote psychoanalysis as a method of treating patients, as a theory of abnormal behavior, and as a system of psychology. Freud and Jung traveled together to the United States in 1909 to give lectures at Clark University in Worcester, Mass. The International Psychoanalytic Association was founded in 1910 to advance psychoanalysis throughout the world. Jung was its first president.

Dissension broke out among the three men; Adler, in 1911, and Jung, in 1914, broke with Freud and started their own schools of psychoanalysis. Under the leadership of Freud, however, the movement prospered. New recruits were attracted and institutes for the training of psychoanalysts were established in many cities. Freud had been named professor in the University of Vienna in 1902, but his chief work consisted of treating patients and expanding and revising his views.

In spite of a heavy practice which occupied his days, Freud was a prodigious writer. His complete psychological writings are published in an English edition of 24 volumes. Among his best-known books, in addition to *The Interpretation of Dreams*, are *The Psychopathology of Everyday Life* (1901), which explains the unconscious significance of forgetting, mistakes, and accidents; *Three Essays on the*

Theory of Sexuality (1905), which traces the development of the sex impulse and its aberrations; *Jokes and Their Relation to the Unconscious* (1905); *Introductory Lectures on Psychoanalysis* (1916–17); *Beyond the Pleasure Principle* (1920), which postulates the existence in man of a death instinct as well as a life instinct; *The Future of an Illusion* (1927), which is a psychoanalytic study of religion; *Civilization and Its Discontents* (1930), in which he examines the reasons for modern man's unhappiness, and *New Introductory Lectures on Psychoanalysis* (1933). His style of writing is lively and lucid and reflects his highly developed sense of humor and his broad knowledge of literature. He was awarded the Goethe Prize in 1930.

In contrast to his scientific life, in which his ideas were violently opposed by many other scientists and during which many of his followers broke with him, Freud's domestic life was quiet and uneventful. He was married to Martha Bernays in 1886 and they had six children. Only one of his children, Anna, became a psychoanalyst. The Freud family lived in a flat at 19 Bergstrasse, Vienna, for 47 years. Freud had his consulting rooms in the same building. Freud's main interest outside of his family and work was archeology, and he made numerous trips to Italy in pursuit of this interest.

In 1923 the first signs of cancer in his upper jaw and palate were detected and during the rest of his life Freud suffered from the progressive ravages of the disease, for which he underwent 33 operations. Although he was preoccupied by the thought of death, he continued to write and to see patients to the very end of his life.

Freud died in exile in London. In 1938, after the Nazi take over in Austria, he realized his dangerous position (the Nazis had banned and burned his books). Although his home was searched and later seized, and his daughter and son interrogated by the Gestapo, Freud and his family were finally allowed to leave Austria in safety, aided by the efforts of Princess Marie Bonaparte, William Bullitt, American ambassador to France, and others.

Freud's impact upon psychiatry and psychology has been enormous. He emphasized the powerful unconscious and irrational forces which motivate and shape man's behavior and developed a pessimistic image of man as a more or less helpless victim of these forces. The influence of his ideas extends into the domains of art, literature, politics, economics, sociology, religion, anthropology, and philosophy. Probably no other man has so profoundly affected the intellectual currents of the 20th century.

See also Psychoanalysis; Psychotherapy.

FROMM, ERICH (1900–), psychoanalyst. Born in Frankfurt, Germany, he took his Ph.D. at Heidelberg and later studied at the University of Munich and at Berlin's Psychoanalytic Institute. He lectured at Bennington College from 1941 to 1950 and was a professor in the National University of Mexico after 1951 and concurrently a professor at Michigan State University after 1957. One of the better-known revisers of Freudian psychology, he developed the concept that many neuroses result from the insecurity created by the increased freedom of choice in complex modern society, as opposed to the rigid, but secure, conditions of earlier times. Among his published

works are *Escape From Freedom* (1941), *The Forgotten Language* (1951), and *The Art of Loving* (1956).

FRUSTRATION AND AGGRESSION. Frustration is normally considered to exist for an individual when temporary or semipermanent interference gets between him and a goal. Such interference may arise from within the person (for example, moral conflict), or from his physical or social environment (for example, from a competitor or some physical barrier). Thus frustration is a response, emotional in nature, that is presumed to be made by a person when his motivated behavior is interfered with; whether or not frustration does arise is best determined from his subsequent behavior. Aggression is often taken as evidence of frustration when the conditions of interference are apparent.

In scientific psychology the following would be acceptable as a definition of frustration: that it exists when interference with a person's ongoing behavior leads to aggression. Unfortunately, however, aggressive acts themselves are often considered sufficient evidence of frustration, particularly when no other obvious explanation is available. When this is done, frustration becomes simply "that which induces aggression," and in this role the term serves no useful purpose.

Aggression, then, which is characterized by forceful or harmful acts, or both, against a person or object, is often taken as a sign of frustration. Juvenile delinquency, when seen as aggression against society, is commonly thought to result from frustration, and efforts are made to identify sources of frustration in the juvenile's environment. It should be noted, however, that the frustration-aggression dependency is merely a hypothesis and that aggression might reasonably arise in the absence of interference with ongoing behavior. Thus, for example, Sigmund Freud saw aggressive behavior as an indicator of a death wish that he imputed to all people. Also, at least in some animals, aggression seems to be occasioned by what more suitably might be called fear. Some young people become delinquent even though they seem to be facing no frustrations more serious than those endured by nondelinquent children.

FUGUE, in psychiatry, an episode of abnormal behavior marked by aimless wandering and possibly confusion, agitation, and amnesia. The fugue is considered to be a form of dissociation—the tendency to detach portions of the mental life from the main stream of the personality. It usually develops from a desire to escape from an intolerable situation. In short fugues the patient may be highly emotional and disoriented. In long fugues he may travel far from his normal surroundings, and appear normal in all respects. Upon emerging from the fugue the patient may have amnesia for the period of the fugue or for his entire past life.

FUNCTIONAL PSYCHOLOGY, school of psychology frequently considered to have been founded by John Dewey, though its development was actually the work of others as well, both before and after Dewey's first writing. It stressed the utility or function of mental activity and thus the adaptive nature of behavior. A functionalist was concerned with mental processes rather than with structure or content of the mind; he sought to explain the "why" of observed behavioral phenomena.

Historically, functionalism was a forerunner of behaviorism. It also provided an appropriate climate for Edward L. Thorndike's law of effect, the principle that learning can be explained in terms of the effect of actions—those reactions that produce satisfying states are learned readily, whereas those that produce displeasing states are learned slowly or not at all. Functionalism was itself significantly influenced by evolutionary theory. In contemporary psychology such a school is no longer readily discernible; an interest in the "why" of behavior exists beyond the bounds of any school, and points of view in psychology differ largely on issues not specifically raised by functionalism. *See also* BEHAVIORISM.

G

GANG, group of persons acting in common, generally for criminal purposes. It is also a special term designating youthful groups whose members are intensely loyal to each other and whose behavior and attitudes are strongly exclusive and even hostile to outsiders, whether adults or other adolescents. Ordinarily regarded as a separate entity characterized by antisocial and delinquent practices, the gang illustrates a universal tendency of adolescents to form closely knit groups.

The typical boys' gang, largely an urban phenomenon, identifies itself closely with a few city blocks, regarded as its territory. This is the so-called "turf," which the gang defends against the real or imagined inroads of outsiders. Each new group in urban slums produces its own gangs, similar but distinguished by ethnic and racial differences.

The romanticized names designating the group and its leadership express the adolescent's sense of adventure and bravado, as well as his imaginative effort to rise above the surroundings. Thus, such names as the Gaylords, the Chaplains, and other colorful epithets, describe the groups, and the leaders hold such honorifics as Overlord, King, and President. A significant aspect of the development of boys' gangs since the end of World War II has been the tendency toward an apparently formal organization, with acknowledged leadership and membership responsibilities. The growth of urban gangs has been accompanied by the formation of affiliated groups of those too young for membership and of loosely associated groups of girl affiliates, or "Debs."

Social agencies, accepting the principle that, for slum youths, these gangs satisfy a natural and deeply implanted need, have attempted to work with them through "detached street workers." These workers are trained in social work procedures, which they employ in attempting to divert gang activity into constructive channels. They meet and work with the gang largely in its own milieu—the local candy store, gymnasium, or pool hall—to overcome initial resistance to their acceptance by the gang boy.

Since the end of World War II virtually every major city in North and South America, Europe, Africa, and Asia has been characterized by the seemingly spontaneous development of gang behavior among adolescents. Herbert A. Bloch and Arthur Niederhoffer, in *The Gang: A Study in Adolescent Behavior* (1958), an extensive study of gang behavior in a large variety of cultures, interpret this development as an effort by adolescents to achieve the status of adulthood under conditions of great strain in the face of efforts by different societies to postpone conferring it. The similarities in many of the excesses of adolescent and gang behavior among youths and groups from different societies are striking, as is the resemblance of this behavior to much of that among the so-called normal middle-class teen-age groups. Frederic M. Thrasher,

in a study entitled *The Gang* (1927), investigated 1,313 gangs and detected wide similarities in the developmental stages in the organization of gang groups. Albert K. Cohen in his work, *Delinquent Boys: The Culture of the Gang* (1955), interpreted the delinquent gang of the working-class youth as a protest against his inability to achieve the objectives of middle-class society. In Cohen's view, such behavior is marked by the culturally ingrained inability to defer the gratification of wants. Walter Miller in a study, *Lower Class Culture as a Generating Milieu of Gang Delinquency* (1958), analyzed gang behavior as reflecting the predominant "focal concerns" of the working class: preoccupation with toughness, smartness, excitement, and freedom from constraint. Richard A. Cloward and Lloyd E. Ohlin, in a joint investigation entitled *Delinquency and Opportunity: A Theory of Delinquent Gangs* (1960), concluded that whether gang behavior leads to "criminalistic," "conflict," or "retreatist" behavior depends upon access to opportunities provided by the slum environment. *See also* JUVENILE DELINQUENCY.

GESELL [gə-zĕl'], **ARNOLD LUCIUS** (1880–1961), American psychologist and pediatrician. He joined the Yale faculty in 1911, establishing the clinic later known as the Yale Clinic of Child Development. Director of this clinic from 1911 to 1948, he also studied medicine (receiving his M.D. degree in 1915) and was professor of child hygiene from 1915 to 1948. After 1950 he was a consultant to the Gesell Institute of Child Development. He is noted for studies of the growth and development of children. His books, written in collaboration with Frances Ilg and others, include *Infant and Child in the Culture of Today* (1943), *How a Baby Grows* (1945), *The Child from Five to Ten* (1946), *Vision: Its Development in Infant and Child* (1949), *Infant Development* (1952), and *Youth: The Years from Ten to Sixteen* (1956).

GESTALT [gə-shtält'] **PSYCHOLOGY,** the view that mental phenomena are organized wholes, that experience consists not in bundles of discrete stimuli but in undivided structures which are more than just the sum of their physical components. A melody is more than a collection of tones. In fact, the form or structure of experience (*Gestalt*, a German word, is often translated "form") is considered to be independent of the particular stimulus components that give rise to it. Thus, for example, a circle is a circle even though the particular stimulus is a ball, the mouth of a bottle, or a group of children holding hands.

This view was first elaborated by Max Wertheimer in Germany (1912). Wolfgang Köhler and Kurt Koffka were also major figures in the development of Gestalt theory, which arose in Europe, partly to combat Wilhelm Wundt's sensationism (analysis of experience into component sensations), at the same time that behaviorism was being enunciated in America. The influence of Gestalt psychology has waned, but many of its principles, such as organization of the perceptual field and relativity of sensory experience, have been recognized as important concepts. *See also* BEHAVIORISM.

GROUP THERAPY, treatment of emotional disturbances based on the conviction that group relationships form the key to living. Through the group, the patient may repair his inappropriate ways of making social contact. He can also experience genuine human relations to provide him with the resources for a natural psychological recovery.

Group discussion of problems started at the beginning of this century, not in psychiatry, but with tuberculosis patients. Later, psychosomatic disorders were treated in this way. After World War II especially, group psychotherapy, incorporating psychoanalytic viewpoints, became an accepted psychiatric technique. In the psychiatric hospital, or in psychiatric wards of general hospitals, all ward patients and staff may meet daily or weekly for a general discussion. Most of the time, management of ward patients is discussed spontaneously. The therapist plays a largely passive role, if necessary discussing particular problem areas, or guiding group discussion of an individual's behavior. In this form, group therapy serves as preparation or adjunct to other psychiatric treatment approaches, such as individual psychotherapy, psychopharmacology, and physical therapies.

Specific group therapy is done in groups of no more than 10 or 20 patients, who meet once or twice a week with one or more therapists. In such groups, the discussion of personal problems is actively encouraged by the therapist. Because the group usually remains constant for long periods of time, sometimes years, group members become strongly involved. Such groups may be indicated for patients who fear or distrust individual therapies, for emotional disorders that do not require a psychiatrist, or those for which extensive psychiatric attention is not indicated.

Many nonclinical therapeutic groups, such as Alcoholics Anonymous and training groups (T-groups), have also come into existence. There are inspirational support groups, with or without confessions, and didactic, counseling, or mutual-experiencing groups. In each, the leader, who may change from session to session, tries to guide the group members to greater mutual acceptance, thereby increasing their freedom of genuine expression. After this acceptance of each other as individuals, the group members may be able to experience communality of goals and interests, without fear of losing their identity. *See also* PSYCHOTHERAPY.

GUIDANCE AND COUNSELING, EDUCATIONAL. The term "guidance" is sometimes used broadly to refer to advising or helping an individual with any kind of educational, vocational, or personal problem. In this sense, guidance is provided by families, schools, colleges, churches, organizations, employers, clinics, doctors, publications, and other sources. This meaning is so broad that the distinction from the general process of education, that is, of learning to live in a culture, is not clear. For the purposes of this article, "guidance" is used in the more spe-

cific sense of programs provided by the schools to help young people with their problems of adjustment. The layman often uses the terms guidance and counseling interchangeably. To the professional, however, there is distinct difference. A guidance program, particularly in a school or college, offers a set of services consisting of occupational information, placement, testing, orientation, and counseling. In this context then, counseling is essential to a comprehensive guidance program.

Guidance Services in the United States. The guidance movement in the United States can be said to have started with the work of Frank Parsons in Boston and Eli Weaver in New York in the early years of the 20th century. Parsons was concerned with vocational guidance—helping young people to choose careers, get started in them, and progress in them. Boys and girls usually received their first counseling toward the end of high school. After a while experience began to show that guidance was being offered too late in some cases. One student might find that the courses he had taken did not fit him for any specific job. Another might decide that the career for which he had been training did not match his real talents or interests. Accordingly, educational guidance was introduced into school systems as a means of helping young people plan their school courses to lead toward selected kinds of work. Since vocational guidance was being offered at the 12th-grade level, the natural progression was downward, introducing guidance in the 11th, 10th, and lower grades.

Not only did guidance services expand in the sense of being made available to more grades, they also began to take in a wider range of problems. Boys and girls showed a need for help with personal and social problems in addition to problems of career planning. In the early days of guidance programs, the training of personnel stressed job information (the jobs available and future employment trends) and methods of testing individuals to determine

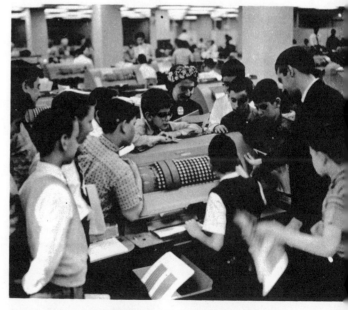

As part of a vocational guidance program, a counselor and a group of students tour a large business office. (NEW YORK CITY BOARD OF EDUCATION)

special aptitudes and interests. But as young people tended to seek help with other problems—matters of physical and mental health, for example, or difficulties in relations with parents or with friends—training programs for counselors were enlarged to include courses in psychology and psychotherapy in addition to courses on occupational trends and aptitude testing.

The demand for all kinds of services increased so rapidly that by the early 1960's there were not nearly enough trained counselors to meet the demand for guidance in the public schools. This situation created a problem for the schools. In some cases counselors were the only trained and informed persons available to help boys and girls with exceptional problems or handicaps, and the schools did not like to cut off this source of aid. On the other hand, problems not directly related to schoolwork were making great demands on the counselors' time. Many educators concluded that it was not feasible to expect guidance counselors to become specialists in such diverse areas as mental and physical handicaps and emotional and social problems. Counselors should, however, have enough knowledge of such fields to work with specialists. A child with a severe emotional disturbance, for example, might be referred to a psychologist or a psychiatrist, who would help the child and work with the counselor and teacher to plan the child's educational program. A number of states have put guidance within a larger organization, often called pupil personnel or special education services. This bureau has medical, psychological, and other specialized divisions to deal with physically handicapped, mentally retarded, speech-handicapped, and other exceptional children.

In so far as possible, a counselor is available, full-time or part-time, in each school. The counselor, working with groups and with individuals, does his best to advise all students. A great deal of the normal work of the counselor involves planning a course of study that will prepare a boy or girl for a desired career. Counseling may be undertaken at any point in a child's schooling, but the most intensive planning often takes place at the time of transition from the 6th grade to the junior high school, from the junior to the senior high school, or from the 8th grade to the senior high school. In high school a student has to select one of several curriculums, or "tracks," which may be labeled college preparatory; general; business, secretarial, or commercial; or vocational, technical, or industrial. Counselor and student may work together for many hours on the choice of a program. While it is usually possible to change from one track to another if it becomes apparent that a better choice can be made, the initial decision should be made as carefully as possible. The counselor uses all available information about the student's health, physique, and school record as well as test results. Experience shows that final choices are most satisfactory when student, counselor, and parents co-operate but the student makes the decision. Self-determined goals are usually the ones that young people work hardest to attain. (For further discussion of career planning, see VOCATIONAL GUIDANCE.)

Students who plan on further education after high school face the problem of choosing one of the thousands of institutions—business schools, technical schools, junior colleges, colleges, and universities—in the country. Providing information and direction in making this choice is a major task of the counselor. The work of the high school counselor does not end when a student enters a more advanced school or takes a job. Follow-up studies are conducted as a means of evaluating the instructional and guidance work of the school.

Educational guidance is an important service at the college level. Entering students face new surroundings and often find that academic competition is stiffer than ever before. Help with these problems is provided by faculty members with a variety of titles, examples being dean of men, dean of women, director of student personnel, or co-ordinator of student affairs. If a student has entered college without a clearly defined goal, the counselor will help him select an area of major study. Other students start college with definite careers in mind but find after a few months that they do not have the ability or interests to stay with the original choice. In such cases guidance experts help the student select another field or, if necessary, another college. One major goal of college guidance services is to reduce the percentage of failure to graduate.

Guidance Services in Other Countries. In the sense of advice on vocational, educational, social, and moral behavior, guidance is given wherever there is education. Specific guidance services are available in the schools of many countries. Most common, perhaps, are special services for exceptional children, often including school psychologists or psychology clinics. Counseling is often left to teachers and administrators.

There are exceptions, however. In English schools voca-

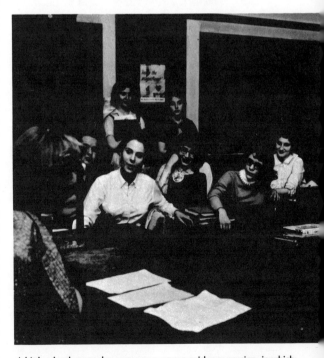

A high school counselor oversees a group guidance session, in which students' problems are discussed. (NEW YORK CITY BOARD OF EDUCATION)

tional counseling, originally one of the responsibilities of headmasters and housemasters, was often delegated to a careers' master. Under a law of 1948 a Youth Employment Service was set up. Specially trained Youth Employment Officers provide vocational guidance and placement services. In certain countries—France and the Soviet Union, for example—boys and girls are directed into designated "tracks" on the basis of estimates of their abilities. Relatively few are selected for higher education. Comparison with other countries points up two features of guidance in the United States. One is the fact that young people have an unusual degree of freedom to make their own decisions about careers and to continue their educations as long as they can pass courses and pay costs. The other is that counseling has developed as a major professional field in education; specialists have tended to take the place of informal advisers.

Guidance as a Career. At the present time in schools and colleges, teaching and counseling are closely related. Most counselors employed in educational institutions must have a teaching credential, in order to be employed as a counselor.

During the administration of President Lyndon Johnson, much legislation was passed aimed at bringing the economic and culturally disadvantaged segment of the population into the main stream of American life. The various agencies responsible for carrying out this "war on poverty" have employed many counselors, which has caused the shortage of trained counselors to become more acute. As many of these agencies are not directly connected with the educational system, they often do not require teaching experience as a requisite to employment. Also, the formal training necessary with these agencies is not as extensive.

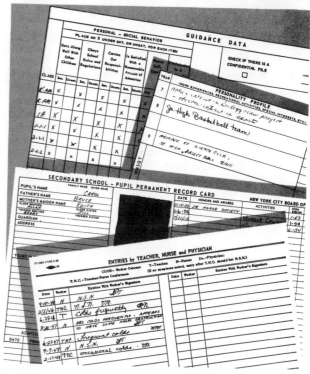

Guidance data, personality profiles, records of school activities, and health reports are helpful in counseling. (NEW YORK CITY BOARD OF EDUCATION)

See also:
EXCEPTIONAL CHILDREN
TESTING, PSYCHOLOGICAL AND EDUCATIONAL
VOCATIONAL GUIDANCE

H

HALL, GRANVILLE STANLEY (1844–1924), American psychologist and educator. He received a Ph.D. degree from Harvard and studied in Germany with Wilhelm Wundt. While professor at Johns Hopkins (1883–88) he founded the first psychological laboratory in the United States. From 1889 to 1919 he was president of Clark University, also serving as professor of psychology. He founded the *American Journal of Psychology*, first American periodical in the field, and was first president of the American Psychological Association (1891). His interest in child and adolescent psychology is shown in *The Contents of Children's Minds* (1883) and *Adolescence* (2 vols., 1904). His other works include *Morals* (1920) and *Senescence* (1922).

HALLUCINATIONS [hə-lŌō-sə-nā'shənz] are errors of perception in which the individual sees, hears, feels, smells, or tastes objects which are not present. Although hallucinations occur principally in persons suffering from mental illness, relatively normal persons may experience them under certain circumstances.

The most common hallucinations are voices and sounds heard by mental patients (*see* SCHIZOPHRENIA). Visual hallucinations are frequently seen in alcoholics suffering from delirium tremens. Hallucinatory smells and tastes, which are comparatively rare, are seen in certain brain diseases. Children with schizophrenia often report voices and objects residing within their own bodies. A special type of hallucination occurs in normal persons in the twilight state between waking and sleeping.

HEAD, SIR HENRY (1861–1940), English neurologist known for his studies on language defects (aphasia) and sensation. Among his numerous contributions to neurology were a description of the role of the vagus nerve in breathing, studies on the effects of injuries to peripheral nerves, investigations on pain (referred pain), and a classic two-volume work on aphasia, *Aphasia and Kindred Disorders of Speech* (1926). He lectured at the Royal College of Physicians and was knighted in 1927.

HERBART [hĕr'bärt], **JOHANN FRIEDRICH** (1776–1841) German philosopher, psychologist, and educator. Born in Oldenburg, he was educated at Jena, and from 1797 to 1800 he was a tutor in Switzerland, where he first became interested in the pedagogical theories of J. H. Pestalozzi. In 1802 he became a lecturer at Göttingen, and in 1805 a professor. In 1809 he moved to Königsberg as professor of pedagogy and philosophy, but in 1833 returned to Göttingen.

In philosophy Herbart formulated a metaphysical system called *pluralistic realism*, which presented reality as composed of many reals, both psychic and nonpsychic.

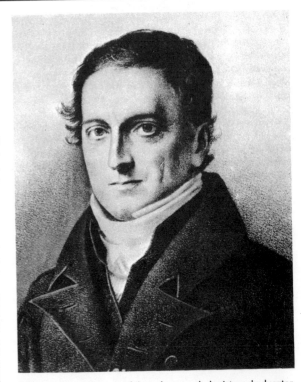

Johann Herbart, German philosopher, psychologist, and educator. (THE BETTMANN ARCHIVE)

The reals are Kantian things-in-themselves. Each real is simple, indivisible, unchangeable, self-sufficient, independent, and ultimately unknowable.

Some psychologists honor Herbart as the founder of scientific psychology and the discoverer of the "unconscious," but reject his thesis that psychology is rooted in metaphysics. According to Herbart's theory, the pure Ego (Soul) is a single psychic real, but the *self*, of which we are aware in self-consciousness, is a changing complex of ideas. Each item of consciousness is an "idea." The ideas differ in time, intensity, and quality, and the active opposition among ideas suppresses some below the threshold (limen) of consciousness. Only those adapted to the unity of consciousness rise above the threshold.

In his theory of education Herbart maintained that education should promote personal morality and the social adjustment of the individual. He saw the importance of arousing the student's interest, and formulated a theory of instruction which was developed by his followers into the famous five steps of teaching: preparation, presentation, comparison and abstraction, generalization, and application.

HEROIN [hĕr′ō-ĭn], a narcotic derived from morphine. Heroin is several times more potent than morphine as a pain reliever, but is also more depressing to the nervous system. Its principal danger lies in its exceptional ability to produce an intense feeling of well-being which leads to a particularly serious addiction. The importation, manufacture, and sale of heroin are prohibited in the United States by the Harrison Narcotic Act. However, it is still legally available in some countries.
See also DRUG ADDICTION; NARCOTICS.

HOMESICKNESS. When a young person is away from home and feels such yearning for home that it disrupts his daily behavior, he is said to be homesick. Homesickness is regressive behavior, in that the individual wishes to return to a pattern of life found satisfying in his earlier years. This earlier period seems especially attractive as compared to his present away-from-home situation because there is a common tendency to remember only the pleasant experiences of the past. Such dwelling on the past indicates an inability to use past experiences as realistic guides for meeting new situations.

Because homesickness is often highly emotional, it may result in such disturbances as loss of appetite, digestive upsets, and vomiting. The homesick individual is often depressed, and homesickness is not to be taken lightly. On the other hand, it is a fairly common reaction to being away from home, and a mild amount of homesickness is not unusual the first night in camp or the first week of freshman year in college. Most people work out a satisfactory solution in a short time.

Homesickness is not a consequence of love in the home, but rather of overindulgence and overprotection, leading to emotional dependence on the parents. The basic preventive, or treatment, is psychological weaning, or emancipation; that is, the young person must outgrow family domination. Sometimes as he is becoming psychologically weaned he may be rebellious, may adopt an "It's none of your business" attitude, may belittle his parents, and may reject some of their social values. In order to show his independence, he may deliberately commit acts of which he knows they disapprove. The period of psychological weaning is often a trying one both for the young person and for his parents, but the process is a necessary step in growing up.

Psychological weaning does not imply a lessening of the genuine love relationship between a child and his parents, but an ending of the childhood relationship of protection and supervision. With the achievement of psychological weaning, the basic cause of homesickness is removed, as are other harmful effects of clinging to parents.
See also ADOLESCENCE.

HORNEY [hôr′nī], **KAREN** (1885–1952), psychoanalyst. Born and educated in Germany, she emigrated to the United States in 1932 and became a controversial figure through her writings on psychoanalysis. She disputed the Freudian doctrine that neurosis resulted from suppression of sexual and other instinctual drives and from disturbances of parent-child relationships. She argued instead that anxiety and mental stress were produced by social pressures, and that the basic human motivation was not sex, but the drive to obtain safety and security. Among her published works are *New Ways in Psychoanalysis* (1939) and *Neurosis and Human Growth* (1950).

HYPERVENTILATION SYNDROME, condition caused by overbreathing, usually resulting from emotional stress and anxiety in persons suffering from psychoneurotic disorders. The patient is usually not aware that he is overbreathing; over a period of time the concentration of carbon dioxide in the blood is altered, leading to the characteristic symptoms which include dizziness, breathlessness, and numbness and tingling sensations in the fingers, toes, and lips. If overbreathing continues, the patient may lose consciousness or develop convulsions. The attack can be halted by having the patient breathe in and out of a paper bag to elevate the carbon dioxide level of the blood. Further treatment consists of psychotherapy.

HYPNOSIS [hĭp-nō′sĭs], a psychological state of altered attention and awareness in which the individual is unusually receptive and responsive to suggestions.

In the latter half of the 18th century the Austrian physician Anton Mesmer obtained remarkable cures of difficult conditions by making passes with magnets over his patients. While these cures apparently resulted from some form of hypnotic suggestion, Mesmer attributed his results to the effect of "animal magnetism," an intangible force or influence which allegedly passed from physician to patient. Mesmer's claims were investigated by a committee appointed by the French Academy of Science, which admitted the effectiveness of his treatment but disputed his theoretical claims and prohibited him from practicing in Paris.

The word "hypnosis," from the Greek *hypnos*, "sleep," was later coined by James Braid, an English surgeon who considered the phenomenon to be artificial sleep.

In 1878 the famous French neurologist J. M. Charcot and his students demonstrated that there were several stages of hypnosis. The French physician Bernheim emphasized the importance of suggestion in the hypnotic state. Sigmund Freud began his investigations into psychoanalysis using hypnosis as a means to explore forgotten experiences; however, Freud later abandoned the use of hypnosis when he encountered difficulty in applying it to some subjects.

Following World War II the study of hypnosis was intensified. In 1955 the British Medical Association approved the use of hypnosis in medicine, and the American Medical Association followed suit in 1958.

Theories of hypnosis are numerous but no single theory is generally accepted as completely explaining all aspects of hypnosis. One of the oldest theories regards hypnosis to be a form of sleep. This concept originated in 1784 and was further developed by the Russian physiologist Ivan Pavlov, who is known for his work on conditioned reflexes. Pavlov noted that the repetition of certain stimulations induced sleep in experimental animals. Before the animal lapsed into sleep, however, it passed through a drowsy state which Pavlov identified as a hypnotic trance. This theory is contradicted by evidence which indicates that the hypnotized person is not asleep: the knee reflex, which is absent in sleep, is present in the hypnotic state.

and recordings of brain waves show the typical patterns of the waking state.

In 1909 the noted psychoanalyst Sandor Ferenczi explained hypnosis as a parent-child relationship, with the hypnotized subject as the child and the hypnotist as the parent. In Ferenczi's view the subject might regard the hypnotist as a stern father or a soft-spoken, gentle mother. Earlier, Freud had advanced the idea that the subject-hypnotist relation was similar to being in love.

In 1941 the psychologist Robert W. White described hypnotized persons as trying to behave in the way in which they believed a hypnotized person should act.

Inducing Hypnosis. There are as many techniques of inducing hypnosis as there are doctors who use hypnosis. The commonest method involves *eye fixation:* the subject is asked to fixate his eyes while the hypnotist suggests that the eyelids are becoming tired and heavy, and are closing. Another widely used technique is *hand levitation:* the hypnotist suggests to the subject that he is feeling various sensations in the fingers and hands and that the hand is rising into the air. So-called "disguised" techniques have also been described which are alleged to hypnotize the patient while he is unaware. It is generally agreed, however, that since the subject is conscious, even while under hypnosis, he is aware that hypnosis is being attempted and cannot be hypnotized against his will.

The Hypnotic State. Perhaps the most outstanding characteristic of the hypnotic state is the suggestibility of the subject. He readily accepts and responds to ideas offered by the hypnotist. He may even carry out suggestions offered to him while in hypnosis after he emerges from hypnosis. This is known as posthypnotic suggestion.

The hypnotized person may be in a light, medium, or deep trance. In the light trance the eyes are closed, breathing becomes slower, the facial muscles are fixed, and the subject is able to carry out simple posthypnotic suggestions. In the medium trance there is a partial amnesia, and simple hallucinations can be induced. The deep trance, or somnambulistic state, is characterized by the subject's ability to maintain the trance with the eyes open; a total amnesia; control over physiological functions, such as the pulse rate and blood pressure; and the ability to anesthetize a part of the body. There is also a *plenary* or *stuporous* trance in which the subject remains absolutely quiet and responds only to suggestions of the hypnotist. This state is achieved in only a small number of subjects and requires considerable effort to produce.

Contrary to popular belief, there is no possibility of the subject not awakening as a result of an accident to the hypnotist. It is also not true that a hypnotized subject is under the will or power of the hypnotist. As has already been noted, hypnosis is a co-operative venture between the subject and the hypnotist: no control can be exercised without the subject's implied or actual consent.

Applications. Hypnosis is used in dentistry, obstetrics, and in surgery to achieve anesthesia. Psychiatrists occasionally use hypnosis to enable the patient to recall early painful experiences he might otherwise not recall.

Hypnosis has also been used to overcome undesirable habits, such as excessive smoking, overeating, and nail biting. A valuable adjunct to this treatment is autohypnosis: the subject is taught to induce a trance by himself. This technique reinforces the suggestions of the doctor and reduces the number of office visits required.

HYPNOTICS [hĭp-nŏt'ĭks], drugs which induce sleep. They depress the activity of the brain, producing sedation when given in small dosages and sleep when given in larger amounts. A hypnotic should ideally induce sleep quickly and reliably without upsetting the stomach or causing a preliminary period of excitation. It should act over a sufficiently long period and in addition should not be toxic or addicting. Although a number of excellent hypnotics are available, none fully meets all of these criteria.

The most important and widely used hypnotic drugs are the barbiturates, of which there are close to 20 in clinical use. They are available as pills and vary in the speed and duration of their action. The shorter-acting barbiturates, such as secobarbital, act for less than three hours; the longer-acting barbital and phenobarbital act for six hours or longer. Patients who have difficulty in falling asleeep may be given the short-duration barbiturates, while those who tend to wake repeatedly during the night may be given the longer-acting variety. Barbiturates can be habit-forming and addicting. They may produce confusion and disorientation in elderly patients.

Chloral hydrate was the most frequently used hypnotic prior to the introduction of the barbiturates. The drug is taken orally as a liquid or in a capsule and quickly produces a long-lasting sleep, usually without unpleasant aftereffects. It is quite irritating to the stomach and unless well diluted may cause abdominal pain and uneasiness.

Paraldehyde is an efficient hypnotic which is also available in liquid form. It produces sleep rapidly, even in persons with marked insomnia and in agitated individuals, but is irritating to the stomach and lungs and has a powerful, pungent odor. An addiction to paraldehyde is possible; symptoms resemble those seen in alcoholism.

Glutethimide (Doriden) is a newer hypnotic which is similar to the intermediate or shorter-acting barbiturates in its action. It is available in tablets and may occasionally produce hang-over, dizziness, and lightheadedness on the following day. A troublesome skin rash may appear, and in some cases addiction has been reported from its use.

Ethchlorvynol (Placidyl), also a newer hypnotic, is a quick-acting drug of short duration. It is available in soft gelatin capsules. Skin inflammation, nausea, and hangover have followed its use.

The availability of specific hypnotics such as those mentioned above tends to obscure the value of aspirin, antihistamines, and other drugs which, although usually used for other purposes, are occasionally effective as sleep-inducing agents.

HYPOCHONDRIASIS [hī-pō-kŏn-drī'ə-sĭs], a term describing persons who are unusually preoccupied with their physical health, dwelling on symptoms that most persons would ignore. At times, fatigue, slight palpitations, or other minor variations in body activity may provoke an attack of anxiety. Hypochondriasis may be seen in senile persons, in those suffering from brain damage, or in certain forms of neurosis and psychosis.

HYSTERIA, in psychiatry, an emotional illness which

mimics physical illness without organic disease. The word is derived from the Greek *hystera*, meaning "uterus," because Hippocrates believed hysterical symptoms occurred only in women. People suffering from hysteria were also believed to be possessed by the devil. Good descriptions of the consequences of such beliefs are given in Aldous Huxley's *The Devils of Loudon* (1952) and Arthur Miller's *The Crucible* (1953). It is now known that hysteric manifestations can occur in both sexes, at all ages; but more often among people with little education, especially in those in early adulthood or during periods of great stress, such as war.

Hysterical symptoms are preceded by an anxiety-producing situation, and serve as a solution to underlying psychic conflict concerning sexual roles, job frustrations, or family relationships. After physical symptoms appear, the hysteric is typically calm and tranquil, a state called *la belle indifférence* ("beautiful indifference"). Symptoms fall into five main groups: (1) Disturbances of consciousness and mental processes. In extreme cases the patient may experience fugue states, with memory loss for parts of his life and experiences. The patient may lead a totally different life, and should he regain knowledge of his prior life, he may be forgetful of anything he experienced during the fugue. Stevenson's *Dr. Jekyll and Mr. Hyde* is an example of such alternating states of consciousness, resulting in a multiple personality. (2) Convulsive hysteria, resembling epilepsy. (3) Psychomotor symptoms, with partial paralysis or involuntary movements, such as panic reaction. (4) Sensory disturbances, with hypersensitivity or insensitivity to pain and touch. (5) Affective disturbances, ranging from depression to mania.

With increasing education, classical hysteria—gross signs of dissociation and conversion reactions—have diminished in the Western world. More subtle hysteric manifestations are, however, still very common as reactions to interpersonal and cultural stresses.

See also AMNESIA; FUGUE; NEUROSIS.

I

ID, in psychoanalytic theory (as developed by Freud), the primitive, unconscious portion of the mind which contains the basic biological drives. The id operates on the "pleasure principle," that is it seeks immediate and complete satisfaction of desires. According to Freud, this is seen most clearly in the infant whose mind is virtually all id. Later as the real world becomes more and more restricting, the ego develops from the id to negotiate between the basic desire of the id and the practical possibilities of satisfying these desires in the real world. In this way the ego operates on the "reality principle." Freud likened the id to a tempestuous horse and the ego to the rider who controls and directs the horse.

See also PSYCHOANALYSIS.

IMAGINATION, a term referring generally to the ability of the conscious mind to call up images. Most people can call up at will images of either a visual or auditory nature, such as a friend's face or a familiar tune. Such deliberate imagery is usually a recollection or simple reorganization of past experience. Often images come to mind involuntarily, however, especially just before falling asleep (hypnagogic images) or while sleeping (dream images). Certain drugs and plants can lead to vivid spontaneous images resembling the hallucinations of psychosis. However, the mental patient usually considers his hallucinations to be reality, while the user of drugs continues to realize that his hallucinatory images are induced by the drug.

Some individuals, especially young people, have a great capacity for experiencing detailed and vivid images, mostly visual, called eidetic images. The occurrence of eidetic images is interesting from a legal viewpoint, since witnesses may testify convincingly on the basis of extraordinary detailed eidetic images, which may not be based on reality.

Imagination is also used to denote an aspect of creative ability. Creative imagination is defined as the mind's ability to create images of things or events not previously experienced but only hinted at. Here imagination has a role in acquiring knowledge, in sympathetic understanding (empathy), and in intuition. Creative imagination, consciously and unconsciously forming partly new images, or making new combinations of previous images, is free to some extent from objective restraints. To be effective, however, imagination must be combined with discipline and critical judgment. One whose imaginings violate the elementary laws of thought, or ignore the principles of practical possibility is usually regarded as insane.

Sometimes creative imagination arises in daydreaming, although most daydreaming is reproductive imagination. In fantasy a boy may lead a space exploration, a girl picture herself as a ballerina, or a frustrated adult escape from boring work by daydreaming of a fishing trip, a new car, or a better job. If the dreamer prefers fantasies to actual living, his mental health may be in danger. Imaginative daydreaming, however, may be a productive phase of thinking, as when an engineer "dreams up" a new design or a writer, a story plot.

Although little is known about the process of creative imagination, scientists, writers, and artists have described their work processes. Based on such descriptions, four stages in the creative process have been defined: (1) Preparation. During this period, often one of long and hard work, past attempts at handling the problem or topic are reviewed, facts are gathered and studied, and experience from related areas is considered. (2) Incubation. Concerted work at the conscious level seems to stop, and the materials "lie fallow." Thinking about the project presumably goes on without full awareness on the thinker's part. (3) Inspiration or illumination. There is a "flash of insight." A possible solution to a scientific problem or a pattern for a work of art suddenly appears. (4) Verification. The insight is tried out. A scientific theory is tested by experiment, or an artistic concept is expressed in words or paint or another medium. This sequence is an ideal formulation of a process that actually remains a mystery awaiting further illumination.

See also DREAMS; HALLUCINATIONS; PSYCHOPHARMACOLOGY; THINKING.

INFERIORITY COMPLEX, term used by the psychiatrist Alfred Adler for a repressed system of desires and memories associated with concern about real or imagined inferiority of a person's physical, social, or psychological characteristics. The inferiority complex must be distinguished from inferiority feelings, which are conscious self-judgments. The complex, by definition, means that the feelings of inferiority have been repressed so that the individual is no longer conscious of them. The complex is created because the individual's real or imagined difficulties make him unable to cope effectively with the world around him. Distorted or neurotic behavior is the usual outcome, frequently taking the form of defensive or aggressive acts. These acts are presumed to be unconsciously determined.

See also ADLER, ALFRED.

INSANITY, LEGAL. The meaning and test of insanity in the field of law are largely determined by the nature of the particular proceeding in question. Thus in a criminal prosecution the *right and wrong test* (M'Naghten rule), which refers to the ability to distinguish between "right" and "wrong" with respect to a particular act, has generally been applied. A similar test is used when insanity is interposed as a defense in divorce cases. On the other hand, statutes frequently make a person subject to guardianship if his mental incompetency is evident from "his incapability of managing his own affairs."

Under constitutional and statutory provisions in the various states of the United States, custody and care of insane and other incompetent persons are vested in the courts. State statutes determine the form of the proceeding for the commitment of a person alleged to be insane. Generally there must be a condition of actual insanity, that is, danger to life, person, or property, or at least a need for care and treatment and a trial of these issues before an individual may be committed. Statutes providing for the commitment of insane persons in judicial proceedings have been held to be a proper exercise of the police power of the state. The writ of habeas corpus is available to one who is confined as an insane person and wishes to test the validity of his confinement. If necessary for the protection and management of the property of a person who has been adjudged incompetent (because of insanity or habitual drunkenness), a receiver or guardian (curator) may be appointed by the court to take charge of such property.

The law presumes sanity. The burden of establishing insanity rests with the party who alleges it. Under statutes the application for the inquiry into the sanity of a person (lunacy proceeding) must usually be made by a relative or friend of the alleged lunatic. Insanity or mental incompetency is not sufficiently shown by mere eccentricity or abnormality in personality, or by advanced age, thriftlessness, or the mere fact of suicide.

Contracts, other than purchases of necessaries, made by an insane person under guardianship are generally regarded as void. Any contract, including that of marriage, made by such person prior to an adjudication of his insanity is not void, but only voidable if disaffirmed by him. An insane person, like a sane person, may acquire title to property and may sue or be sued if he is not under guardianship or has not been otherwise adjudged incompetent to manage his affairs.

Statutes of limitations frequently determine the number of years during which an action may be maintained after the removal of the disability of insanity. In such cases the disability must have existed at the time when the cause of action arose.

At common law an insane person was not competent to testify. Today most courts permit him to do so if he has sufficient understanding of the nature of an oath and is able to give a sensible account of the facts at issue. Contrary to the civil law rule, an insane person is generally liable in the common law countries (because of considerations of public policy) for an injury caused by his tortious acts (negligence, trespass) except when malice or intent to injure is a necessary element of the tort.

If a person is found to have been insane at the time of the commission of the crime, he must be acquitted by reason of insanity. If a person is found to be insane after the commission of the crime or after conviction, he will be committed to an asylum until recovery. An insane person cannot be tried or sentenced while he is in such condition, but only afterward if he becomes sane again.

In accordance with recent developments in the field of psychiatry, some courts have discarded the traditional right and wrong test of insanity in a criminal prosecution and have instead attempted to determine whether or not the accused was suffering from a diseased or defective mental condition at the time he committed the criminal act charged, and, if so, whether or not the act was the product of such mental abnormality (Durham rule). The courts disagree as to whether an irresistible impulse to commit an act (murder, sex act, kleptomania, pyromania) or an insane delusion can, apart from the right and wrong test or the Durham rule, constitute a defense against a criminal charge. Statutes occasionally provide for the sterilization of sexual psychopaths, other persons afflicted with serious mental defects, and habitual criminals.
See also MENTAL ILLNESS; PSYCHIATRY; SCHIZOPHRENIA.

INSOMNIA, sleeplessness, the inability to sleep. Some individuals, especially as they grow older, may need very little sleep, but sleeplessness may lead to complaints, especially among the elderly and the mentally diseased. Causes of insomia vary, but research has led to generally applicable explanations of the condition in healthy people who claim to sleep very little. Such people produce normal brain wave patterns during sleep, but are subject to unusually vivid, realistic dream images, which they may mistake for wakeful thought and thus maintain that they slept very little.

Children may fear falling asleep after a nightmare. Most persons occasionally experience difficulty in falling asleep because of legitimate concern over business, school, health, or personal affairs. When this condition occurs regularly, the subject may resort to sleeping pills. If he becomes dependent on them he has established an undesirable drug habit. A brisk walk or television before bed time is more advisable. Physical illness, especially when it is accompanied by pain or discomfort, causes insomnia. Often insomnia is the first sign of a depression, neurosis, or other mental disorder.
See also DRUG ADDICTION; NEUROSIS; SLEEP.

INSTINCT [ĭn'stĭngkt], term most frequently used to refer to those components of behavior patterns that are unlearned, appear uniformly in members of a species, and are normally adaptive. Nest building, seasonal migration, mating behavior, patterns of maternal care, and manner of food gathering are examples of activities with instinctive components. Although individual differences in execution of these acts may be acquired through learning or departures from usual living conditions, the instinctive aspect of behavior is determined through evolutionarily selected genetic variables that are remarkably uniform for a given species.

The concept of instinct has had a long history which has given rise to a number of common but incorrect usages of the term. Acts so well practiced that they can be executed without deliberate thought, such as typing or playing a musical instrument, are mistakenly termed "instinctive," even though it is clear that much learning and practice are necessary conditions for such performances. A more subtle error lies in conceiving of instincts as inherent urges or desires that drive an animal to activity independently of internal and external stimulus conditions. Finally, it is erroneous to make a sharp distinction between instinctive and learned modes of behavior. All inherent patterns are modified by practice, and all acquired habits are dependent upon and are organized on the basis of inherited structural possibilities and limitations.

To illustrate several of these points, it is a common practice to say that dogs instinctively chase cats and that cats instinctively kill mice and rats. An experiment with cats and mice reared together led to the conclusion that cats do not usually kill rodents unless they have learned this behavior as a result of seeing older cats killing mice. At the same time, the body structure of cats, an inherited and not a learned factor, is good equipment for catching and killing mice.

While much remains to be learned about instinctive behavior, certain facts are clear. The appearance of such behavior is dependent on particular combinations of internal chemical states and external releasing, or instigating, stimuli. Migration in birds starts only when particular internal nutritional and hormonal states and external light and temperature conditions occur. Cocoon spinning in caterpillars is similarly dependent on particular endocrine mechanisms coupled with specific classes of external stimuli. The nervous system is so organized, in a way as yet obscure, that these correct conditions initiate a sequence of behavior, and this behavior is as much a consequence of the way the animal is structured as is its external appearance or any other species-specific characteristic.

Some of the apparent mystery of these inherent properties of behavior may be dispelled by thinking of a continuum from the simplest possible action to the most complex. At the bottom would be the *reflexes*, such as the knee jerk and the constriction of the pupil of the eye in response to bright light. These responses depend upon simple nerve connections between a sense organ and a muscle, and such invariable connections are a part of our inherited structure. More complicated, but still relatively constant from member to member of a species, are the *tropisms* and *taxes*. These are responses of the whole organism toward or away from classes of simple or pervasive stimuli. Examples would be the flight of some insects, notably moths, toward a bright light or the turning of flowers toward the sun. These species-characteristic responses are also functions of inherited structure and, like the reflexes, are also dependent upon appropriate stimulation for their appearance. *Habits*, which may be the most complex of living activities, are individually acquired ways of behaving, but are just as dependent upon adequate nervous system structure (which is inherited) and are called forth by stimulation of a particular kind, just as are the reflexes and the tropisms. *Instinctive* behavior, then, would fall somewhere between tropisms and habits. Like the former it depends on inherited structures characteristic of species; like habits, it displays individual variability. *See also* REFLEX.

INTELLIGENCE [ĭn-tĕl′ə-jəns], has been defined in many different ways, and writers on the topic are still in wide disagreement. Originally, the term was used synonymously with "intellect," which was defined as the "faculty or capacity of knowing." Present-day concepts of intelligence are broader, concerned more with adaptive human behavior, and sometimes cover so-called nonintellective factors of intelligence. Most definitions of intelligence emphasize certain capacities as basic to general intelligence. The three most often mentioned are the ability to learn, the ability to educe relations (abstract reasoning ability), and the ability to profit from experience. A fourth capacity is frequently added, the ability to envisage and solve problems. If one examines the instruments by which intelligence is appraised—namely, the tests used to measure it—one finds that not only these but other abilities as well are tapped. The current view is that general intelligence involves not only learning, adapting, reasoning, and problem solving, but also a variety of capacities which in one way or another enable the individual to cope effectively with his environment.

Factors. In order to identify more precisely the abilities that enter into intelligence as well as to explain the different ways in which intelligence manifests itself, psychologists have employed a special technique known as factor analysis, which is a statistical method used to study various interrelationships among test scores. Although "factor" is in the strict sense a statistical term, it has been extended to designate any basic trait or ability that influences performance on tests. The resulting studies have given rise to two major theories. The first, associated with the name of Charles Edward Spearman, is the Bifactor Theory, according to which all intellectual ability may be expressed as a result of the operation of two factors. One of these is a general intellectual factor (g) which is common to all abilities; the other is a specific factor (s) which is specific to any particular ability but different in every case. The specifics tend to cancel each other, so that in the long run most of what accounts for an individual's intelligence is determined by g. In contrast to Spearman's view there is the Multifactor Theory of intelligence associated most often with the name of L. L. Thurstone. According to this theory, intelligence is not determined primarily by a single general factor but by a variable number of similarly broad factors. Each of these is important in certain respects, and all are considered necessary to account for differences encountered in the performance of individuals on different kinds of intelligence tests. Thurstone's factors are construed as aspects or components of mental function, corresponding in a rough way to the different kinds of sensation—vision, touch, and the like. Much of the work of factor analysis has been devoted to discovery and identification of the different factors, or "vectors," of the mind.

Depending upon the kind and number of tests used in measuring intelligence, a greater or lesser number of factors can be discovered. Among the most often reported are the following five: verbal meaning, or the ability to understand ideas expressed in words; perceptual speed, or the ability to recognize likenesses and differences in objects and symbols; a number factor, or the ability to understand the meaning of numbers and the capacity to manipulate them; a memory factor, or the ability to retain and recall acquired information; and a space factor, or the ability to visualize or think about objects in two or three dimensions. However, though these or similar factors are found in most tests of intelligence, they are not as independent as investigators at first assumed; in actuality, they correlate with each other to a significant degree. This finding tends to support Spearman's concept of an ever-present, single general factor, even though other broad factors must also be assumed in order to account for whatever enters into general intelligence.

While intellectual ability cannot be localized in any specific part of the brain, effective mental functioning depends upon the intactness of the brain as a whole. Recognition of this fact once gave rise to the belief that intelligence could be correlated with the size of the brain. This has proved incorrect. What has been found is that individuals with markedly undersized brains (technically known as microcephalic brains, less than 750 grams) turn out to be mental defectives. However, brains above the average weight (1,400 grams for males) are not related to higher levels of intelligence.

One of the recurrent questions regarding intelligence, as measured by tests, is the degree to which it may be influenced by racial and cultural factors. Here again there is much difference of opinion. The bare facts are as follows: A large number of studies in which comparisons have been made between groups of different racial or national origin have shown significant differences between mean test scores of the compared groups. The magnitude of these differences has varied both with the character of the groups compared and the type of test used. In most instances it is not altogether clear to what extent the findings may be due to differences in culture and educational opportunities rather than to differences in native endowment. Anthropologists point out that it is almost impossible to arrange a comparison of test scores for groups in which cultural influences are identical but genetic (racial) make-ups are clearly distinguishable. Hence, any conclusion on the problem of race and intelligence is highly tentative in the present state of knowledge. The influence of cultural factors is generally considered great. Test scores of intelligence have been found to correlate significantly both with socioeconomic and educational status, particularly the latter. There is a considerable relationship between intelligence test scores and level of income as well as grade reached at school. Group differences often persist even after allowance for some of these factors is made, but the overlap is generally so wide that established differences between groups cannot be used to predict performance of individuals within groups.

Testing. The high correlation between educational level and intelligence test scores has led to the wide use of intelligence tests for grade placement in U.S. schools. This is a very helpful procedure provided that the decision on placement takes account of other criteria. There is much evidence that the intelligence quotient, or its equivalent, is the best single predictor of scholastic achievement, but in individual cases other factors need to be taken into account in evaluating a child's basic potential.

Intelligence test scores have been used profitably in areas of vocational guidance and personnel selection. Their use here depends largely on the fact that different occupations may call for different levels of intellectual ability. When tests are administered to large groups in varied occupations, systematic differences, and often large ones, are found between the mean scores of individuals in the various occupations. Accountants and engineers as groups score among the highest on intelligence tests, whereas persons in service occupations and unskilled

laborers score lowest. This statement applies to members of these occupations in general; it does not mean that every laborer scores below the lowest engineer. The predominantly higher scores of those in certain occupations may be interpreted as meaning that such jobs call for higher levels of intelligence or that by virtue of their requirements they are progressively selective. At the same time, it is important to remember that admission to any particular profession or trade, and success in it, may depend on a variety of other factors, among which motivation and opportunity are often very important.

See also INTELLIGENCE QUOTIENT; INTELLIGENCE TEST; TESTING, PSYCHOLOGICAL AND EDUCATIONAL; VOCATIONAL GUIDANCE.

INTELLIGENCE QUOTIENT (IQ). Intelligence quotients are a range of numbers employed by psychologists and educators to define relative mental ability as measured by standard tests of intelligence. IQ's are arrived at by comparing a person's score with the average score of individuals of the same age. In the case of children IQ's may be computed by dividing the subject's mental age (MA) score by his chronological age (CA). The result is multiplied by 100 to eliminate a decimal point. The formula, then, is $IQ = \dfrac{MA}{CA} \times 100$. If an individual gets a mental age score of 12 on a test and his chronological age is 10, his IQ is 120. In the case of adults the CA denominator used is not the subject's actual age but an age beyond which test scores cease to increase significantly with advancing years. In most cases this turns out to be about 16. In recent years this ratio method for calculating IQ's has been increasingly replaced by other methods which, though involving different statistical procedures, serve the same purpose. The deviation quotient, or deviation IQ, is based on the difference between the score an individual obtains on a test and the score that is considered normal for that age level. It is expressed as a number and is considered comparable to the ratio IQ.

One of the important questions concerning the IQ is whether it remains constant, that is, whether it continues unchanged over the years. There is considerable difference of opinion on this point. Results of studies depend upon the age at which a child is first tested, his co-operativeness at the time, the length of the interval between successive testings, and the nature of the test used. If one considers 5 to 10 points an allowable variation, then the IQ may be said to be relatively constant for most ages. It is surprisingly constant in the case of retested adults and fairly constant in the case of children aged 6 to 16, provided that the retest interval is not much more than two to three years. On the other hand, IQ's obtained from infants and very young children (under 5) often show shifts of as much as 20 points or more. This does not invalidate all IQ's obtained at these early ages but does imply the need for using supplementary criteria when the intelligence of very young children is evaluated. Again, IQ's obtained on emotionally and mentally disturbed individuals cannot always be taken at face value. For these reasons, psychologists are generally loathe to reveal IQ's to other than qualified professional persons.

The most important application of IQ's is their use in

defining grades of intelligence. These are generally based on the distribution of IQ's of the population as a whole and depend in some degree upon the particular test employed. Below are intelligence classifications based on IQ's devised from two widely used tests, the Stanford-Binet and Wechsler Scales.

Any classification of IQ's is arbitrary, and it cannot be assumed that a difference of a few points distinguishes superior from average mental ability or average from borderline. The value of a classification is in showing where any individual score falls in relation to the normal or average range (90–109). Close to half of the general population falls in this average range. The terms "superior" or "gifted" are applied to persons significantly above average. This range may be considered to start at 120, or at a higher level, depending on the tests used and the criteria for giftedness. The term "genius" has sometimes been applied to the small percentage of persons with IQ's of 140 and above, but the nature of genius seems to depend on additional factors such as creativity and unique or rare ability in a given field and not on intellectual ability alone. Concerning those at the lower end of the scale, a further breakdown of the mentally retarded is often employed. Thus a "moron" is a person whose IQ falls in the range from 50 to around 70. Usually he cannot be expected to do much better than fourth- or fifth-grade schoolwork, but he can learn to do useful work. Below the moron level of intelligence are those individuals with still greater intellectual deficit, often designated "imbeciles" and in recent years referred to by some workers in the field as "trainable mentally retarded." An imbecile is an individual whose mentality will not develop beyond that of a child of seven or eight years and whose IQ falls in the range from 25 to 49. Lowest on the scale is the "idiot," who seldom exceeds the mental development of a normal child of two and usually requires custodial care in an institution. On standard intelligence scales idiots are defined as individuals whose IQ is below 25.

INTELLIGENCE CLASSIFICATION ACCORDING TO IQ'S*

Classification	IQ	Per Cent of Population
Very Superior	140 and above	1
Superior or Gifted	130–139	2.5
	120–129	8
High Average	110–119	16
Normal or Average	100–109	45
	90–99	
Low Average	80–99	16
Borderline	70–79	8
Mentally Retarded	60–69	2.5
	59 and below	1

* Based on data from *A Glossary of 100 Measurement Terms*, published by Harcourt, Brace & World, Inc.

INTELLIGENCE TEST, a set task or series of tasks designed to measure a person's mental ability in different areas, and thereby to make it possible to appraise his level of intelligence. The abilities tested may vary from scale to scale. Tests that make use primarily of items of general information, of ability to understand ideas expressed in words, and of ability to comprehend and deal with numbers and symbols and the like are called verbal tests; tests measuring perceptual functions, manipulative abilities, and comprehension of pictorial materials are called performance tests. *See also* BINET, ALFRED; INTELLIGENCE; INTELLIGENCE QUOTIENT (IQ); MENTAL AGE (MA); TESTING PSYCHOLOGICAL AND EDUCATIONAL.

INTROSPECTIVE PSYCHOLOGY, a school or system of psychological inquiry in which the basic data are obtained by self-observation. An introspector endeavors to report the content of consciousness, which is considered to derive from sensations (sight, hearing, and the like) and to include images and feelings. The content psychology (also called structural psychology) of Wilhelm Wundt, as well as the classical experiments on memory by Hermann Ebbinghaus, depended on introspection as their method of inquiry. Introspective psychology as a point of view concerning the subject matter of the psychological science underwent its final great development at the hands of E. B. Titchener in America in the early 20th century.

Contemporary American psychology generally considers the method of introspection unscientific, subjective, and a fruitless attempt to deal with "private" experience and has turned toward various forms of behaviorism for its methods of inquiry. Research in the areas of sensation and perception, however, still relies heavily on observers as a source of data.

INTROVERSION-EXTROVERSION, expression for a range, or scale, used in describing personality. The terms "introvert" and "extrovert" were originated by Carl Jung to label what he considered types of personality. People whose actions were largely determined by subjective, personal, inner values were described as introverts by nature. Those whose behavior was guided by external things rather than by their own thought processes were classed as extroverts.

To most psychologists such a system of types is too rigid to match the realities of human personality, which displays almost infinite variety. Nevertheless, habitual ways of reacting to particular situations can be observed. Some individuals tend to turn their interests inward, to daydream, to be shy in social relationships, and to be secretive, as compared with others who direct their energies outward toward things and people, are extremely sociable, and are open about thoughts and dealings. The man who tends to enjoy the face-to-face relationships involved in salesmanship could be described as belonging, in this respect, toward the extroverted end of the scale, whereas a man who prefers solitary research and writing could be put toward the introverted end. Neither man would necessarily fall toward the same end of the scale in all forms of behavior. In modern usage the adjectives "introverted" and "extroverted" (or "extraverted") are preferred to the nouns "introvert" and "extrovert." The term "ambiversion" is sometimes used to indicate a personality that tends to be balanced between introversion and extroversion.

Many clinical psychologists have used the introversion-extroversion dimension as one convenient means for describing personality. They do not fully agree, however, on what behavior is to be classed as introverted or extroverted. For some, introversion is almost synonymous with neurotic behavior, but in general use introversion does not imply an abnormal condition.

J

JAMES, WILLIAM (1842–1910), American psychologist and philosopher. He taught at Harvard from 1872 to 1907. His two-volume *Principles of Psychology* (1890) collected and interpreted almost all the information available on what was then a new science, and was the standard reference in psychology for many years. Later James's interests were directed more to philosophy, where some of his best-known works are *The Will to Believe and Other Essays* (1896); *The Varieties of Religious Experience* (1902), the Gifford Lectures at the University of Edinburgh; and *A Pluralistic Universe* (1909), the Hibbert Lectures at Oxford.

James is probably most widely known for his advocacy of pragmatism, of which his book *Pragmatism* (1907) is one of the classic statements. In *The Meaning of Truth* (1909) he developed his famous pragmatic theory of truth, according to which if one asserts that a given idea is true, all that one is saying is that if we act upon the idea it will work successfully as a plan of action. For example, to say that one has a true idea of how to get an astronaut into space is to say that if one acts upon his idea one will succeed in launching a manned satellite. Truth is simply a name for the mundane process of workability.

JANET [zhà-nĕ'], **PIERRE MARIE FÉLIX** (1859–1947), French psychiatrist well known for his studies of hysteria and his concept of "dissociation." This idea considered certain forms of mental disturbances (for example, hysteria, multiple personalities) to result from a splitting-off, or dissociation, of segments of mental activity from the main stream of consciousness. Janet taught psychiatry at the Collège de France and directed the psychological laboratory at La Salpêtrière.

JUNG [yo͝ong], **CARL GUSTAV** (1875–1961), Swiss psychiatrist and founder of analytic psychology. An early disciple of Sigmund Freud, Jung broke with Freud over what he considered the latter's excessive emphasis on sexual instinct as a regulator of human conduct and a cause of neurotic disorders. Jung's analytic psychology postulates two types of unconscious influences on the mind: the personal unconscious, containing the life experiences of the individual, and the racial, or collective unconscious, containing the accumulated memories of preceding generations.

The most distinctive feature of Jung's view of man is that it acknowledges future as well as past determinants of behavior. Jung attributes aims and aspirations to personality. Both the past as actuality and the future as potentiality guide present behavior. Man is characterized by self-actualization. He searches for wholeness and his behavior is not conditioned by his individual and racial histories alone. Jung stressed the role of archetypes and the problem-solving and compensatory aspects of dreams in man's search for destiny and purpose in life.

In his development of word association, Jung showed the existence of psychic complexes, or groups of thoughts or perceptions, connected to a strong affect. Eliciting such emotion-laden material is the basic principle of modern lie detector tests. His famous book *Psychological Types* (1923) introduced the concepts of introversion and extroversion into psychology. Most psychologists consider Jung overly mystical in his explanation of symbolic thought. Although his analytic psychology did not achieve the influence of Freud's psychoanalysis, it remains one of the most challenging approaches to self-knowledge.

JUVENILE DELINQUENCY, those acts of the young which the children's court codes of various jurisdictions consider dangerous to the young person, to his family, or to the community. Contrary to popular opinion, the child or youth designated as a delinquent by the children's courts is not a "junior criminal," although the behavior which brings him before a court may be of a criminal type.

Definitions. Delinquency thus encompasses a variety of youthful behaviors regarded as maladjusted, of which only a few may be considered criminal. The juvenile courts, accordingly, have enormous latitude in determining whether a given child shall be adjudged delinquent. An examination of the codes defining delinquency in the various American states reveals their great similarity, despite differences in respect to certain particulars, and their common failure to give precise meaning to delinquent behavior as contrasted with their careful definition of criminal acts. Criminal acts must be characterized by the criminal intention to commit such acts, the classical *mens rea*, or guilty mind, and there must be an exact designation of the nature of the act performed. Neither of these conditions applies to the acts of children regarded as delinquent. With few exceptions, such as in the case of a capital offense, an offense punishable under the criminal statutes by a sentence of life imprisonment or death, the child committing a delinquent act is judged on the basis of his status *as a child* and not on the basis of the act committed. This distinction under law between *adjudication by status*, as applicable to children and youths under a certain age, and prosecution of an individual *on the basis of the act he has committed,* probably constitutes the most basic distinction between juvenile adjudication and criminal justice.

Accordingly, the children's codes in most states are quite loose and tenuous in their determination of what constitutes a delinquent child. The courts are asked, in effect, to impose their own judgment as to when a child's behavior is dangerous to himself, to others, and to constituted authority. The result is extreme variation among the more than 3,000 jurisdictions (cities, counties, and court districts) in the United States regarding the circumstances in which a child may be properly judged a delinquent. Added to the considerable difficulty of the courts in arriving at uniform and unequivocal standards of delinquency is the fact that children's courts have wider jurisdiction than cases legally specified as delinquent. The children's courts may also exercise jurisdiction in cases of neglect, those cases in which the parents or legal custodians of the child are unable, unqualified, or unwilling to assume the rightful burden of customary and legal child care. Since the distinctions between the so-called neglected child and the delinquent child are often difficult to determine, the children's courts are asked to decide questions in which sentiment, bias, and predilection, rather than the strict judicial appraisal of evidence, are frequently crucial factors. Studies of the psychological, social, and behavioral characteristics of both neglected and delinquent children who appear before the nation's courts reveal little basic difference between the .two groups. The appellation "delinquent" as contrasted with "neglected," however, involves considerable difference in public and official attitudes and in the subsequent course of treatment.

Children's Courts. While acknowledging criminal behavior as a form of delinquency, the law simply specifies broad categories within which such behavior may fall. Thus, the law states that a child may be adjudged a delinquent if he commits an act which, if committed by an adult, would be considered criminal. Furthermore, the law ordinarily states that a child may be adjudged delinquent if he engages in occupations or frequents premises which are regarded as illegal under the criminal statutes. Other than these broad stipulations concerning behavior which the law may regard as criminal, the statutes are generally concerned with descriptive categories lacking common substantive meaning. Thus, a child may be adjudged delinquent if he is "incorrigible" or "ungovernable," judgments reflecting different attitudes prevailing in various jurisdictions and expressive of the personalities of different children's court judges. A child may also be officially adjudicated delinquent if he is habitually truant, runs away from home, solicits alms in public places, deports himself in such a way as to injure or endanger the morals or health of himself or others, and even, in rare cases, if he uses obscene or profane language. The children's court is not a court of law in the usual sense; it is a social agency through which certain judicial functions concerning children may be exercised.

It is this peculiar mixture of court and social agency embodied in the children's courts which creates difficulty and considerable misunderstanding concerning the entire problem of delinquency. When the first juvenile court was established in 1899 in Cook County, Ill., to serve the city of Chicago, the court was conceived as a means of assisting children and not punishing them; but recent significant trends have led to serious questioning of some of the assumptions involved in the original working philosophy of children's courts. Recognizing the ambiguities involved in the legal definitions of delinquency, the National Council on Crime and Delinquency (formerly the National Probation and Parole Association), in its efforts to establish a Standard Children's Court Act as a model for the states to follow, has recommended that the term "delinquent"

be reserved for those children who violate the regular criminal statutes. The proposed Standard Act tends to avoid the use of the term "delinquency," and suggests that many acts presently conceived as delinquency, such as truancy, be handled by nonjudicial agencies. Commitment to training schools (popularly referred to as "reform schools") should be confined, according to the model act, to those children who actually break the law.

British juvenile courts, in their efforts to safeguard the legal rights of the child and his parents, have been accused of being unduly "legalistic," while American courts frequently have been charged with overlooking legal scruples in the desire to aid the child. The problem of maintaining full legal safeguards for children has arisen from the fact that children's courts in the United States have been preeminently concerned with maintaining their function as a *protective* children's agency while, at the same time, adjudicating the cases that come before them in accordance with legal process. It has been charged that legal responsibilities have often been neglected in the attempt to maintain this dual responsibility.

The states vary widely in respect to the age of children over whom the juvenile courts may exercise jurisdiction. While there tends to be broad agreement that the age of seven, when, according to traditional British common law, the child gives rudimentary evidence of the capacity to reason, constitutes an appropriate minimum age for jurisdiction, there is considerable diversity concerning a legally appropriate upper age limit for handling by the children's courts. The question of when a child ceases to be a child and becomes an adult for legal purposes has never been satisfactorily decided, and reflects historical differences of tradition and social practice in various states. Several states regard a person as adult when he has passed his 16th birthday; others have, with some variations, constituted the 17th birthday as the upper limit of juvenile status. A few states have established different age levels for boys and girls. The majority have established 18 years or higher as the legal dividing line between juvenile and adult status. In addition, certain states have enacted legislation permitting the courts to deal with certain types of offenses outside the regular children's courts for children falling within the legally prescribed juvenile age categories. Such differential handling is frequently based upon sexual differences. The laws of certain states provide for special handling of youths falling beyond the legally prescribed age categories. In New York State, for example, the Youthful Offender and Wayward Minor laws, while not regarded as statutes dealing with delinquency, provide preferential and protective treatment for youths who commit criminal acts between the ages of 16 and 19 and 16 and 21, respectively. Such protective legislation, designed to benefit the youthful offender falling outside the beneficent provisions of the delinquency codes, is applicable to youths who have no record of a previous criminal conviction, have not committed a capital offense, and who give evidence of reformative potentialities.

Whether or not a youth who violates the law or who may be otherwise guilty of a delinquency infraction in a given community is adjudicated before the courts depends upon the following contributory conditions: (1) the jurisdictional policy of a given children's court, itself a highly variable condition; (2) the number, range, and scope of private and public social agencies available in the area to assist the youth; (3) the organization of the local police department and the character of its youth division; and (4) the nature and degree of family disorganization within the given area and local tolerance toward delinquent behavior. Since delinquency assumes such a variety of expressions, many of which may be construed as forms of adolescent prankishness or maladjustment, children and youths engaging in a continuing or chronic type of delinquent behavior may be placed in the following five categories: (1) the official or adjudicated delinquents, those who have been processed by the courts; (2) the unofficial delinquents, those who have appeared before the courts but for whom no official dispensation has been made; (3) the police cases, those who are handled by some police agency but who are not brought before the courts; (4) children handled by some nonpunitive social-work agency; and (5) children informally treated by the schools, a religious counsellor, a friend, neighbor, or relative.

Prevalence of Delinquency. Because of the variable nature of delinquency and the fact that much delinquent behavior is hidden, it is almost impossible to measure the scope of the problem and determine whether or not it is increasing. The general impression, based upon official or adjudicated court statistics, is that the problem of delinquency has increased, especially in the United States since the close of World War II. This increase is not confined to the United States. Recent evidence seems to confirm the impression that delinquency has become a problem of increasing magnitude in many other parts of the world, including Southeast Asia and the Far East, where the problem was relatively unknown until the last two decades. Since 1948 the annual volume of delinquency in the United States has attained a level of approximately 600,000 cases officially adjudicated in the courts. At the same time, the yearly volume of police arrests of juveniles is in excess of 1,700,000, although only approximately one-third of this number are brought before the courts. While in the decade 1930–40 the annual percentage volume of officially adjudicated cases of delinquency was approximately 1% of all youths between the ages of 10 and 17, the annual percentage since the end of World War II amounts to almost 2.5%. If the large number of children and youths who are not adjudicated but whose behavior is sufficiently delinquent to warrant handling by some public or private agency is considered, the annual percentage volume of delinquency would need to be regarded as well over 5%. If a so-called prevalence rate, or a rate including the percentage of all children between 10 and 17 who have been involved in at least one court appearance during their adolescence, is used to measure delinquency, the rate may be as high as 12%.

More than 75% of the children adjudicated as delinquents are over 14 years old. Annual variations in the relative rates of adjudication of male delinquents as compared to female delinquents range from 4:1 to 5:1. The principal reasons for the referral of male delinquents to court have been stealing and acts of carelessness or mischief, while in the case of females the chief reasons have been ungovernable behavior, running away from home, and sex offenses. Significantly high rates of delinquency have been associated with minority and immigrant groups in the United States. High rates for previous immigrant groups have subsided as such groups have risen from the lowest socioeconomic levels, moved away from slum areas, and become assimilated into American cultural patterns. While delinquency rates in urban areas still exceed those in rural areas by ratios of approximately 3.5:1, rural rates have shown a fairly rapid increase since World War II, especially in areas where industry is becoming established. State and national police officials also report significant increases in youth delinquency, both in the number of offenses and the gravity of crimes committed, in suburban areas among the children of the so-called white-collar classes.

The Search for Causes. Since the range of delinquency varies from criminal or antisocial acts to behavioral evidences of emotional disorder, there is no common causal process to account for the different behaviors called delinquent. Past attempts to identify single causes of delinquency, whether some psychological defect in the personality or some stress in the environment such as bad housing, deficient schooling, or inadequate parents, have all proved futile. Modern explanations of delinquency acknowledge different etiologies for various types of delinquency. Such explanations tend to find the source of delinquency in the character of the adaptation of a certain type of individual within a specific kind of environment, placing prior emphasis upon neither psychological conditions nor environmental stress, but upon the mutual reinforcement of both factors.

Recent explanatory hypotheses have attempted to identify specific types of delinquency and the underlying social and cultural conditions. The American sociologists Herbert Bloch and Arthur Niederhoffer, in a study entitled *The Gang: A Study in Adolescent Behavior* (1958), have set forth and partially validated the hypothesis that delinquency results from tension between the growing adolescent and the adult world. Delinquent strains occur as a result of social and cultural barriers imposed upon adolescents in the attainment of normal adulthood. In another study, *Delinquency: The Juvenile Offender in America Today* (1956), Herbert Bloch and Frank Flynn have attempted to identify special psychological types of delinquency, indicating their linkages to crucial social configurations within the home and neighborhood.

Broad-based programs for delinquency prevention and control are of little value unless the variable sources and the different types of delinquency are adequately envisaged. Effective programs must acknowledge the differences between communities and attempt to ameliorate the situation in terms of specific conditions within a given area, as these are revealed by research and investigation. Because of its broad outreach through the local community and the patterns of American culture, adequate control involves concerted social planning, frequently of a long-range character. Since, as Bradley Buell and his associates have shown in the study *Community Planning for Human Services* (1952), the "hard core" of delinquency is concentrated within less than 5% of the families studied in given areas, concerted and co-ordinated attacks must be made upon the focal and multiple problems of such families. The early identification of the predelinquent child, as indicated in the claimed prognostic device, the Social Prediction table of Sheldon and Eleanor Glueck, may pave the way for the institution of preventive measures for the vulnerable or delinquent-prone child and his family.

See also ADOLESCENCE; CRIMINOLOGY; GANG.

K

KLEPTOMANIA, compulsive stealing, obsessive desire to steal. In most cases the objects stolen are petty and useless, although they may have symbolic value. This behavior, through which the person tries to get attention, can be seen as a symptom of neurosis and often occurs in children. The act is compulsively repeated and so clumsy that it cannot escape notice. The kleptomaniac ensures being caught, wants to be punished, and looks forward to the attention given him in a trial, or by parents and relatives. Kleptomania occasionally occurs in a sociopathic personality who may become an expert shoplifter. Such persons show no meaningful motivation for their antisocial acts, which are characteristic of a personality disturbance. They seem indifferent to being caught, while trying to talk their way out of trouble. Often they are intelligent and have good technical ability.

KOFFKA [kôf'kə], **KURT** (1886–1941), American psychologist. Born in Berlin, Koffka received his Ph.D. at the University of Berlin (1908). Arriving in America in 1924, he was a visiting professor at Cornell, Chicago, Wisconsin, and finally at Smith (1927), where he remained as professor of psychology after 1932. One of the founders of the Gestalt school of psychology, Koffka conducted research in perception. His best-known books are *The Growth of the Mind* (Eng. trans., 1924), written originally in German and translated into English, Spanish, Chinese, Japanese, and Russian, and *The Principles of Gestalt Psychology* (1935).

KÖHLER [kû'lər], **WOLFGANG** (1887–1967), German psychologist, a founder of the Gestalt School of psychology. Born in Reval, Estonia, he was educated at German universities, receiving his Ph.D. from Berlin in 1909. Interned in the Canary Islands during World War I, he conducted his now classic experiments on the intelligence of apes. He was professor of psychology at Göttingen (1921–22) and Berlin (1922–35). In 1935 he moved to the United States and became associated with Swarthmore College. From 1955 to 1956 he was a member of the Institute for Advanced Study, Princeton, N.J. Outstanding among his books are *The Mentality of Apes* (1925) and *Gestalt Psychology* (1947).
See also GESTALT PSYCHOLOGY.

KORSAKOFF'S PSYCHOSIS, also called amnestic confabulatory syndrome, a severe mental disturbance seen mainly in chronic alcoholics. The disorder is characterized by degeneration of nervous tissue, extensive loss of memory, and a tendency to fabricate stories to fill in the gaps of memory. The individual may be confused as to his identity and his surroundings. There may be pain and tenderness in the legs and a loss of normal reflexes. The actual cause of the condition may be a deficiency of the B-complex vitamins, particularly thiamine (vitamin B_1). This view is supported by the appearance of the psychosis in nonalcoholics and the frequent occurrence of vitamin deficiencies among chronic alcoholics. The condition sometimes improves with treatment. A complete cure is rare.

KRAEPELIN [krâ-pə-lēn], **EMIL** (1856–1926), German psychiatrist known for his classification of mental diseases. He grouped mental ailments on the basis of their symptoms, course, and outcome. This classification introduced order into what had previously been chaos in psychiatric thinking, and made possible the scientific observation and study of mental diseases.

KRAFFT-EBING [kräft'ā'bĭng], **BARON RICHARD VON** (1840–1902), German psychiatrist and neurologist known for his studies of sexual perversions. His *Psychopathology of Sex* (1892), is still an important reference work.

KRETSCHMER [krĕch'mər], **ERNST** (1888–1964), German neurologist and psychiatrist, known for his attempt to correlate body type with temperament and characteristics of mental illness. In *Physique and Character* (Eng. trans., 1925), he distinguishes three constitutional types—pyknik, athletic, and asthenic, or leptosome—and relates them to personality types. The pyknik generally has a rounded body build, believed to be associated with cyclothymia, a tendency to alternating periods of low activity and sadness with times of elation, common in patients with manic-depressive psychosis. The athletic type has a well-proportioned body with strong muscular development, related to a deliberate and slow temperament, possibly associated with epilepsy. The asthenic, with long, slender body build, is said to be associated with schizoid tendencies, such as withdrawal and avoidance of close personal relationships, prevalent in schizophrenic patients. In addition there is a less clearly defined group, the dysplastics, who show abnormal development, mostly with glandular derangements, and mixed personality characteristics.

See also BODY TYPES.

L

LAUGHTER in man is a complex reflex of the muscles of respiration, face, and throat. It usually involves a series of involuntary spasmodic contractions of abdominal muscles, accompanied by contractions of cheek muscles (the smile) and semiarticulate sounds. The response may undergo modification in that facial expressions or vocalizations are altered or absent, hence the expressions "silent laughter," or "sardonic laughter." The essential characteristic of laughter, therefore, seems to be the serial abdominal contractions with expirations of air from the lungs. With minimal contraction of the vocal muscles the result is the familiar "ha-ha-ha"; marked contraction produces the "he-he-he."

Laughter has been regarded by most authors as peculiar to man, but this is debatable. The essence of laughter may be observed in many other species, and much has been written of the laughing crow, gull, hyena, and jackass. Moreover, most and possibly all of the monkeys and apes exhibit the fundamental characteristics of laughter.

The neurophysiology of laughter has received little study beyond the human clinic. There it has been learned that involuntary laughter may be produced by mild anesthetics such as nitrous oxide (laughing gas) or may be the result of various forms of accident or disease in the brain. One of these neurological disorders (pseudobulbar palsy) is even known as "laughing sickness." A person with this disorder may laugh but feel sad, or he may cry but feel happy. The most common form of psychosis, schizophrenia, often includes involuntary mirthless laughter.

One theory attempts to explain laughing sickness and laughing gas. It holds that with both there has been an interference in nervous impulses from outer brain tissue (cortex) to mid-brain and related structures (especially the thalamus). It holds that the cortex has an inhibitory effect on the thalamus; thus, if the inhibition is removed, the lower brain centers are more free to react.

Normal laughter in man occurs first in the early months of life. One investigator has reported it as early as 12 weeks, and another reports smiling at birth. It seems that smiling precedes laughter but that, later, they combine into an ordered behavior pattern: smiling, silent laughter, vocalized laughter.

There is less agreement about what is laughable. Beyond tickling, laughter depends for the most part on learning, but there are some common features. Numerous authors have tried to catalog them. D. H. Monro lists four main classes: (1) feelings of superiority—for example, the attempt to aggrandize one's self; (2) incongruity—that is, a response to the novel or bizarre; (3) release from restraint—as with the tendency to laugh after relief of frustration or pain; and (4) ambivalence—for instance, the "giggle," so common in situations of embarrassment, where no clear course of action is perceived.

Monro's classification is probably incomplete, and Florence Justin, another student of this field, lists more categories: surprise and defeated expectation; joy, pleasure, play; and social stimulation. Moreover, she cites laughter as a possible defense mechanism, as a means to subconscious gratification, and as an energistic mechanism—that is, we feel better after laughing.

It is obvious that human laughter becomes a learned response to many situations, and there are many theories to account for the facts (in particular those of Henri Bergson, Max Eastman, Sigmund Freud, and N. R. F. Maier). None seems entirely satisfactory, and the explanation of the nature of laughter must await further research.

LEARNING generally is said to occur when an organism changes its behavior as a result of experience—as when a dog learns to recognize its master or when a wolf learns to avoid snares. In man virtually all complex activities are learned, ranging from learning how to swing a baseball bat to the learning of language and the acquisition of the values and culture of society.

Several major psychological theories have been built around learning as a central topic. To some extent this emphasis can be understood as growing out of the psychologist's concern with the scientific status of his subject, and the desire to develop methods of investigation similar to those used in other sciences, such as physics. The problem of learning seemed to offer the possibility of an objective study of human behavior, particularly as it was developed by the Russian physiologist Pavlov.

Pavlov found that a dog could be "taught" to salivate upon hearing a bell. The dog would normally salivate when presented with food. If a bell were sounded each time food was presented, eventually the bell alone would cause salivation. The model of learning was thus stimulus (bell)—response (salivation). Both elements, the stimulus and the response, could be observed and measured and thus satisfied the desire of the psychologist to avoid dealing in inaccessible internal processes, such as "ideas" and "images," which could be neither seen nor measured. While many "S-R" (for "stimulus-response") psychologists adhered to this model, others modified the scheme to include processes which could not be observed, so-called "mediating" processes. "Cognitive" psychologists, particularly those of the "Gestalt" school, were unwilling to accept stimulus-response links as an explanation of all learning. They claimed that most learning involves understanding and that only a small part of human learning can be understood in S-R terms. As an example, the Gestaltists cite the situation of reading and understanding a map which has never been seen before. In such a case, they argue, stimulus-response links have not been developed and therefore reading the map and choosing a correct route must depend upon more complex mental processes (cognitive processes).

These opposing views of learning—divided roughly into the Gestaltists (*cognitive learning*) and the behaviorists (*stimulus-response learning*)—generated a vast amount of experimentation accounting for a considerable bulk of the psychological literature. Certain principles of learning have emerged from these experiments, but in reviewing them it should be kept in mind that they arise from particular types of experimentation and that, since most of the studies were carried out on animals, they should be viewed with caution when applied to the human organism.

The Principles of Learning. Learning theorists of the behaviorist (stimulus-response) tradition distinguish between two types of learning (or conditioning), *classical* and *operant*.

Classical conditioning refers to the type of learning described above in the case of Pavlov's dog. This is characterized by the fact that a stimulus (here the bell) which originally does not produce a response (the flow of saliva) eventually acquires the power to evoke the response by being associated with a stimulus that can produce the response (the sight of food). In this situation the bell is the *conditioned stimulus* and the food is the *unconditioned stimulus*.

In *operant*, or *instrumental*, conditioning the order of events is reversed—the response brings about the stimulus. The model for learning of this type is the *Skinner box* (named after its originator, B. F. Skinner), a device in which a rat obtains pellets of food by pressing a lever. The response is the act of pressing the lever and is followed by *reinforcement* (the pellet of food). A *primary reinforcer* (such as food) is able to "stamp in" a response in its own right, possibly because it satisfies a basic need, such as hunger. A *secondary reinforcer* is a stimulus which originally has no reinforcing power, but acquires such after repeated association with a primary reinforcer. For example, if a light flashes as the food pellet (the primary reinforcer) is delivered, the rat will eventually press the lever even if he is "rewarded" only with the light (which is now a secondary reinforcer). According to Skinner and his supporters, most human activities involve operant rather than classical conditioning.

Certain principles of learning are associated with these conditioning experiments. *Generalization* refers to the tendency of the subject to respond in the same way to similar stimuli (for example, as a child may call all four-legged animals "dogs"). *Discrimination* describes the reverse phenomena, whereby different responses are applied to different stimuli (calling one type of birds "owls" and another type "crows"). *Extinction* applies to the disappearance of a response when it is no longer reinforced. Thus, if the rat's bar pressing no longer produces food pellets, the rat will eventually stop pressing the bar. However, if the rat is placed in the same cage some time after extinction has taken place, it is likely that it will press the bar again. This is called *spontaneous recovery*.

Early experiments on human learning utilized *nonsense syllables* (such as "zog," "bef," "xeh," and so forth) presented on a specially constructed moving drum. Other experiments on human subjects dealt with the mastery of manual skills and the transfer of training from one task to another. Among the conclusions of these studies were the following: (1) Learning is more efficient when distributed over several periods rather than when "crammed" into one long period. (2) Learning is more efficient when the subject is actively intent on learning rather than when he is exposed to the material in the course of some other activity (*intentional* versus *incidental* learning). (3) Learning is enhanced when the subject is kept informed of his performance, as, for example, when students are given their test grades. (4) Competition usually enhances learning if it is not too intense. (5) Learning does not take place during sleep. (6) Transfer of training may facilitate learning of a new task (*positive transfer*) or interfere (*negative transfer*). Transfer effects depend upon the similarities of the two tasks—for example, knowledge of French may aid in the study of Italian. Conversely, responses learned in one situation may interfere with learning new habits. This is frequently observed by dancing instructors, who would prefer to teach beginners in preference to those who have been dancing incorrectly for many years and who must thus unlearn old habits before they can master new ones.

Experiments on learning in reference to problem solving have led to the concepts of "trial-and-error" versus "insightful" learning. A frequently cited example of trial-and-error learning is that of the cat in the problem box, from which it can escape by releasing a trigger mechanism. In this situation the animal was observed to make random movements until it accidentally succeeded in releasing the escape mechanism. On succeeding trials the animal would escape more and more easily until it could smoothly activate the device whenever placed in the box. This type of learning in problem solving is accepted by behaviorists as fitting within the stimulus-response model and is opposed by Gestalt psychologists, who suggest that most human learning involves insight. A familiar example of insightful problem solving is the one experienced while working on a puzzle, when after hours of fruitless groping the answer is seen suddenly in a moment. Some behaviorist psychologists do not accept the concept of insight as an adequate description of any learning and claim that it can be interpreted as a variety of trial-and-error learning.

The Status of Learning Theories Today. As can be seen from the above discussion, there is no general agreement among psychologists on a single theory of learning. Some points of controversy are:

(1) Is human learning similar to animal learning? Most stimulus-response psychologists feel that legitimate inferences concerning human learning can be derived from animal experimentation. Gestalt and cognitive psychologists are not convinced that such inferences are valid.

(2) Among stimulus-response theorists there is disagreement as to how the link between stimulus and response is forged. The *reinforcement* theorists believe that the link is "stamped in" by events following the stimulus-response act, such as a food pellet being delivered. The *contiguity* theorists believe that the close occurrence of stimulus and response within a short time interval is sufficient to connect them. *Cognitive* theorists suggest that the bond may occur because of "understanding" the relation between stimulus and response. To them, the bell would come to mean food to the dog.

(3) There is also disagreement as to the relationship

between primary and secondary reinforcement and as to whether secondary reinforcers play a central part in the establishment of permanent learned habits.

(4) The *continuity-discontinuity* argument concerns whether learning occurs "gradually," step by step, or suddenly, when the total situation is grasped (as in the problem-solving experiments described above).

(5) Finally, the question is often asked as to whether there is one or several kinds of learning.

Applications of Learning Theory. One of the earliest applications of learning theory was in education. The American psychologist Edward Thorndike prepared dictionaries for teachers on the basis of word frequency and investigated transfer with respect to specific educational problems, such as whether training in one subject (as Latin) developed skills useful in other subjects (as mathematics, science, or English). He concluded that transfer occurred only where the two subjects shared common elements: Latin aided English because of the large number of Latin roots in the English language.

The best-known modern application of learning research to education has been the teaching machine, based upon Skinner's studies of *operant* conditioning. Written material is presented in a sequence designed to produce the desired response, which is then reinforced when the student confirms his answer. This has also led to the burgeoning field of *programmed instruction*, which uses the same principles, but without use of the machine as a means of presentation.

Skinner's principles have also been used to treat withdrawn hospital patients. These patients are given machines which will provide a variety of reinforcements, such as candy or pictures, if operated correctly by pulling or pushing handles similar to those used in popular candy machines. This method has had some success in stimulating the patients to relate to their immediate surroundings.

Conditioning techniques have also been utilized in training in motor skills for telegraphers, pilots, and workers in other occupations. Some learning theorists have attempted to use their methods to bring psychoanalytic concepts under laboratory study and thus to unify psychological theory.

See also PSYCHOLOGY; THINKING.

LIBIDO [lĭ-bē′dō, lĭ-bī′dō], concept of Freudian psychoanalytic theory, which originally described the psychic energy derived from the sexual instincts. Later Freud applied libido to the energy of the instincts associated with self-preservation as well (the ego instincts). Libido has been widely used by writers and other lay persons to describe sexual urges. In this sense the public retains the earlier exclusively sexual emphasis of the term.

See also PSYCHOANALYSIS.

LOBOTOMY [lō-bŏt′ə-mē], also called prefrontal lobotomy, or leucotomy, is a surgical method of treating certain mental disorders, which was introduced by the Portuguese physician Egas Moniz in 1936. The operation severs some of the connections between the frontal lobes of the cerebrum (the highest part of the brain) and the thalamus (a nerve relay station which lies below the cerebrum).

A great variety of techniques has been used to perform lobotomies. The early procedures consisted of introducing a cutting instrument through holes drilled in the skull. Other methods involve shaving off portions of the upper brain layer, approaching the brain through the eye cavity (transorbital leucotomy), injecting hot water or alcohol into the brain, or focusing ultrasonic beams on the thalamus.

The Effects of Lobotomy. Immediately after the operation the patient may be severely confused for a few days. Subsequently he may lose normal social habits and may soil himself, eat voraciously, and become noisy and unruly. In a few months these reactions subside and the effects of the operation can be assessed.

In some as yet unknown way, the quality of the patient's emotional experience is apparently altered, so that, although certain severe symptoms may persist, they no longer disturb the patient. A similar effect is observed in some cases in the patient's reaction to pain—the pain is still felt but ceases to be annoying. The intelligence of the patient is also subtly affected. He loses some capacity for higher thinking and cannot easily apply past experience to the solution of present problems. In considering the effects of lobotomy it should be kept in mind that the operation is performed on the most poorly understood part of the brain—the so-called "silent" areas of the cerebral cortex.

In the most successful cases, the patient is able to return to a useful life outside the hospital, and may even assume positions of responsibility though he may lose a certain degree of creativity. A less fortunate outcome is the "frontal-lobe personality," marked by selfishness, quick temper, inability to exercise good judgment, and often, mania.

The Present State of Psychosurgery. After many years of performing operations and modifying the original techniques, most physicians have concluded that the small number of good results does not justify the use of surgery in most cases of functional mental disorders. At present lobotomies are generally limited to patients with severe anxiety, incapacitating schizophrenic processes that do not respond to other forms of treatment, and to patients suffering from intractable pain, especially in the region of the head and neck.

LORENZ, KONRAD (1903–   ), Austrian zoologist, one of the founders of modern ethology, the study of animal behavior in its natural state. His detailed observations of animals provided a more precise understanding of the bases of instinctive behavior. Lorenz also introduced several key concepts in ethology, including those of imprinting and releaser mechanisms. His studies showed that imprinting was a form of instantaneous learning whereby young animals form social preferences that remain intact for life. He also described the role of a releaser or "sign stimulus," such as a color, in triggering an instinctive response in an animal. Born in Vienna, he received an M.D. degree in 1928 and a Ph.D. in 1933, both from the University of Vienna. He became the director of the Max Planck Institute for Physiology of Behavior in West Germany. He presented his findings in such popular works as *King Solomon's Ring* (1952) and *On Aggression* (1966).

LSD or LYSERGIC ACID DIETHYLAMIDE, an alkaloid made by a simple chemical modification of lysergic acid, which is obtained from the fungus *Claviceps purpurea*. Lysergic acid itself is not a hallucinogen (which produces mood changes and hallucinations of space, time, and vision) but its diethylamide derivative (LSD) is. LSD is the most potent hallucinogen known, being active in dosages of 100 to 200 micrograms. One to 3 hours after ingestion LSD produces profound effects. Colors are enormously vivid and a variety of intense hallucinations may occur, some pleasant and some unpleasant. Typically, the individual seems to lose his normal identification as "I" and to fuse with inanimate aspects of his environment. This sense of ego destruction and distortion of the body image may induce a severe panic reaction. Often the hallucinatory content is erotic and frequently religious figures and images are seen. The experience characteristically lasts 4 to 12 hours but may be far more prolonged.

LSD has potential medical use in treating severe alcoholism, childhood schizophrenia, psychoneurosis, sexual deviancy, and in aiding terminal patients with severe pain.

When LSD is taken under nonmedical supervision, many claims are made for it including the capacity to augment esthetic sensitivity, increase insight, enhance creativity, and increase the individual's capacity to love. None of these claims is substantiated; indeed, what evidence is available indicates that these claims are spurious.

The dangers of LSD taken under promiscuous or illicit circumstances are enormous. It can produce psychosis, acting out of antisocial impulses, acting out of homosexual impulses, inadvertent or intentional suicide attempts, uncontrolled aggression (including attempts at homicide), epileptic seizures, and overwhelming panic. Equally important, LSD can unequivocally produce such long-term effects as chronic psychosis, extended panic reactions, and recurrence of hallucinations as long as one year after their appearance even if no additional LSD is taken in the interim. Chronic use of LSD often is associated with complete withdrawal from society into a passive and self-centered cocoon. Additionally, recent studies suggest that LSD can produce genetic damage, raising the specter of an adverse hereditary effect.

See also DRUG ADDICTION; DRUGS;
PSYCHOPHARMACOLOGY.

M

McDOUGALL, WILLIAM (1871–1938), British psychologist, pioneer in social and abnormal psychology. As a medical student at Cambridge, he became interested in psychology while on an anthropological expedition in Australia in 1899. He returned to Europe to study with G. E. Muller at Göttingen, Germany. McDougall's background in biology influenced his psychological views and led him to the belief that life processes have goal-seeking natures. His pronouncements on the subject upset the official materialistic psychology of the time.

In 1902 he founded a laboratory for experimental psychology in London. From 1904 to 1920 he taught at Oxford. Among his influential works are *An Introduction to Social Psychology* (1908) and *Psychology: The Study of Human Behavior* (1912). In the United States after 1920, he was professor of psychology at Harvard until 1927, afterward holding that position at Duke University. Rejecting behaviorism during the era of Watsonian behaviorism, McDougall developed the psychological concept that all behavior was purposive, directed toward a goal. He also stressed the primacy of instincts. Although these theories were unpopular in the United States, he gained an international reputation as a major theorist.

In 1927 McDougall brought J. B. Rhine to Duke to direct the parapsychology laboratory that was to do much for the scientific study of paranormal phenomena. McDougall's stature was somewhat diminished later in his life by his adherence to a questionable hypothesis. He believed he had proven the Lamarckian theory that acquired characteristics are inheritable.

See also PARAPSYCHOLOGY; PSYCHOLOGY; RHINE, JOSEPH BANKS.

MANIC-DEPRESSIVE [măn'ĭk-dĭ-prĕs'ĭv] **PSYCHOSIS,** a psychotic disorder characterized by moods of extreme elation or depression, or an alternation of both. Its most common age of onset is between the ages of 25 and 35. Females are more susceptible than males. There is a strong tendency for the condition to appear in several members of the same family.

Depression is the most common mood. In the mild forms the individual is fatigued, lacks confidence, and withdraws from society. As the depression progresses, physical symptoms appear. The patient loses weight and cannot sleep. Vague pains arise in the chest or stomach, and he may feel that these physical complaints are the cause of his mental distress. In the severe stage the depression advances into a stupor in which the patient does not speak or move.

The manic form usually begins as an acceleration of all normal activities. The patient is buoyant and happy. His ideas move rapidly. He is playful and full of grand schemes that he quickly abandons. He may squander his money and write large checks for both friends and strangers.

The patient usually recovers from the moods of depression and mania, only to fall ill again at a later date. In the cyclic form of the psychosis the manic and depressive states follow one another.

See also PSYCHOSIS.

MAUDSLEY, HENRY (1835–1918), English psychiatrist. Shortly after receiving his M.D. from the University of London Maudsley became medical superintendent of the Manchester Royal Hospital for the Insane in 1859. He taught medical jurisprudence at the University of London and founded Maudsley Hospital in London (now united with Bethlehem Royal Hospital). In his well-known work, *Physiology and Pathology of the Mind* (1867), he advanced the idea that mental diseases resulted from abnormalities of brain tissue.

MELANCHOLIA [mĕl-ən-kō'lē-ə], in psychiatry, a term describing mental disorders in which depression is the major symptom. These include neurotic depression, the depressive phase of manic-depressive psychosis, and involutional melancholia. The last condition occurs primarily in women in the age group 40 to 60. Affected persons are usually orderly, conscientious individuals who are basically insecure and have a highly developed sense of duty and responsibility. With the decline in physical vigor which accompanies aging and particularly with the changes in sexual functioning, these persons (who are often repressed sexually) may feel that life has passed them by. They withdraw from the world, narrowing their interests and activities and developing hypochondria, insomnia, loss of appetite, and a haunting fear of death. Characteristically, they awaken before dawn and lie in bed in the morning, unable to arise because of fatigue. The patient may attempt suicide.

Because of the association of melancholia with the menopause, hormone therapy was tried, but has proved unsuccessful. Electric shock therapy, alone or in combination with psychotherapy to reorient the patient's attitudes toward aging, has been helpful in many cases. Several antidepressive drugs have also been of value.

MEMORY involves the reappearance or reinstatement of some previously learned behavior. Thus we may remember how to roller skate, remember a poem that we have learned or a movie we have seen, or recall that we went to the store. It was at one time widely held that memory was a special mental faculty which could be improved through exercise, as a muscle might be. This view is not held by modern psychologists, to whom memory is not a thing but rather a relation between stimuli and responses.

The reinstatement of a learned response depends on many things, among which are the following:

(1) The response must have been learned in the first place. Many times when we say that we have forgotten something, the truth is more nearly that it was never adequately learned. Many studies have shown that over-learning—continued study beyond the point of mastery—greatly improves retention.

(2) The time elapsing between the original learning and retention tests is important. Hermann Ebbinghaus showed that learned material is forgotten rapidly at first and then more slowly as the time since learning increases. The shape of this forgetting curve, obtained when results of experiments are graphed, has been repeatedly verified. With human subjects it is very difficult to control what the person does between learning and testing, which activity may be as important a factor as the amount of time that elapses. While it is not true that elephants never forget, animals do show remarkable retention for learned behavior when the living conditions in the retention interval are kept different from those in the training situation. Pigeons that have been trained to peck at a translucent disk have been shown to retain this response with remarkably little loss for four years. When tested, they responded to the disk within two seconds of its presentation.

(3) The kind of activity within the retention interval is perhaps the most important variable in memory. For example, if a person sleeps in the interval between learning and testing he is likely to remember more than if he is awake. This is not because of the beneficial properties of sleep but rather because of the lack of opportunity to learn additional responses that might be confusing or interfering. This tendency of later learning to interfere with earlier learning is called retroactive inhibition. It is greatest when the interpolated activity is similar to but not identical with the learned behavior. Thus, if a student has learned to speak French, forgetting is likely to be more rapid if he subsequently learns Spanish than if he later learns Hindu because of the differing degrees of similarity to the original learning. Bicycle riding shows great retention over many years, probably because few things are subsequently learned that are similar to the riding behavior.

(4) Forgetting may be motivated. As Freud has pointed out, events that are associated with painful or disturbing circumstances are likely to be forgotten. Thus, we may forget a dental appointment or an embarrassing experience because remembering reinstates painful stimuli, which are often avoided.

Memory Training. So-called memory training does not consist of exercise of the memory faculty. William James, the pioneer American psychologist, demonstrated the futility of such exercise in a heroic experiment in which he memorized portions of Victor Hugo's *Satyr* before and after memorizing the entire first book of Milton's *Paradise Lost*. The lines from the Hugo poem were not more easily or speedily learned after this exercise than before.

Memory systems and mnemonic devices are techniques for helping the individual to provide himself with the stimulus for the correct response. These are often chains of behavior which, once started, lead to the correct response. Well-known examples are "Thirty days hath September..." and "*i* before *e* except after *c*..." Such devices were apparently familiar to the ancient Greek orators, who would memorize orations by associating various parts of the text with different parts of a house. Point one would be associated with, say, a hallway—hence the expression "In the first place..." Modern memory systems can be elaborate. A typical one calls for associating numbers with sounds ($t = 1$, $n = 2$, and so on.) These in turn are associated with words. The 22d word, for example, would be "noon" (n--n, 2--2). Then in learning a list of items the 22d word on the list is learned in a sentence that contains both the word "noon" and the word to be learned. The 22d item can then be remembered by the learned sentence. Such devices may facilitate remarkable feats of memorization, but they are useful for stunts rather than for mastery of logical material. Students, for example, cannot expect to retain information and ideas by means of mnemonic systems.

MENNINGER [měn'ing-ər], **KARL AUGUSTUS** (1893–), American psychiatrist well known for his association with the Menninger Foundation of Topeka, Kans. Menninger established a psychiatric clinic with his father and brother. This eventually became the Menninger Foundation, a nonprofit center for education, research, and treatment in the field of mental disease. The foundation, which employs 650 persons, has a budget of $5,000,-000 and is the core of a unique affiliation of federal, state, and community mental health agencies. Under Menninger's guidance, Kansas reorganized and modernized its mental hospitals, a program later emulated by other states.

MENOPAUSE [měn'ə-pôz], period of gradual decline in the activity of the female reproductive organs, usually occurring between the ages of 42 and 52 years (average 47.5 years). During this time menstruation becomes irregular and finally ceases. Fertility declines, and it has been estimated that about 99 out of every 100 women are infertile one year after menstruation has ceased completely. The tissues of the breasts, womb, and vagina shrink and lose their elasticity, and the skin becomes thin and dry. Body activity generally declines, so that the menopausal woman burns fewer calories and tends to gain weight on a diet which formerly was not fattening. Disturbances in the nervous control of the blood vessels may cause hot flushes and sweating. Depression, heightened irritability, and other emotional responses are often seen at this time. The head hair thins, but this does not usually become evident until about the age of 60. In rare cases, there is an excessive growth of body hair (hirsutism) during the menopause. The extent of these symptoms varies greatly from woman to woman, and in some cases virtually no changes may be seen.

An "artificial menopause," with many of the above changes, may occur in younger women following surgical removal of the ovaries in certain diseases.

Female hormones may help relieve the hot flushes which are often disturbing. Hormones in the form of creams are applied locally to the vagina to restore the tissues to their earlier condition. *See also* MELANCHOLIA.

MENSTRUATION [měn-stroo-ā'shən], cyclic activity of the female reproductive organs associated with female fertility. The principal events underlying menstruation occur in three parts of the body: (1) the pituitary gland, which lies on the underside of the brain; (2) the ovaries, which contain the eggs; and (3) the uterus.

The pituitary gland initiates the cycle by secreting a hormone (follicle-stimulating hormone, FSH) which stimulates one of the egg-containing follicles in the ovary to mature. As the follicle ripens under this influence, the ovaries step up their production of the female sex hormone, estrogen. The latter stimulates growth in the cells lining the uterus. Around the 14th day of the cycle the egg ruptures from its follicle and is expelled from the ovary. The egg then travels down the fallopian tube and finally reaches the uterus. Shortly before the egg leaves the ovary, the pituitary gland begins to secrete a "luteinizing" hormone. This stimulates the ruptured follicle, which has been left behind in the ovary, to become the corpus luteum (literally, "yellow body"). The corpus luteum secretes progesterone, a hormone which continues the stimulation of the uterine lining and prevents further eggs from maturing in the ovaries. The final stage of menstruation is apparently triggered by the interaction of progesterone with the pituitary gland. When the blood concentration of progesterone reaches a certain level it inhibits further secretion of the luteinizing hormone by the pituitary gland. This results in degeneration of the corpus luteum and a sudden fall in the progesterone content of the blood. As the progesterone is withdrawn, the lining of the uterus is sloughed off as the menstrual flow, carrying the egg with it. If, however, the egg is fertilized before this time, the corpus luteum does not degenerate but continues to secrete progesterone for a period. This inhibits menstruation and prevents new eggs from ripening in the ovaries. In this way progesterone maintains pregnancy.

Characteristics of the Menstrual Cycle

The menarche, or beginning of menstruation, ordinarily occurs around the age of 13 or 14 in the temperate zones and about 9 or 10 in the tropics. In some families there may be an inherited tendency to an especially early or late menarche.

The average menstrual cycle ranges from 26 to 30 days. The menstrual flow usually lasts for four days. Prior to the flow various signs appear, such as swelling of the breasts, congestion of the reproductive organs, and irritability and nervousness ("pre-menstrual tension"). The normal blood loss is small and is not significant.

Menstrual Regularity. Though the great majority of women have regular menstrual cycles, the regularity may be upset by stress, anxiety, fever, colds, or other factors which act through the pituitary gland—which, as we have seen earlier, exercises an important control over menstruation. This regulation can be extremely precise: cases have been noted in which a dive into a cold pool started or halted menstruation. Climate may also affect the cycle: women raised in temperate climates may note an increase in the frequency of the menstrual cycle if they move to the tropics.

Menstruation and Pregnancy. The earliest sign of pregnancy appears in the pattern of changes in the basal body temperature. Normally, the temperature drops sharply when the follicle ruptures (ovulation) and then rises about a degree higher than the pre-ovulatory temperature. Pregnancy is likely if the temperature is maintained at this elevated level, meaning that a new ovulation is not taking place.

Menstruation has been known to occur during the first few months of pregnancy and in rare cases has continued throughout pregnancy.

Menstrual Disorders. These include absence of menstruation (amenorrhea), scanty menstruation (oligomenorrhea), excessive bleeding (menorrhagia), or painful menstruation (dysmenorrhea). These disorders may be caused by tumors or abnormalities of the reproductive organs, or by pelvic infections or hormonal imbalances. Most cases of primary dysmenorrhea (appearing with the first menstruation) are caused by emotional stress.

MENTAL AGE (MA), measure of level of intellectual ability, expressed in years and months. Specifically, it is a mode of evaluating intelligence test scores so that the average mental age score of the average individual of a given age is equal to his chronological age. Thus an MA of 7 is the intellectual level of an average child of 7, and an MA of 10 years 6 months that of a child of 10 years and 6 months, and so on. Intelligence quotients (IQ's) are computed by relating an individual's mental age to his chronological age. Mental age scores increase with chronological age to about 16 or 18 years, depending on the tests used. Beyond this age, increments in score are negligible and not useful as measures of intellectual levels. *See also* INTELLIGENCE QUOTIENT (IQ).

MENTAL DEFICIENCY, also called mental retardation, feeble-mindedness, or amentia, may be inherited or be caused by abnormal development, or by disease or injury in prenatal life or in infancy.

In the inherited types numerous abnormalities, including skin lesions, epilepsy, tumors, and stunted bone growth, accompany the mental defect. Some cases involve disorders of body chemistry in which specific substances (for example, amino acids) cannot be normally processed.

Noninherited forms of mental deficiency can be caused by injury or disease before birth (syphilis, German measles), by birth injury (cerebral palsy), or by disturbances appearing in infancy (encephalitis, lead poisoning, head injury).

Familiar types of mental deficiency include:

Idiopathic, also called physiological mental deficiency. This includes the vast majority of defectives. In these cases no specific cause of the deficiency can be identified.

Mongolism, which occurs approximately once in every 5,000 births and receives its name from the presence of certain features of the Mongolian race, such as slanted eyes and a fold over the inner corner of the eye. Mongolism has been shown to result from a developmental abnormality which results in the presence of an extra chromosome (one of the structures which transmit inheritance) in the cells of the child.

Cretinism, a form of mental deficiency caused by undersecretion of thyroid hormone. This may be inherited or result from a deficiency of iodine in the diet. The latter type, called endemic cretinism, is seen in certain areas such as the Alps, where the iodine content of the soil is low. The typical cretin has a low, wrinkled forehead, puffy eyes, wide and flattened nose, thick lips, and a large protruding tongue. Early diagnosis and treatment with thyroid hormone can produce much improvement in these cases.

Microcephaly, an inherited disorder marked by an undersized brain. The face is of normal size, but the forehead tapers markedly, giving a characteristic "pinhead" appearance.

Phenylpyruvic oligophrenia, an inherited disorder of body chemistry in which the body lacks a key chemical needed to process phenylalanine (one of the amino acids found in protein foods). Treatment of infants with low phenylalanine diets has been tried in this disorder.

Cerebral palsy, which results from brain injury at birth. Mental deficiency of varying degree is present in 50%–60% of these cases.

The Extent of Retardation. Mental defectives are generally classified in three groups, based upon performance on IQ tests. The *severely retarded* (idiots: 0–19 IQ) remain below the mental age of three and are entirely dependent on others for their needs. The mental age of the *moderately retarded* group (imbeciles: 20–49 IQ) is between three and seven years and while they too are largely dependent on others, they can be trained to a limited extent. The largest group (75%) of mental defectives are the *mildly retarded* (morons: 50–69 IQ) whose mental age extends beyond the eight-year-old level. These individuals can participate in elementary academic activities and can be gainfully employed in certain lines of work.

Social and Educational Problems of the Mentally Retarded. The early attitude of hopelessness which characterized the approach to the mentally retarded has been replaced by a feeling that much can be done for them. Efforts are now made to keep the defective child in as normal a setting as possible (preferably the home), and to develop his maximum potential. To this end, some communities have established special classes for the retarded, and some "sheltered" workshops have been made available in which the retarded person can develop vocational skills in a noncompetitive atmosphere. The emotional problems of the retarded child and his family have also received attention from the psychologist, psychiatrist, and social worker—indeed, the field has virtually become a psychiatric subspecialty.

See also EXCEPTIONAL CHILDREN.

MENTAL HEALTH. The treatment of mental illness and the preservation of mental health have been called the number one public health problem in the United States, Canada, and other nations. This fact is evidence of a major change in the attitudes of citizens and governments —a change that has taken place in the 20th century.

From ancient times through the 19th century the mentally ill were called "crazy people" or "lunatics" and were feared, ridiculed, or shunned. Their condition was considered to be the result of "seizure by demons" or control by "evil spirits." At times they were even thought to be witches. They were persecuted and jailed or at best sent to poorhouses.

Reform Movements. The first notable effort to change these views about the mentally ill came in Europe and the United States during the last part of the 18th century. The American and French revolutions stirred reform movements in many areas, including concern for the sick and even for the "insane." In the United States, Benjamin Rush, a signer of the Declaration of Independence and a physician, became a champion of humanitarian care for these afflicted people and for their treatment as sick people. He was able to put his theories into practice as a physician in the Pennsylvania Hospital. In Europe another physician, Philippe Pinel, started a reform movement in 1792 with the then radical method of "striking the chains" from the "madmen" at two "lunatic asylums" in Paris. Similar movements for reform in the treatment of the "insane" took place around the same period in Italy and in England. The physician Vincenzo Chiarugi, not so well known as Pinel, in 1788 instituted medical treatment and abolished all forms of restraint as director of the Bonifacio Asylum in Florence, Italy. William Tuke, physician and founder, in 1792, of the York Retreat at York, England, became well known for the humane and successful treatment of mental patients.

Though these reform movements had an immediate effect, they soon gave way to opposition and, only a decade or two later, treatment of the mentally ill fell back into its medieval state. In 1840 a new reform movement was initiated in the United States by Dorothea Lynde Dix, a Massachusetts schoolteacher. As a result of her appeals, a number of asylums were built in the United States, Canada, and Europe, and in these institutions the mentally ill received somewhat better care than formerly. Nevertheless the typical "insane asylum" at the end of the century was a place to keep people confined rather than a center for treatment. More and more doctors and psychologists were concerned with mental illness, but the public and governments were not.

Sustained and successful efforts to make mental health a matter of widespread public concern can be dated from as recently as 1908. In that year a U.S. citizen, Clifford Whittingham Beers, took the lead in organizing a mental hygiene society to promote public efforts to deal with mental illness medically. Beers had himself been mentally ill, had been committed to a number of mental institutions, and had experienced and observed neglect, brutality, and the complete absence of psychiatric care for the mentally ill in these institutions.

Societies for Mental Hygiene

The group that met with Beers, including such men as William James, Adolf Meyer, and Anson Phelps Stokes, formed the Connecticut Society for Mental Hygiene. This society had as one of its purposes the enlistment of public interest to improve conditions in mental institutions. But the members did not believe that this would be enough. They wanted "insanity" to be regarded as illness and the "insane" as sick people in need of treatment. They further believed that medical science should give more attention to identifying the different mental illnesses, probing into their causes, and finding ways to prevent them.

The word "hygiene" in the name of the society shows the importance with which the founders regarded prevention. In this respect the aim of the society was identical with the long-range goal in other health fields—to find ways to prevent illness and ultimately to wipe it out.

In 1909 Beers organized the National Committee for Mental Hygiene, with headquarters in New York City. Nationwide voluntary health and welfare agencies did not exist at this time. It was only as the National Committee was able to bring about the organization of mental hygiene societies in the various states that such a movement began to come into being. Among the pioneer state mental hygiene societies following the Connecticut Society were the Illinois Society (1909), the New York State Society (1910), and the Maryland, Massachusetts, and Pennsylvania societies (1913).

The National Association for Mental Health. The development of state groups in the United States, and eventually of hundreds of local groups, all operating more or less independently, continued until 1950. In that year the National Committee for Mental Hygiene merged with two other national organizations—the National Mental Health Foundation and the Psychiatric Foundation—to form the National Association for Mental Health. Immediately after it was formed the National Association for Mental Health undertook to bring together all these independent state and local mental health associations into one united, national, voluntary organization. Today the National Association for Mental Health has state divisions in nearly every state and local chapters in some 1,000 communities. It has more than 1,000,000 enrolled members and volunteers.

Prevention of Mental Illness Through Education. During the early years of the mental health movement a great deal of attention was given to the principle that adult personality development is dependent, to a large extent, on childhood influences and that adult mental illness has its roots in emotional disturbances of early childhood. From this principle it follows that the prevention of mental illness must start in early childhood. One way to do this is to eliminate or reduce the kinds of stressful emotional experiences assumed to be among the causes of mental illness. The other is to provide treatment services for emotionally disturbed children so that they can get psychiatric help as soon as their problems are detected.

The first of these two objectives—prevention of mental illness through the reduction or elimination of stressful childhood experiences—resulted in the development of widespread parent-education programs. The aim of these programs was to acquaint parents with the things they could do to help the child develop good mental health and the things to avoid doing in order not to injure the child's mentally healthy development.

A number of mental health principles were developed, including the following: (1) In order to grow up in good mental health, a child needs to feel that his parents love him and that they love him just for himself. (2) A child also needs parental guidance and control so that he can learn how to control his own behavior and his own emotions. (3) A child needs a certain amount of independence in growing up. He needs to be allowed to make his own mistakes and undergo his own trials and even suffering and pain. He needs to grow up in his own way, not according to a fixed pattern that his parents have set for him. (4) Overprotection of a child is as harmful to his mental health as are indifference and neglect. (5) Inconsistency can be harmful to the child's mental health: punishing him for something one day and ignoring it the next, or showing excessive love to the child one day and treating him with coldness or indifference the next.

Programs of mental health education were considered important not only for parents but also for others who had an influence on the child's emotional life, especially teachers. The teaching of mental hygiene and mental health principles became an important part of the training of teachers. In addition, in the late 1930's and early 1940's counseling and guidance programs began to be established in the schools. One aim of these programs is to help pupils work out emotional problems which otherwise might develop into more serious mental disturbances.

Mental Health Clinics. Parallel with the development of the mental health education movement was the development of the mental health clinic movement. Child guidance clinics—clinics where children are given psychiatric treatment for emotional problems—started out as clinics to prevent delinquency. The first of them was set up in St. Louis in 1922. In the next five years similar clinics were set up in Norfolk, Dallas, Minneapolis, Los Angeles, Cleveland, and Philadelphia.

From experience with this project—conducted by the National Committee for Mental Hygiene—it was evident that the child guidance clinics had a much broader use than prevention of juvenile delinquency. They were, indeed, centers for the treatment of all mental and emotional disorders cropping up in childhood. Hence the National Committee, working with state and local mental health associations, began to set up such clinics all over the country. The standard pattern was to have each clinic staffed by a psychiatrist, a psychologist, and a social worker. These clinics treated anywhere from 50 to 500 children a year. By the early 1960's there were more than 1,500 of these clinics, most of which treat adults as well as children. Because of the very great need (it is estimated that one child in every ten is in need of psychiatric treatment) all of these clinics have long waiting lists. They now treat about 300,000 children each year.

Government Programs for Mental Health

The work of private societies produced good results at the local level. Until the 1940's, however, mental illness was not generally recognized as a national problem of the first rank. Most people considered the incidence of mental and emotional illness to be relatively low. The mental health movement continued to concentrate on the gradual development of education for mental health and on prevention through counseling and guidance in the schools and treatment of children in the clinics.

Then came World War II and the awakening. By the time the Selective Service Administration had completed its work, nearly 1,000,000 men between the ages of 18 and 37 had been disqualified for service because of mental and emotional disorders—about 20% of the 5,000,000 rejected for all causes. Mental illness also took a high toll of people already in service. Between 1941 and 1945,

460,000 men were given medical discharges because of mental disorders. This constituted 36% of the 1,250,000 men who received medical discharges.

Almost simultaneously came the disclosures that there were about 500,000 patients in state mental hospitals, that the great majority of these patients were receiving nothing but custodial care, and that in a large number of these hospitals the patients were being subjected to brutal treatment, starvation, overcrowding, and insanitary conditions. It was apparent that mental illness was a national problem of such proportions that it could no longer be dealt with through limited programs of education and prevention. Certainly these must continue and be expanded. But something had to be done about the hundreds of thousands of patients in the mental hospitals who were getting little or no help at all. And something had to be done to expand the facilities for treatment, and to improve them, so that the additional millions of people who needed psychiatric help could get it—in hospitals, clinics, and private treatment. There was a shortage of professional personnel, and this required a large expansion in training programs for psychiatrists, clinical psychologists, psychiatric social workers, and psychiatric nurses. In addition, there was an obvious need to step up research on the causes and treatment of mental illness.

The National Institute of Mental Health. In 1946 Congress passed the National Mental Health Act. As a result, the National Institute of Mental Health came into being in 1947 as one of the seven institutes in the U.S. Public Health Service. The growing importance of the National Institute of Mental Health is reflected in its budget. The first year of its operation, 1947, the NIMH had a budget of $7,500,000. In 1962 Congress appropriated $143,000,-000 for this agency's work, including $58,000,000 for research, $49,000,000 for training, and $11,000,000 to help finance state community mental health services.

Action at the State and Local Level. Government concern began to show itself in the postwar period on the state and community level too. In 1949 the Governors' Conference directed the Council of State Governments to make a study of the care and treatment of the mentally ill in all states. The study revealed that the average doctor-patient ratio in mental hospitals was about 1 to 400 and the average daily expenditure per patient was less than $2.75. The hospitals were about 25% overcrowded. Many of them were unfit for habitation and were reminiscent of conditions in Clifford Beers's day. This report touched off ever-widening circles of activity, resulting in eventual improvement of many of the conditions cited.

In 1953 the Governors' Conference directed the Council of State Governments to undertake a new study dealing primarily with training of personnel and development of research. In 1954 the Governors' Conference devoted its entire proceedings to the subject of mental health. Out of these three conferences there emerged an Interstate Clearing House on Mental Health (within the Council of State Governments) to permit the exchange between states of information on care, treatment and prevention, training, and research.

Not long after the 1954 Governors' Conference, New York State introduced a completely new concept and practice in the mental health field—state responsibility and support for the development of community mental health services. Under the provisions of the Community Mental Health Act state funds were offered to help a local area inaugurate the services with which the act was mainly concerned: mental health clinics, psychiatric services in general hospitals, rehabilitation services, and preventive education. Other states followed New York's lead quickly.

The Joint Commission on Mental Illness and Health. In 1955 Congress directed the Joint Commission on Mental Illness and Health to investigate this problem—by then officially called "the nation's number one health problem"—and to make recommendations for a national policy to deal with it. The commission, made up of representatives of 36 national agencies concerned with mental health, issued its final report in 1961, titled *Action for Mental Health*. This report noted that medical science had already made available measures for treating many mental illnesses, including tranquilizing and antidepressant drugs, as well as individual and group psychotherapy. Most mental patients, however, were unable to have the benefit of these measures because the mental hospitals were severely short of staff.

Among the many recommendations of the commission were these: sharply increased training programs for psychiatrists, psychiatric social workers, and psychiatric nurses; tripling of government expenditures for the treatment of the mentally ill by 1970; reduction in the size of state mental hospitals to 1,000 beds or fewer as against the current national average of 5,000 beds; increase in research; and increase in community facilities for the treatment and prevention of mental illness and rehabilitation of the mentally ill. The commission noted that in hospitals where patients were getting intensive treatment, as many as 85% could be released, partially or fully recovered, within three to six months after admission. Without intensive treatment the discharge rate was 50% or less. The commission also urged that communities develop facilities to treat patients in the communities near their relatives and friends, rather than in far-off institutions.

New Trends in Treatment

At the time of the commission's report a trend had already begun to develop for treatment of mental illness, even the most serious mental illness, right in the community. By 1962 more than 20% of the general hospitals in the United States had already established psychiatric units where they treated patients with psychoses. These patients were admitted to these general hospitals just like medical and surgical patients and without the necessity of legal commitment. In many hospitals they were treated in separate psychiatric wards, but in some they were treated in the same wards as the other patients.

In June, 1962, the American Medical Association declared mental illness to be America's most pressing and complex health problem and voted to involve its entire membership, as professional people and as citizens, in action to deal with this vast problem. The American Psychiatric Association had been active in this work for half a century. These two major professional organizations and the National Association for Mental Health emphasized four main lines of action:

(1) **Continued Improvement in the State Mental Hospitals.** In the early 1960's these hospitals housed 85% of the nation's 800,000 mental hospital patients. Most state hospitals were able to give intensive treatment only to the new patients, being forced to neglect those who were "chronic patients." It was found that some patients who had been in hospitals 10, 20, and even 30 years could achieve partial or total recovery with intensive treatment. The goal set was intensive treatment for all.

(2) **Increased Community Facilities.** Since it had been shown that even the most seriously sick mental patients could be treated in the general hospitals in the community, efforts were made to get most or all general hospitals to set up psychiatric sections. Some doctors hoped that in 10 or 20 years all mental patients would first get treatment in a general hospital and that only those who did not respond to intensive treatment there would be sent to specialized mental hospitals for treatment as chronic cases.

Efforts were also made to increase the number of psychiatric clinics and all-purpose mental health centers. These mental health centers provide inpatient care as well as outpatient care, and their services include diagnosis, treatment, and rehabilitation. Emphasis was also given to the establishment of 24-hour emergency psychiatric services in general hospitals, similar to the emergency services for medical and surgical cases.

(3) **Rehabilitation.** Many patients discharged from mental hospitals were found to need help in finding a place to live, finding a job, and obtaining follow-up medical care. Research showed that the relapse rate for discharged mental hospital patients could be cut from 35% to 10% through rehabilitation services.

As treatment of mental illness improved, the number of patients discharged increased. In 1956, for the first time in 50 years, mental hospital rolls stopped climbing and began to drop. The decline, while still very small, continued into the 1960's. This did not mean that fewer people were in need of help. As a matter of fact, mental hospital admissions increased sharply, but improved treatment permitted a greater turnover, with the resultant decline in the total number in hospitals. The large number treated and released make the need for rehabilitation services more urgent.

(4) **Treatment of Mentally Ill Children.** Surveys in the early 1960's indicated that there were at least 500,000 children with serious mental illness (psychosis) in the United States. About 4,000 of these, ranging in age from 5 to 16, were in the state mental hospitals. An additional 2,000 were being cared for in small residential treatment centers and day care centers in the communities. In 1963 the National Association for Mental Health absorbed the smaller National Organization for Mentally Ill Children. As a result of the consolidation, intensified efforts were made to assure separate and special treatment for children in the state mental hospitals and to increase vastly the treatment services in local communities.

World-wide Mental Health Programs

Canada. The mental health movement in Canada followed a pattern similar to that in the United States. The first leader in the movement, a physician named Clarence Meredith Hincks, was influenced by Clifford Beers's program. Hincks established the first mental health clinic in Canada. In 1918 he founded the Canadian National Committee for Mental Hygiene, with assistance from Beers. This committee worked to reform and expand treatment of mental illness throughout Canada. After World War II the name was changed to the Canadian Mental Health Association.

By the 1950's mental illness had come to be regarded as Canada's top priority health problem. Public interest and government actions resulted in improved programs of treatment. Canada experienced the same problems—such as a lack of doctors and nurses—as the United States. Canadian programs stressed such services as increasing the number of mental health clinics and giving treatment locally rather than in large asylumlike institutions.

The World Federation for Mental Health. The pioneers in the mental hygiene movement in Canada and the United States hoped to extend their programs to all nations. Hincks and Beers established the International Committee for Mental Hygiene in 1920. In the next 10 years mental health associations were formed in many countries, and the first International Congress on Mental Hygiene was held in 1930. In 1948 the International Committee adopted a new name, the World Federation for Mental Health. The U.S. and Canadian associations are charter members, and total membership is more than 140 organizations in 46 nations and 2 dependencies. The U.N. World Health Organization works with the World Federation on problems of mental health.

See also EXCEPTIONAL CHILDREN; GUIDANCE AND
    COUNSELING, EDUCATIONAL; MENTAL ILLNESS;
    PSYCHIATRY; PSYCHOTHERAPY.

MENTAL ILLNESS may be caused by changes in the structure or chemical function of the brain, or by psychological stress. The interrelation between the physical and psychic components that are believed to cause particular mental disorders, such as schizophrenia, is the subject of considerable debate and controversy.

Organic Mental Illness

Mental disturbances of organic, or physical, origin may result from infection, injury, poisoning, or other assaults on the structural and chemical integrity of the brain. Chemical poisoning caused by substances such as lead, mercury, carbon disulfide, or carbon monoxide may produce mental symptoms. Alcohol may cause a variety of mental disorders, ranging from the temporary derangement of pathological intoxication, seen in persons especially sensitive to alcohol, to Korsakoff's psychosis, which is marked by memory loss and degeneration of nervous tissue. Injury to the head may produce concussion, coma, and possibly long-lasting mental impairment resulting from brain damage. A decrease in the brain's blood supply, commonly seen in elderly persons with "hardening of the arteries" (arterio- or atherosclerosis), is thought to lead to changes in brain substance and a gradual loss of mental alertness. In certain disorders of the endocrine glands, personality changes may be observed. Deficiencies of certain vitamins of the B complex group (niacin and thiamine) frequently cause mental disturbance. Syphilis may cause insidious personality changes some 20 to 30 years after the original infection. The list of organic bases of disturbed mental function is rounded out by tumors, and diseases of the nervous system such as multiple sclerosis. Organic illnesses are regarded as acute, if they are reversible, and chronic, if they persist.

Functional, or Psychogenic, Illness

In contrast to the above group, functional mental illnesses are believed to be caused by psychological factors. The fact that no known structural or physiological changes are associated with these illnesses does not necessarily mean that such changes may not be present. The division of mental disorders into organic and functional groups may merely reflect present ignorance of the detailed chemical and physiological functioning of the brain. This possibility has been emphasized by the ability of certain chemicals (for example, LSD) to create psychoticlike reactions in normal persons, and by the effectiveness of some drugs (for example, tranquilizers) in relieving some of the severe symptoms of functional disorders.

The functional disorders include psychoneuroses, psychotic reactions, psychosomatic disorders, and character disorders. To various degrees, these are all assumed to result from disturbances in interpersonal relations, and to have anxiety as an important component. The psychotic disorders, which include schizophrenic and manic-depressive psychoses, frequently require hospitalization. The individual loses contact with reality and is unable to function effectively at work, in school, or with his family and friends. In psychoneurotic disturbances the person can function better, but is troubled by rigid patterns of behavior, such as unreasonable fears (phobias) or obsessions, which he is powerless to control. The personality, or character, disorders are a varied group, and include schizoid personality types, who are withdrawn and emotionally detached, and cyclothymic types, who alternate between states of elation and sadness.

Treatment of Mental Disorders

The principal therapeutic tool of the psychiatrist is psychotherapy, which may be supplemented by tranquilizing drugs, shock therapies, and, less often, psychosurgery. Psychotherapy basically involves talking about one's problems and experiences with a specially trained person. This type of treatment is usually reserved for neurotics, persons with character disorders, and certain types of psychotic patients. Hospitalization is indicated when it becomes necessary to help a patient get relief from the many stresses of daily living, as well as in the rarer cases where there is need to protect the patient from harming himself or others.

It should be emphasized that many mentally ill people are able to function without being treated. In support of this are reports which indicate that the incidence of mental illness is much higher than one would be led to believe on the basis of mental hospital admissions and the number of patients being treated by private practitioners. Many persons who might objectively be considered to be neurotic and to function at a level somewhat less than their full potential do not consider themselves sick and usually do not come to the attention of a psychiatrist unless some great personal or general stress intervenes.

Unfortunately many people still regard mental illness as a stigma and often block efforts to give prompt treatment to themselves or to members of their family. Many individuals who would not hesitate to seek prompt medical attention for a physical ailment, procrastinate until mental symptoms become so severe that help is often too late to be most effective.

An encouraging development, however, is the increasing tendency to regard the psychotic person not as a criminal, but as a victim of illness. Hospital planners are designing smaller buildings that will offer more privacy and avoid the depressing atmosphere of many currently used hospitals. There is also greater flexibility in allowing week-end passes and home visits; the time of hospitalization has been shortened and after-care programs are being established to help the patient when he returns home. Another innovation is the day hospital, where patients are treated during the day but are given the opportunity to live with their families at night. The oft-mentioned belief that "once you go to a state hospital, it is for life," is adequately refuted by the increasing number of discharges. *See also* Neurosis; Psychiatry; Psychoanalysis; Psychotherapy.

MENTALLY RETARDED, THE, persons classified as having lower than average intelligence. In terms of tests of intellectual ability, their intelligence quotients are below 70. They may be classed, in descending order of IQ's, as educable mentally retarded, trainable mentally retarded, and custodial mentally retarded, or as morons, imbeciles, and idiots. *See* Exceptional Children; Intelligence; Intelligence Quotient (IQ); Mental Deficiency.

MENTAL TEST. *See* Intelligence Test; Testing, Psychological and Educational.

MESCALINE [měs′kə-lēn], an alkaloid drug obtained from the peyote (also known as peyotl or mescal), a cactus plant found in Mexico and the southwestern United States. Mescaline has been of interest to psychiatrists and pharmacologists as a tool for the experimental investigation of schizophrenia. It produces vivid hallucinations, consisting usually of brightly colored lights, animals, and geometric patterns. In sufficient doses it produces disturbances of thought and perception which appear to resemble those seen in schizophrenia. The peyote plant has been used for generations by the Indians of the southwestern United States as part of their religious rituals. Most authorities agree that it causes no harmful effects or addiction. An interesting subjective acount of the effects of mescaline is given in Aldous Huxley's *Doors of Perception* (1954).

MIND sometimes means "the set of mental states associated with a particular individual" and sometimes, "the active principle which *produces* the mental states associated with the particular individual." Philosophers like Descartes often identify "mind" with "soul" and both of these with "self" or "person." Others, like Aristotle and Aquinas, while identifying "self" with "person," have held that soul (as form) plus body (as matter) constitute the person and that "mind" is the name for a whole set of powers of the person (where reason and will are elementary factors). Still others, such as Berkeley, have identified "mind" with "spirit" and have denied the existence of nonmental being, being which does not derive its existence from being a mind or an event in a mind. Spinoza held that mind and matter are just two among an infinite number of attributes of God.

Twentieth-century investigators of the mind-body problem tend to treat "mind" as the set of events we call mental, and "body" as the set of correlated physical events, asking such questions as: Are mind and body two aspects or powers of a third thing, or are they independent substances united to form an accidental whole? Could there be a mind without a self whose mind it is? Can there be and are there any disembodied minds, and, if so, how are they distinguished? Is there any conclusive argument to show that there are minds besides my own?

Ancient aspects of this question, still disputed, are: If mind and body are different substances, how can they interact? What is immortality and is anything immortal? These and other problems, as well as new difficulties suggested by depth psychology and advances in the study of human and animal learning, have made the mind-body problem a live, challenging, and complex philosophical issue.

MORGAN, CONWY LLOYD (1852–1936), British biologist and psychologist, considered the founder of scientific comparative (animal) psychology. After teaching in South Africa Morgan was associated with University College, Bristol, and from 1909 to 1919 with the new University of Bristol. His lectures at Harvard and Clark universities influenced the development of comparative psychology in the United States. Rejecting earlier anecdotal reporting of animal behavior and particularly the tendency toward anthropomorphic treatment of animal behavior (attributing humanlike thinking to animals), Morgan insisted on scientific experimentation. His statement that no behavior should be interpreted as a product of higher mental faculties if it could result from simpler processes is known as Lloyd Morgan's canon.

MORPHINE [*môr′fēn*], the principal active ingredient of opium, the dried juice of the oriental white poppy plant. Morphine acts principally on the central nervous system—it relieves pain and induces sleep. It also slows breathing, and may cause constipation, nausea, or vomiting. In recognition of its unrivaled ability to control pain, morphine has been called "God's own medicine." Morphine tends to produce addiction, and for this reason it is used only in cases where other pain-relieving agents fail. Codeine, apomorphine, heroin, and several other narcotics are chemical modifications of morphine.
See also CODEINE; DRUG ADDICTION; HEROIN; NARCOTICS; OPIUM.

MULTIPLE PERSONALITY, a condition in which an individual leads distinct and separate existences. Each personality may have a different name, different memories, and radically different attitudes toward life. Frequently the familiar everyday, or primary, personality is aware of the secondary personality, but the reverse does not hold true. A classic example of multiple personality is that described in Robert Louis Stevenson's *Dr. Jekyll and Mr. Hyde*. The multiple personality is thought to be an extreme expression of the tendency to repress and detach unacceptable aspects of oneself from conscious awareness.
See also HYSTERIA.

N

NARCISSISM [när-sĭs'ĭz-əm], a concept of psychoanalytic theory denoting a stage of development in which the libido (primitive psychic or sexual energy) of the infant is directed toward his own body. This is termed *primary narcissism*. Later in life *secondary narcissism* may occur, associated with mental illness, in which the libido is withdrawn from objects or other persons and redirected toward the self. In developing this concept Freud related narcissism to the "purest and truest feminine type" of love. He argued that beautiful women, especially, direct their libido toward their own bodies in a narcissistic fashion and consequently expect to receive, but not to give, love.

NARCOTICS [när-kŏt'ĭks], a group of drugs of varied chemical nature that relieve pain, produce drowsiness and sleep, and cause addiction. The term "narcotic" is also sometimes used more broadly to include the stupor- or sleep-producing properties of any drug, as in referring to the "narcosis" produced by ether. Narcotics are divided into two classes: the natural and the synthetic narcotics.

Natural Narcotics. The major source of the natural narcotics is the unripe seed capsule of the poppy, *Papaver somniferum*, a plant cultivated in the Middle and Far East. The milky juice which exudes when the poppy capsule is cut is dried to a brown powder known as opium. This substance has been used for thousands of years for its sleep-producing and pain-relieving (analgesic) action. Throughout the centuries when truly curative drugs and surgery were unknown, the analgesic action of opium was one of the few real services the physician could provide. In addition to its pain-relieving and sedative effects, opium and morphine (its major component) tend to produce a state of euphoria, or well-being.

In small doses morphine relieves pain, in large doses it induces deep sleep, and in still larger doses it produces coma and halts breathing. The principal toxic action of morphine is interference with breathing, caused by depression of the respiratory center of the brain. Morphine may also cause nausea, vomiting, and constipation.

Another well-known narcotic found in opium is codeine, which is chemically similar to morphine, but is less potent and not as dangerous. Codeine is widely used in medicine to relieve moderate pains and as a cough-suppressant.

Synthetic and "Semisynthetic" Narcotics. A group of narcotic analgesics can be prepared by chemically modifying the natural alkaloids, morphine or codeine. The most notorious member of this class of "semisynthetic" narcotics is heroin, prepared from morphine. This drug is not used in modern medicine. It is a major item in illegal narcotic traffic. Other derivatives of morphine are dihydromorphinone (Dilaudid), ethyl morphine, and nalorphine. The latter compound is of considerable interest because it acts as an antagonist of morphine and is an important antidote for acute morphine poisoning.

The strictly synthetic narcotic analgesics differ chemically from morphine. Most of these drugs, which include meperidine (Demerol), methadone, and levorphanol, were developed during or after World War II. They are similar to the natural narcotics, both in their analgesic effects and their tendency to produce addiction.

The Harrison Narcotic Act. Although the narcotic analgesics are the major drugs generally included under narcotics, this term is sometimes also used in a legal sense to include drugs which are listed and controlled by the Harrison Narcotic Act (1914). One such drug is cocaine, an alkaloid prepared from the coca leaf. This compound is not a sedative, but is, on the contrary, a stimulant which can produce marked restlessness and even convulsions.

Drug Addiction in the United States. The use of narcotics did not become a problem in the United States until after the Civil War, when drug addiction became known as the "army disease." In 1919, under the terms of the Harrison Act, the U.S. Treasury Department won several court cases against physicians accused of prescribing opiates indiscriminately. The convictions were interpreted as denying physicians the right to prescribe narcotics to relieve the suffering of addicts. Although the Supreme Court reversed the decision in 1925, it was too late for a redefinition of the addict as a sick person rather than a criminal; the way was left open for the illicit drug peddler.

Estimates of the extent of drug addiction in the United States are, at best, approximations. In general, an addict is identified as such only when he is arrested or seeks treatment. There are a number of signs by which the drug user can be identified—hypodermic needle punctures, for example—but definite evidence of addiction can be established only through chemical tests or by the appearance of the abstinence syndrome after drug withdrawal. Therefore, statistics of arrests for drug offenses cannot properly be interpreted as statistics on addicts, even though a majority of those arrested are drug users.

U.S. Treatment of Addicts. In 1914 the passage of a federal law, known as the Harrison Act, provided for the strict regulation of traffic in opiates and cocaine. This and other legislative acts that followed declared the sale and use of narcotic drugs illegal and subject to rigorous punishment. An exception was the granting of legal rights to physicians to prescribe narcotic drugs in limited amounts. It did not provide, however, that a physician could supply a known addict with progressively smaller and smaller amounts of a drug so that he might co-operate with the drug user in breaking the habit. Consequently, the addict has to turn to the narcotics trade or to underworld characters for relief. The situation was somewhat relieved in 1927 by a

Supreme Court decision (*Bush* v. *United States*) in which the court held: "A physician may give an addict moderate amounts of drugs for self-administration, if he does so in good faith and according to fair medical standards."

Another obstacle to rehabilitation is that it is difficult under existing legislation to obtain clearance on parole and probation for drug addicts. Drug users who are sent to the federal narcotics hospitals at Lexington, Ky., and at Fort Worth, Tex., enter as criminal cases. The law requires that these hospitals give priority to addicted prisoners and probationers who were convicted of violations of the federal narcotics laws. Other addicts who wish to attempt a cure may be admitted only when facilities permit. While individual hospitals are very active in the treatment of addiction, the number of cases treated is small compared to the number of existing addicts, and the cost of the treatment is quite expensive. Studies indicate that an unusually high percentage of persons who have been under treatment for drug addiction in the federal hospitals resume the use of drugs sooner or later.

New treatment procedures usually involve keeping the patient in a drug-free environment. When necessary, the patient is administered decreasing dosages of drugs. Sometimes, other drugs of nonnarcotic type are used to break the addict's interest in the habit. The treatment thus becomes a medical, physiological, psychiatric, and social problem. Obviously, the best approach to the problem is prevention of the addiction.

British Treatment of Addicts. Prior to 1920 narcotics users could buy drugs from local chemists. A British Dangerous Drugs Act was passed in 1920 which placed responsibility for the prescription of drugs for addicts upon physicians. Control of drug law enforcement is in the hands of the Home Office of the national government. To clarify the legal limits the physician must observe in supplying, prescribing, or possessing drugs, and to advise Home Office officials and the medical profession on such matters, a medical committee on the interpretation and administration of the law was appointed.

The general policy recommended by the committee is: morphine or heroin may be properly administered to addicts in the following circumstances, namely, (1) where patients are under treatment by the gradual withdrawal method in order to effect a cure, (2) where it has been demonstrated, after a prolonged attempt at cure, that the use of the drug cannot be safely discontinued entirely because of the severity of the withdrawal symptoms produced, and (3) where it has been similarly demonstrated that the patient, while capable of leading a useful and relatively normal life when a certain minimum dose is regularly administered, becomes incapable of this when the drug is entirely discontinued. The availability of narcotic drugs under medical supervision has caused the removal of narcotics from the black market and reduced other forms of illegal trafficking. Costs have been kept to a minimum and therefore much of the profit motive, so characteristic of the drug traffic in America, has been removed. There are very few peddlers and "pushers" in Great Britain, and sentences for drug violations are much less severe than those imposed in the United States.

Addiction and Crime. There was a time when narcotics addiction was thought of only as a personal tragedy for the individual addict. Today narcotics addiction is a threat to the larger society as well. In some New York City neighborhoods where addicts are heavily concentrated, addicts control the neighborhoods and the other residents live in constant fear for their lives and property. In a 1969 study conducted by the Justice Department, it was estimated that "many, perhaps most" of the muggings, burglaries and holdups committed in the United States were the work of addicts who, to supply a heroin habit, for example, need from $50 to $60 in cash every day, or ten times that amount in stolen merchandise. Those favoring reform of the present narcotics laws to permit treatment of addicts as sick people point out that addicts often become criminals because under the present law they cannot become patients. They point out, for example, that if known addicts could be treated with maintenance doses, then the system in which the addict serves as both consumer and distributor for criminal syndicates of narcotics smugglers would probably be destroyed, and the traffic in illegal drugs would no longer be a source of profit to racketeers. *See also* DRUG ADDICTION.

NERVOUS SYSTEM, a system of specialized tissue that controls the internal activities of the organism and regulates its interaction with the environment.

The Evolution of the Nervous System

The evolution of the nervous system was shaped by the basic problems that confront all life forms: How can food be obtained, enemies avoided, and the species reproduced? Primitive nervous systems were geared to detect changes in the environment by analyzing chemical substances, largely through the sense of smell, and were eventually replaced by forms dominated by vision and hearing. These latter senses provided considerable advantage in that the organism could obtain more precise information from the environment over greater distances and in less time. With this, other nervous mechanisms evolved which enabled the organism to associate between past and present events, and thus to profit from past experience. These mechanisms enhanced the prospects for survival.

Rigid Versus Flexible Behavior

Some nervous systems developed complex sequences of behavior that insured the continuation of the species. Such behavior sequences included the elaborate nesting and social habits of insects, birds, and lower mammals. These rigid and inflexible patterns of activity are more or less built into the nervous system and, as methods of survival, suffer the serious disadvantage that they cannot be modified to accommodate even small changes in the environment. Thus, birds that instinctively flee predators of a particular shape and coloring might be easy victims of a new predator of a different species. Such animals, however, might adapt to difficult environmental problems over thousands, or millions, of generations by genetic mutation, combined with the competitive winnowing of the less fit animals that retained older and less adaptive behaviors. Evolution of this type can occur with the relatively rigid simpler nervous systems of lower forms remaining at their same level of complexity.

By contrast, the human nervous system is able to survive by virtue of its capacity for flexible behavior, its ability to explore and modify the environment and to change behavior to suit the needs of the moment. This demands a vastly more complex brain. The human nervous system not only discovers and selects alternative means of action but inquires into problems not directly concerned with survival. This higher inquiry becomes science, art, religion, politics, and many other fields of study. In the cases of some highly dedicated scientists, scholars, and artists the nervous system seems to survive in order to inquire and create. Survival may even be compromised by certain types of thinking, as when individuals sacrifice their lives or personal interests for the preservation of the lives of others, or for an abstract social ideal.

The Cortex, Old and New

What differences in nervous structure can account for the differences in flexibility of behavior described above? The significant developments can be traced in Fig. 1, which compares schematically the brains of the salamander (an amphibian), the tortoise (a reptile), the opossum (a lower mammal), and man.

The primitive brain of the salamander can be roughly divided into two functional units: one which regulates internal activity (visceral functions, for example, control of the heartbeat, regulation of digestive movements); and a second which guides the organism in its dealings with the environment (somatic functions). The activity of the internal organs is controlled by the cells of the hippocampal area located near the midline; these cells integrate the sense of smell with taste and the operation of the digestive and other internal organs of the body. Hippocampal integration is accomplished by the many connections of this structure with a central group of nuclei known as the *hypothalamus*.

In the outer portion of the salamander's brain is a group of cells (in the *piriform area*), which govern the connections between the sense of smell and the senses of touch, sight, and hearing. These cells also control the limb movements of the animal. These somatic functions are aided by a structure called the *thalamus*.

We see therefore that the inner nuclei of the salamander serve visceral control, while the outer nuclei govern somatic functions. These structures have come to be known as the *paleo-*, or "old," cortex. Between them appeared a highly significant evolutionary development, the *neo-*, or "new," cortex. This first appeared in reptiles. The paleocortex continued to regulate the sense of smell and internal body control, while the expanding neocortex permitted more complex integration of touch, hearing, and vision, with body movement. The significance of the enlarging neocortex becomes even clearer in the mammals, as shown in the opossum (Fig. 1). The increased versatility of behavior in the mammals as com-

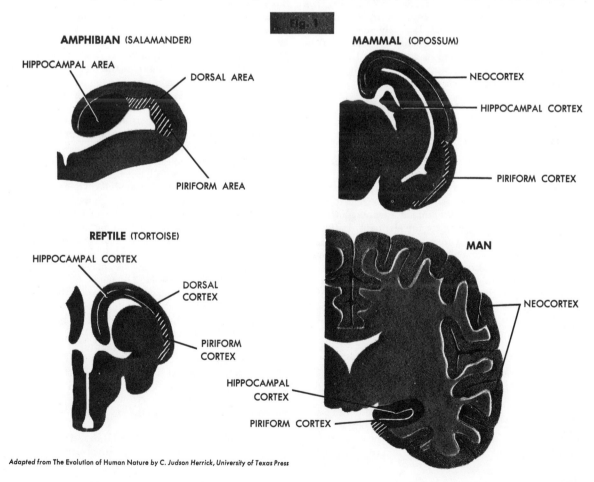

AMPHIBIAN (SALAMANDER)

HIPPOCAMPAL AREA

DORSAL AREA

PIRIFORM AREA

MAMMAL (OPOSSUM)

NEOCORTEX

HIPPOCAMPAL CORTEX

PIRIFORM CORTEX

REPTILE (TORTOISE)

HIPPOCAMPAL CORTEX

DORSAL CORTEX

PIRIFORM CORTEX

MAN

NEOCORTEX

HIPPOCAMPAL CORTEX

PIRIFORM CORTEX

Adapted from The Evolution of Human Nature by C. Judson Herrick, University of Texas Press

pared to the reptiles can be ascribed to the larger neocortex. The paleocortex is also larger in mammals, but the increase is relatively smaller.

In man the extraordinary importance of the neocortex becomes obvious. To be sure, the hippocampus of man is by itself larger than the entire brain of the opossum. Relatively, however, the hippocampus is dwarfed by the enormous increase in the neocortex, to which man owes his great skill with tools, his speech, and his culture and civilization.

From conception to adult life the neocortex expands to eventually dominate all other brain structures. Particularly important is the fact that the human nervous system is not complete at birth, but continues its development in early life under the influence of the environment. There is a great deal of evidence which suggests that the nervous system is "ripe" for particular types of learning early in life, which could not be absorbed later in life. This appears to be the case with language learning; young children acquire language with a facility and permanence which the adult cannot match. Because of the environmental stamp on the developing nervous system, it is often difficult to differentiate between the effects of early experience and a truly innate characteristic of the nervous system. In monkeys the mating behavior that superficially seems to be instinctual and innate, as is found in lower mammals, is really dependent on learning. Monkeys reared in isolation from other monkeys have great difficulty in mating. If a female reared in isolation does bear young, she does not perform any maternal functions. The early isolation blocks the necessary learning for such behavior. This development of the nervous system in early life after birth is called *maturation*, and is advantageous in enabling the organism to better adjust to its environment.

Brain Size as an Index of Intelligence

The evolutionary tendency toward increase in brain size did not always result in a proportionate increase in intelligence. The brains of the elephant (about 10 lb.) and the whale (about 14 lb.) far exceed in size that of man (about 3 lb.).

These larger animals require massive brains to control their enormous bulk. The ratio of brain weight to body weight, however, reveals the human advantage: for the whale, the ratio is 1:10,000; for the elephant, 1:500; for the gorilla, 1:250; and for man, 1:50. But such comparisons still do not accurately reflect brain capacity, since some monkeys have brain-body ratios of 1:50, like that of man. A more accurate ratio is the weight of the brain compared to the weight of the spinal cord. In the frog, the brain weighs less than the spinal cord; in the gorilla, it weighs 15 times more than the cord; in man, the ratio is 50:1.

Function and Structure of the Nervous System

As we have seen, the relations of the body with the environment are governed by the *somatic* nervous system, which notes the position of objects, listens for the sounds they emit, and moves the muscles that guide the body through space. The internal activities of the body are regulated by the *visceral*, or *autonomic*, nervous system that diverts the flow of blood, as needed, and sets the pace of activity of the digestive organs. These systems are complemented by higher structures that blend both autonomic and somatic functions into unified patterns of action. Such higher integrating structures are involved in emotion, thinking, and consciousness.

The Body and the Outside World—Somatic System. The world makes itself known to the mind by physical stimuli, such as light, sound, heat, and pressure on the skin, or by chemical stimuli which excite the senses of taste and smell. Nerve impulses carrying touch, temperature, and pain from the skin ascend to the brain via the spinal cord. Visual, sound, smell, and taste impulses enter the brain at levels above the spinal cord. All sense impulses pass to the neocortex by way of the thalamus, the sole exception being the sense of smell.

The centers of muscle control lie in the neocortex, not far from the cells which receive sense impulses.

Motor pathways from this area pass through the brain stem and spinal cord to the muscles of the arms, legs, head, and trunk. The movements of the body are controlled by these pathways, and are smoothed by groups of nerve cells (basal ganglia, striatum) in the lower brain and by the cerebellum. Much of this regulation of movement depends on precise information about the position of all parts of the body before, during, and after movement. This information originates in the muscles and tendons and goes via the spinal cord back to the centers initiating the movement.

Control of the Internal Organs—Autonomic Nervous System. This part of the nervous system, closely associated with structures of the "old" cortex, has two subdivisions: The *parasympathetic system* tends to slow the heart, lower the blood pressure, increase the movements of the stomach, and promote digestion. The *sympathetic system* is associated with the emotional responses brought on by excitement and action. This system speeds the heartbeat, raises the blood pressure, retards stomach activity, and dilates the pupil of the eye. Important in the functioning of the sympathetic system are the adrenal glands, two small structures situated one astride each kidney. The glands are composed of distinct sections: an outer portion, or *cortex*, and an inner portion, or *medulla*. The relationship between the brain and the adrenal glands illustrates the two methods of long-distance communication in the body: one by electrochemical impulses along nerve fibers; the other by means of chemical messengers (hormones) traveling through the blood.

Sudden or acute emotional stresses may excite the inner portion, or medulla, of the gland by means of sympathetic nerve fibers. When stimulated in this way, the medulla secretes epinephrine and norepinephrine, two hormones which produce the sympathetic effects on the heart, blood vessels, and other structures.

The cortex, or outer layer, of the adrenal gland is responsive to chronic stresses and is activated more indirectly by a hormone (ACTH), secreted by the pituitary gland, which is located at the center of the skull. The adrenal cortical hormones help regulate the composition of the body fluids, and promote the conversion of protein to sugar in the liver.

The medullary hormones, epinephrine and norepinephrine, are also of interest in that they are probably involved

COMPARATIVE BRAIN DEVELOPMENT OF MAN AND LOWER ANIMALS

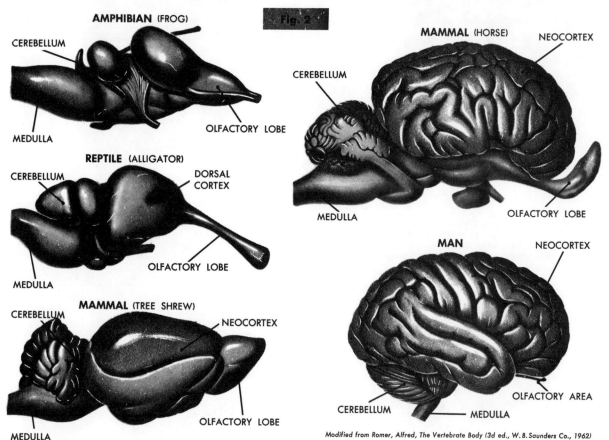

Fig. 2

AMPHIBIAN (FROG)
CEREBELLUM
MEDULLA
OLFACTORY LOBE

REPTILE (ALLIGATOR)
CEREBELLUM
DORSAL CORTEX
OLFACTORY LOBE
MEDULLA

MAMMAL (TREE SHREW)
CEREBELLUM
NEOCORTEX
OLFACTORY LOBE
MEDULLA

MAMMAL (HORSE)
NEOCORTEX
CEREBELLUM
MEDULLA
OLFACTORY LOBE

MAN
NEOCORTEX
OLFACTORY AREA
CEREBELLUM
MEDULLA

Modified from Romer, Alfred, The Vertebrate Body (3d ed., W. B. Saunders Co., 1962)

in the transmission of impulses between some neurons. It might therefore be expected that epinephrine and norepinephrine in the bloodstream would throw many brain cells into chaotic activity. This is prevented by the *blood-brain barrier*, a filtering mechanism that prevents many chemical substances from easily reaching the brain cells.

Co-ordination of the Inner and Outer Worlds. Although we have considered separately the regulation of the internal and external environments (through visceral and somatic functions, respectively), in life these activities are blended together by higher brain structures. Thus, a frightened man running from danger is performing somatic functions (the contractions of the leg and body muscles to run), while, at the same time, sympathetic impulses raise his blood pressure and quicken his heartbeat. In contrast, the parasympathetic system dominates activity during the eating and digestion of food. At this time blood must be diverted from the skeletal muscles of the trunk and extremities to the stomach and intestines.

Higher Integration—Thinking and Consciousness

At one time certain schools of psychology described the brain schematically as a "black box." Impulses were fed into the box (input, or sensation); after a period impulses emerged (output, or muscle control) from the box. The task of psychology was to understand what happened in the box (the brain) between the input and the output. We have here described the input, or sensation; the output, or motor impulses; and the parts of the brain involved in sense activity and motor control. There remain the processes occurring between input and output; these involve the higher, integrating parts of the brain, structures which have no specific sensory or motor functions.

The frontal lobes of the brain are such higher structures. Consequently, it has been presumed that, along with many other parts of the brain, they are involved in higher mental processes, such as abstract thinking. In the operation frontal lobotomy, performed in certain types of mental disease, severance of the connections between these lobes and the thalamus produces certain subtle changes in personality and abstract thought.

A vital part of all co-ordination and integration is the *reticular formation*, a dense network of cells in the central core of the brain. This network extends from the upper reaches of the spinal cord through the brain stem and thalamus and fans out to all parts of the cerebral cortex. All sensory systems (touch, hearing, and so forth) feed into the reticular formation, and can lead it to activate or excite the rest of the nervous system. For this reason, it has become known as the *reticular activating system.*

The system has several distinctive properties which suggest that it is essential to consciousness and is funda-

THE NERVOUS SYSTEM

The major component of the nervous system is the brain, which is the center of intelligence, memory, and personality. The spinal cord, the peripheral nerves, and other nerve structures link the brain with the outside world, and various parts of the body.

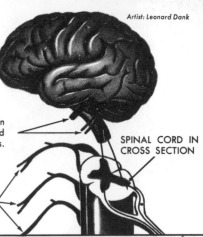

THE BRAIN

The cranial nerves connect the brain directly with the eye, ear, nose, and tongue and various internal organs.

SPINAL CORD IN CROSS SECTION

The peripheral nerves link the spinal cord to the organs and tissues of the body.

CONTACT WITH THE MUSCLES

The voluntary muscles are controlled by the motor area of the cerebral cortex — the convoluted "higher" brain. The nerve circuit shown here illustrates how the nerve fibers controlling the muscles of the arm pass through the brain and out of the spinal cord.

MOTOR AREA OF BRAIN

ASCENDING TRACTS TO BRAIN

AFFERENT NERVES CARRYING SKIN SENSATION

SPINAL CORD

DESCENDING TRACT IN SPINAL CORD

MOTOR NERVE CELL OF SPINAL CORD

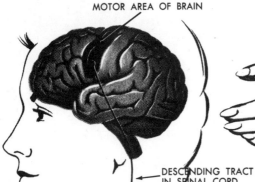

CONTACT WITH THE OUTSIDE WORLD

The eye, ear, and nose receive information about distant objects in the outside world. The taste and skin receptors report to the brain the presence of objects in contact with the body. Impulses are carried to the brain by afferent fibers.

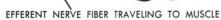

EFFERENT NERVE FIBER TRAVELING TO MUSCLE

CONTACT WITH THE INTERNAL ORGANS

A special branch of the nervous system called the autonomic (or automatic) nervous system regulates the internal activities of the body. The nerve connections of this system to the heart and stomach are shown here. The dotted pathways belong to the *parasympathetic* branch of the system, which slows the heartbeat and stimulates the activity of the digestive organs. The solid pathways are *sympathetic* fibers, which speed the heartbeat and inhibit digestive activity.

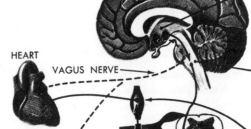

HEART

VAGUS NERVE

STOMACH

The HYPOTHALAMUS of the brain regulates internal activity.

The MEDULLA contains nerve centers for the control of respiration and heartbeat.

GANGLIA: collections of nerve cells outside the brain and spinal cord.

SPINAL CORD

THE NERVE CELL

A CELL OF THE CENTRAL NERVOUS SYSTEM

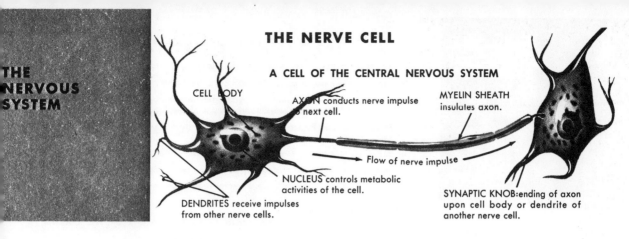

CELL BODY

AXON conducts nerve impulse to next cell.

MYELIN SHEATH insulates axon.

Flow of nerve impulse

NUCLEUS controls metabolic activities of the cell.

DENDRITES receive impulses from other nerve cells.

SYNAPTIC KNOB: ending of axon upon cell body or dendrite of another nerve cell.

THE CONDUCTION OF THE NERVE IMPULSE

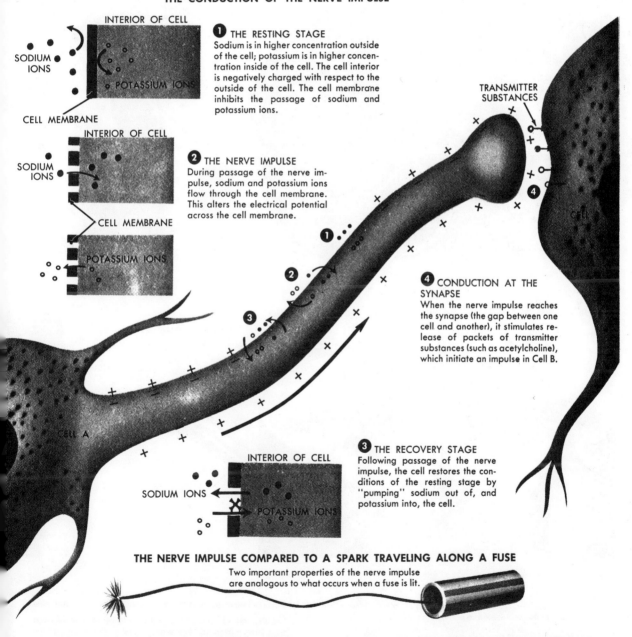

INTERIOR OF CELL

SODIUM IONS

POTASSIUM IONS

CELL MEMBRANE

❶ THE RESTING STAGE
Sodium is in higher concentration outside of the cell; potassium is in higher concentration inside of the cell. The cell interior is negatively charged with respect to the outside of the cell. The cell membrane inhibits the passage of sodium and potassium ions.

INTERIOR OF CELL

SODIUM IONS

CELL MEMBRANE

POTASSIUM IONS

❷ THE NERVE IMPULSE
During passage of the nerve impulse, sodium and potassium ions flow through the cell membrane. This alters the electrical potential across the cell membrane.

TRANSMITTER SUBSTANCES

❹ CONDUCTION AT THE SYNAPSE
When the nerve impulse reaches the synapse (the gap between one cell and another), it stimulates release of packets of transmitter substances (such as acetylcholine), which initiate an impulse in Cell B.

CELL A

❸ THE RECOVERY STAGE
Following passage of the nerve impulse, the cell restores the conditions of the resting stage by "pumping" sodium out of, and potassium into, the cell.

INTERIOR OF CELL

SODIUM IONS

POTASSIUM IONS

THE NERVE IMPULSE COMPARED TO A SPARK TRAVELING ALONG A FUSE

Two important properties of the nerve impulse are analogous to what occurs when a fuse is lit.

(1) As long as the nerve cell is stimulated by an impulse of a certain minimum strength, it makes no difference how strong the exciting impulse is, just as a match or a blowtorch produces the same reaction in a fuse. This is known as the *all-or-none-law*.

(2) The nerve impulse remains at the same strength as it travels along the nerve fiber, just as the spark remains at the same intensity as it moves along the fuse.

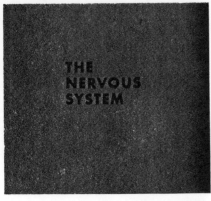

SOME NERVE CIRCUITS

A CIRCUIT FOR THE EXECUTION OF A VOLUNTARY MOVEMENT

(1) Impulse originates in pyramidal cells of parietal lobe of the brain.

(2) Impulse passes along axons of pyramidal cells through pontine nuclei to the cerebellum, the muscle-coordinating center of the brain.

(3) Impulse reaches Purkinje cells of the cerebellum. Pattern of muscle action is selected.

(4) Action pattern passes to dentate nucleus of the cerebellum.

(5) Impulses ascend to red nucleus on way to the cerebrum.

(6) Impulses reach pyramidal cells of motor area of cerebral cortex.

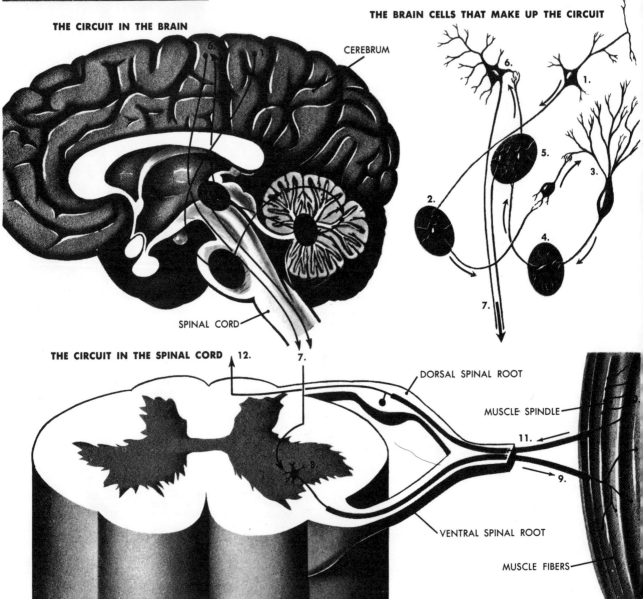

THE BRAIN CELLS THAT MAKE UP THE CIRCUIT

THE CIRCUIT IN THE BRAIN

CEREBRUM

SPINAL CORD

THE CIRCUIT IN THE SPINAL CORD

DORSAL SPINAL ROOT

MUSCLE SPINDLE

VENTRAL SPINAL ROOT

MUSCLE FIBERS

(7) Impulses from the cerebral cortex travel along descending tracts in the spinal cord to activate muscles.

(8) Motor nerve cell in spinal cord is activated.

(9) Impulses pass to muscle via spinal nerve.

(10) Muscle sensory receptor alters firing pattern as muscle contracts.

(11) Sensory impulses from the muscle travel to the spinal cord.

(12) Sensory impulses ascend spinal cord to brain. The information transmitted in this way apprises the brain of the state of muscular contraction, thus making possible coordinated movement.

THE AUTONOMIC NERVOUS SYSTEM

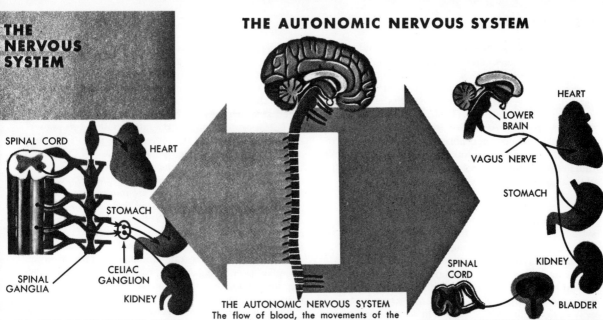

THE NERVOUS SYSTEM

SPINAL CORD
HEART
STOMACH
CELIAC GANGLION
SPINAL GANGLIA
KIDNEY

LOWER BRAIN
HEART
VAGUS NERVE
STOMACH
SPINAL CORD
KIDNEY
BLADDER

THE SYMPATHETIC NERVOUS SYSTEM
During vigorous exercise, sympathetic nerves acting on the blood vessels direct blood from the digestive organs and skin to the muscles of the arms, legs, and trunk. This "emergency," or "alarm," system also increases the heartbeat and inhibits digestive activity.

THE AUTONOMIC NERVOUS SYSTEM
The flow of blood, the movements of the digestive tract, the secretions of the digestive and endocrine glands, and various other internal activities are under the unconscious, automatic control of the autonomic nervous system. The two major divisions of the system are the sympathetic system *(left)* and the parasympathetic system *(right)*.

THE PARASYMPATHETIC NERVOUS SYSTEM
The fibers of the parasympathetic nervous system promote digestion by increasing the movements and secretions of the digestive organs. Parasympathetic stimulation also slows the heartbeat and stimulates the secretions of the glands lining the breathing passages.

THE CELL STRUCTURE AND CHEMISTRY OF THE AUTONOMIC SYSTEM

THE CHEMISTRY OF THE SYMPATHETIC SYSTEM
The impulse traveling via the sympathetic pathway to the heart or any other organ must cross two gaps: (1) between the preganglionic fiber (A) and the ganglion cell and (2) between fiber B and the heart tissue. Two different types of chemicals mediate this passage: (1) cholinergic substances at the first gap and (2) adrenergic substances at the second gap. Since most sympathetic endings are of type 2, sympathetic effects are generally associated with these adrenergic fibers.

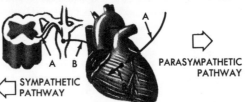

PARASYMPATHETIC PATHWAY
SYMPATHETIC PATHWAY

THE CHEMISTRY OF THE PARASYMPATHETIC SYSTEM
The nerve impulses traveling along the parasympathetic pathway to the heart must cross: (1) the gap between fibers A and B and (2) the gap between fiber B and the heart tissue. A cholinergic substance mediates the passage of the impulse at both points.

THE TWO CELLS OF THE AUTONOMIC SYSTEM
Both parts of the autonomic system have one cell in the brain or spinal cord and another contained in a ganglion outside of these structures. Above, the fibers "A" link the spinal cord and brain with the ganglion. The difference between the two systems can then be seen. The sympathetic cells are located in ganglia adjacent to the spinal cord. The parasympathetic cells are usually found close to, or within, the organ innervated.

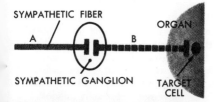

SYMPATHETIC FIBER
A
B
ORGAN
SYMPATHETIC GANGLION
TARGET CELL

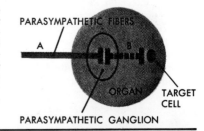

PARASYMPATHETIC FIBERS
A
B
ORGAN
TARGET CELL
PARASYMPATHETIC GANGLION

HOW DRUGS ACT UPON THE AUTONOMIC SYSTEM

LEVARTERENOL (NOREPINEPHRINE) acts upon the cells which are normally stimulated by sympathetic fibers.

ATROPINE blocks the action of cholinergic fibers on the target cells.

PILOCARPINE acts upon the cells which are normally stimulated by parasympathetic fibers.

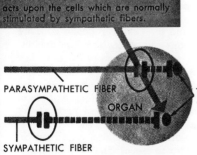

PARASYMPATHETIC FIBER
ORGAN
TARGET CELLS
SYMPATHETIC FIBER

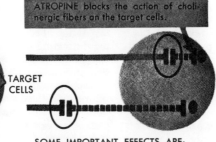

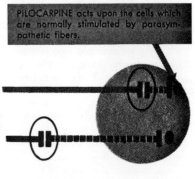

SOME IMPORTANT EFFECTS ARE:
(1) to constrict the small arteries
(2) to elevate the blood pressure.

SOME IMPORTANT EFFECTS ARE:
(1) to dilate the pupils of the eyes and paralyze accommodation
(2) to inhibit secretions of the glands lining the mouth, nose, and upper respiratory passages
(3) to increase the heartbeat rate.

SOME IMPORTANT EFFECTS ARE:
(1) to induce sweating
(2) to induce salivation
(3) to contract the pupil of the eye.

mentally involved in the highest brain functions. It is *nonspecific*, as mentioned above; that is, it is alerted by any incoming sense impulses; it is rich in connections with other parts of the nervous system; it can excite or inhibit nervous activity; and it is connected with the hypothalamus and visceral control mechanisms, which suggest that it is one of the basic structures involved in emotion. Experimental evidence has confirmed the importance of the system in maintaining the waking state: electrical stimulation in this region arouses a sleeping animal; destruction of the region causes permanent sleep.

The Basic Nerve Unit—The Neuron

The neuron is the basic conducting unit of the nervous system. It contains, within the confines of a single cell, the basic properties of the nervous system as a whole. The input enters through a specialized signal-receiving region (dendrites and cell body), and integration between input and output occurs in a central region (the cell body). The output is discharged along the axon, a structure specifically designed for this purpose. The axon of one neuron ends on the dendrite or cell body of another neuron at a junction called a *synapse*.

Nerve impulses travel down the axon to the region of the synapse and there stimulate the release from small packets (vesicles) chemicals (called transmitter substances), which excite the dendritic membrane on the other side of the synapse. The electron microscope reveals some very small filaments crossing the synapse which keep the two sides of the synapse in precise association. This allows for the rapid and well-controlled release and destruction of the transmitter substance. Rapid destruction of the transmitting agent is extremely important, since otherwise the synapse could no longer transmit impulses. The substances most studied as probable transmitter agents are acetylcholine, epinephrine, and norepinephrine.

The Laws of Functioning. Like all physical systems, the nervous system is subject to certain laws of functioning which determine its properties. These can be studied in the region of the synapse. The incoming fiber, the axon, has two choices: it may "fire" (conduct a nerve impulse) or not fire; it cannot adjust the intensity of the nerve impulse. Across the synapse (that is, in the dendrite and cell body) the situation is quite different. It must be emphasized first of all that many axons impinge on a single dendrite.

Some axons may *inhibit* the dendrite; others may *excite* the dendrite. In effect, an incoming axon firing at a synapse may say to the dendrite "react" or "do not react." The dendrite and cell body usually do not fire in response to any single stimulation but average the effects of the activity of many incoming axons. A single quick tap on a hot iron, for example, may not produce the sensation of heat, but several consecutive taps may reveal what one tap fails to elicit. The consecutive taps produce consecutive reactions at the synapse which are added, or summated, over a time interval, to eventually fire the dendrite and cell body. This is known as *temporal summation*. The dendrite may also compute several impulses arriving at adjacent points, as when one compares weights of the same size and shape, one finds that the heavier weights cause more displacement of the skin, bones, and muscles

of the hands, and generate a feeling of greater weight. In this case more impulses arrive at the dendrites and cell bodies simultaneously; this is termed *spatial summation*.

Types of Neurons. Many types of neurons are known; one of the bases for distinguishing among them is the speed at which they can conduct messages. Impulses in the fastest neurons move at the rate of 110 meters per second; in the slowest, at 0.5 meter per second. The speed of conduction is matched by the thickness of the myelin sheath, the insulating material around the axon. The more myelin, the faster the conduction. The slowest conducting fibers have no myelin at all, and are more primitive, since myelinated nerve fibers appeared and became progressively more prominent with the vertebrates as they evolved to higher forms. As brains enlarged, faster long-distance connections became necessary. This bears a striking analogy to the increasing prominence of freeways and turnpikes as cities enlarge, in order to keep the fast-moving, long-distance traffic from getting tangled up with slow-moving local traffic.

Neurons and Nerve Circuits. The complexity of the nervous system derives from the fact that billions of nerve cells are linked in a constantly changing variety of circuits. Despite this complexity, there are basically three types of neurons, again corresponding to the three basic types of function in the nervous system: (1) sensory neurons that conduct impulses to the nervous system (*afferent fibers*); (2) neurons that conduct impulses within the nervous system (association neurons); and (3) motor neurons that conduct impulses away from the nervous system (*efferent fibers*).

One of the simplest nerve circuits is that of the simple reflex. A painful stimulus applied to the skin (for example, touching a hot stove) excites a sensory neuron which conducts the impulse to an association neuron and directly to an effector, or motor cell, which stimulates the arm muscle to contract and draw the arm away from the stove. More than one set of neurons is actually involved in such a reaction. impulses are also transmitted up the spinal cord to alert the brain and generate the sensation of pain.

The Nervous System in Action

Like a polished athlete, the normally functioning nervous system makes the difficult look easy. The football player evading opponents to catch a pass and score a touchdown, moves so surely and naturally that it is difficult to appreciate the staggering complexity of nerve activity which underlies his movements. Literally billions of events are occurring every second: he is alerted through the activity of the reticular formation and has focused attention on tracking the football via the eye and optic nerve to thalamic visual relays and visual neocortex. The thalamus, the cortex, and the central reticular core are facilitating needed actions and perceptions, and inhibiting distracting stimuli, such as the roar of the crowd or pain from a bruised leg. Many other thalamic and neocortical areas are simultaneously co-ordinating running and positioning of the arms for the anticipated point of catch. Information (feedback) on the position of parts of the body comes from muscles, tendons, and the balance organs of the ear, and is correlated with vision and muscle control areas of the cortex to execute the over-all plan of the football player to catch, run, and score. The cerebellum, the basal ganglia, and other structures feed into the primary motor systems to enhance the smoothness of what would otherwise be a jerky and un-co-ordinated muscle action. We often take smoothness of function for granted and it is not until the jerky un-co-ordinated action of muscles appears, with disease of these systems, that we realize how much is necessary to attain smooth co-ordination.

In addition to all this, the nervous system is regulating body function through its control of hormone release: epinephrine and norepinephrine from the adrenal medulla speed the heartbeat; the antidiuretic hormone from the pituitary gland reduces loss of water in the urine to conserve water during the heavy losses from sweating, and so forth. This brief description is only a small sample of the processes underlying such an action.

Research on the Nervous System

Electricity and the Nervous System. Electricity has been a valuable tool in neurophysiology, both as a means of recording the normal electrical activity of nervous tissue and as a method of stimulating the brain.

The electrical activity from individual nerve cells reveals under what conditions neurons fire and how they can be kept from firing. The electrical activity of large numbers of brain cells produces the well-known "brain waves." These are measured in millionths of a volt, and can be recorded from the scalp. The waves are particularly informative in regard to states of arousal or consciousness.

The waves get broader and higher with drowsiness and sleep and become narrower and lower during arousal and periods of concentration, as when working on arithmetic problems. The reticular activating system is fundamental in the regulation of these brain-wave patterns. Abnormal brain-wave patterns are helpful in diagnosing conditions such as epilepsy and brain tumor.

The wave forms are often helpful in following pathways in the nervous system as they are actually functioning. Following a click, evoked responses can be detected as the impulse travels toward the brain: first in the auditory nerves, then the thalamus, and finally the auditory cortex. The activity of the visual and touch systems can be explored in similar fashion.

Changes in brain waves can also be observed in learning. Using the conditioning technique developed by the Russian physiologist Ivan Pavlov, some of the electrical patterns can be brought under experimental control. If a cat is exposed to a particular sound, brain-wave arousal patterns may appear. If the sound is repeated a number of times, it fails to evoke the arousal pattern. The arousal pattern may be induced once more if the animal is taught to expect some food with the sound. It is also known that an electrical pattern much like that accompanying light sleep can be generated in the brain of the cat by stimuli that the cat learns are unassociated with anything, in contrast to those which signal food. From this it has been learned that a mechanism exists in the brain for reducing responses to stimuli that are learned by the subject to be of no significance.

Electrical stimulation of the brain is a time-honored method for analyzing nervous system function. It received much attention following the discovery that a rat or a monkey can be made to work at a furious pace to receive as a reward an electrical impulse in certain parts of the brain. The animal can also be made to stop working by placing the current in certain other areas. When the electrode is placed in "pleasure," or "start," areas, the laboratory rats appear alert and excited. They will solve mazes and cross electrically charged grids to get to the controls for the brain stimulus. With stimulation in nonpleasurable "stop" areas, they appear to be in pain and will work to avoid repetition of the stimulus.

The presumed pleasurable or exciting effects described above may have been produced by electrical stimulation in a few human subjects, but ordinarily such effects are difficult to find. In some persons suffering from epilepsy it is possible to stimulate parts of the temporal cortex and elicit memories which seem to be activated and re-experienced as perceptions in the present, and which continue only so long as the current is applied. It has been postulated that the temporal lobe in some people is a storehouse for memories, but this cannot always be reliably demonstrated.

Chemical Investigations. Research into the chemistry of the nervous system has been stimulated by the discovery that certain drugs can produce profound effects on behavior, to the extent of inducing psychosislike reactions, or calming highly agitated mental patients. The effect of hormones on nervous function has been demonstrated by injecting hormones into areas of the brains of cats to put them into heat. Hormone injections into rats' brains have produced nesting behavior.

Surgical Investigations. Early investigations consisted largely of removing parts of the brain of experimental animals and observing the effects on behavior. A novel technique of surgically separating the two sides of the brain of animals without interfering with sensation and motor control on either side has revealed that it is possible to train each side of the brain independently of the other. The "split-brain" technique makes it possible to train a single animal in conflicting tasks simultaneously, each task being mastered by one-half of the brain.

Psychological Investigations. It is sometimes possible to make inferences about nervous structure and function by observing behavior, without physically acting upon the nervous system. This is illustrated by experiments which show that it is possible to interfere with memory by putting rats to sleep immediately after they have learned something new. On recovering from the immediate sleep they fail to remember the learning experience; when put to sleep 30 minutes after learning, memory is intact. It is evident that for some minutes after a learning experience the rat is consolidating what he has learned for permanent retention. It is this consolidation that can be experimentally manipulated. The experiment clearly suggests that nervous activity continues for an interval after the learning experience.

Understanding of the function of the nervous system is progressing rapidly because of the availability of many more precise, faster responding, and automatic tools. In addition, the large quantities of data obtained can now be computer-analyzed with great saving in time and effort.

For these reasons, researchers in a variety of disciplines, including engineers, physicists, and biochemists, are collaborating with the neurophysiologists and psychologists in the ever-expanding effort of the human nervous system to understand itself.

See also BRAIN; REFLEX.

NEUROSIS. While sensitive and irritable individuals are commonly described as "neurotic," in strict psychiatric usage this term is applied to individuals who adopt certain rigid, repetitious, and fruitless patterns of behavior in an attempt to reduce anxiety.

The central problem of neurosis is anxiety. According to Freud, a combination of constitutional and emotional factors are involved. He felt that neurosis was related to problems in early development, especially those occurring during the period of weaning, toilet-training, and the resolution of the Oedipus conflict (q.v.). Other writers, such as Karen Horney and Harry Stack Sullivan, stress the role of society and difficulties between people in creating anxiety.

Whatever its origins, neurosis is generally agreed to result from efforts to control anxiety. The particular form a neurosis takes is felt to depend upon the way in which the individual deals with his anxiety.

The Types of Neurosis. One method of dealing with anxiety is to surrender one's personal identity. In a *dissociative reaction* the neurosis expresses itself in stupor or forms of amnesia in which the individual avoids anxiety by forgetting who he is.

In some cases anxiety is "converted" into physical symptoms such as paralysis or blindness. This is sometimes called a "conversion reaction." The individual is not consciously aware that his physical distress results from mental conflicts. A classic example of such a reaction is the soldier who develops paralysis of the legs when faced with the prospect of combat. The conflict between duty and fear is unconsciously resolved by the paralysis which yields the individual both escape from the threatening situation and public sympathy.

In *phobic reaction* anxiety is displaced from its real source onto an object or situation which is symbolically related to it. The phobic person recognizes that his fear of such things as going up in an elevator or touching germs on a doorknob is unrealistic, but he may feel powerless whenever confronted with these situations.

Anxiety may also be dealt with by indulging in repetitive patterns of thinking or acting—the obsessive-compulsive reaction. These may take the form of recurring thoughts which plague the patient or of actions which he feels compelled to carry out. He may, against his will, find himself thinking over and over whether he left the lights on or locked the front door, and not be reassured,

even by checking. In the compulsive forms, the individual may repeatedly perform some act, such as washing his hands, 50 or 60 times a day.

Another reaction to an anxiety-producing frustration is the neurotic depression, or *depressive reaction.* Unlike normal grief, which passes with time, neurotic depression lingers and grows, and is usually caused by relatively trivial frustration. Instead of directly expressing anger, the neurotic person becomes depressed, making the target of his anger "sorry."

An *anxiety reaction* is characterized by sleeplessness, irritability, restlessness, and a "free-floating" anxiety which the individual is unable to attribute to any specific cause. As a rule such individuals eventually develop symptoms of one of the other forms of neurosis.

It should be emphasized that few patients fall neatly into any of these categories; "mixed" neuroses are far more prevalent than pure cases. The incidence of the various forms of neuroses has changed considerably. The hand-washing compulsions and conversion reactions which were common when the neuroses were first studied in 19th-century Vienna are now seen less frequently than anxiety reactions.

The neuroses are best treated by psychotherapy.

See also ANXIETY; MENTAL ILLNESS; PSYCHIATRY; PSYCHOANALYSIS; PSYCHOTHERAPY.

NIGHTMARE, dream characterized by fear and anxiety. The dreamer usually awakens during or shortly after the dream, recognizes his surroundings, and can tell about his bad dream. Often he can be calmed in a few minutes.

A more severe condition is the *night terror,* in which the individual shows highly emotional behavior after he appears to be awake. Oftentimes he is unable to recall the dream that has caused his terror.

Nightmares and night terrors are most common in childhood, although the battle dreams of combat soldiers are similar. Such experiences are most likely to occur in individuals who display other symptoms of nervous instability.

Both nightmares and night terrors are probably more likely to occur if the individual goes to bed excited from bloodcurdling stories heard or seen during the evening and if he is not in good health. Anything that can be done during the day to relieve fears and promote an atmosphere of security will probably help eliminate unfortunate dreams. Sedatives should be used only under the direction of a physician. Although a child should be able to go to sleep without having to have a toy in bed or a light in the room, such indulgences may be justified if they help reduce fears.

OBSESSIVE-COMPULSIVE NEUROSIS, a neurosis characterized by unwanted thoughts, or obsessions, and uncontrollable actions, or compulsions. It is seen primarily in meticulous, formal, rigid, perfectionist persons who tend to suppress emotional expression. Their obsessions take the form of persistent, violent, aggressive thoughts, which are distressing and unacceptable to the conscious mind—the patient may be plagued with the idea of slaying his loved ones or setting fire to his house. The compulsions may appear as repeated hand-washing or elaborate rituals before going to bed. As in other forms of neurosis, obsessive-compulsive behavior is regarded as a means of dealing with anxiety.
See also ANXIETY; NEUROSIS; PSYCHOANALYSIS; PSYCHO-
    THERAPY.

OCCUPATIONAL THERAPY, a health service specialty which uses occupational activity to promote emotional and mental stability and to develop the use of weakened or injured limbs. For these purposes occupational therapists teach creative arts such as wood, metal, leather working and clay modeling; and job skills, such as typing and business machine operation. Most therapists work in hospitals, school clinics, sanitariums, or nursing homes. Training consists of a four-year college course leading to a bachelor's degree with a major in occupational therapy. After graduating and completing a period of clinical training, therapists may take the registration examination given by the American Occupational Therapy Association. Those who pass the examination are entitled to use the initials O.T.R. (Occupational Therapist, Registered) after their names.

OEDIPUS COMPLEX, a psychoanalytic concept designating the sexual desire of the male child for his mother or a mother figure and the corresponding hostility toward his father or father substitute. The name derives from the Greek tale of Oedipus, King of Thebes, who slew his father and married his mother. The analogous complex for the female child stems from the myth of Electra, Greek princess who murdered her mother, referred to as the Electra complex.

According to Freud, the manner in which a child resolves the Oedipus complex determines his future relations with both men and women. In psychoanalytic theory, therefore, many personality traits and neurotic illnesses, especially hysteria, are explained by the Oedipus complex; it constitutes a major part of infantile sexuality.

The concept of the Oedipus complex has met with strong opposition from psychologists and the general public, initially because it was difficult to accept the idea of sexual desire in the infant. When this objection was overcome, however, a more serious doubt arose from evidence that the complex exists only in certain types of society and that in these cases the specifics which Freud described are confined to certain types of disturbed personalities. Thus the Oedipus complex and other aspects of psychoanalytic sexual theory have to be reevaluated.
See also PSYCHOANALYSIS.

OPIUM [ō′pē-əm], dried juice of the white poppy, *Papaver somniferum*. This plant, originally native to Asia Minor, was later cultivated in Egypt, India, Greece, and China as the use of opium spread. One of the oldest drugs known to man, opium has been used since prehistoric times, and for many centuries constituted the only effective means of relieving pain. In 1803 the German pharmacist Sertürner isolated morphine, the principal active ingredient of opium. Later codeine, papaverine, and other opium alkaloids were extracted. Morphine has now largely replaced opium in medical practice.
See also DRUG ADDICTION; HEROIN; MORPHINE

OPTICAL ILLUSIONS, misinterpretations of visual impressions that result from physiological or psychological causes, or both.

Natural Illusions. The sun or moon appears much larger near the horizon than when high in the sky, particularly if the horizon is defined by adjacent trees or buildings. Yet the measured diameter of sun or moon is constant regardless of its altitude, except for slight effects of atmospheric refraction. The cause of this illusion is not fully understood, but proximity of familiar objects on the horizon appears to be an important factor.

The rainbow is an illusion in that it appears to be a real structure that touches the earth at definite points. Yet it moves with the observer, and really indicates only a direction in space related to the direction of the sun.

A pond or stream whose bottom is visible deceives an inexperienced wader, who finds that it is deeper than it appears. This illusion is caused by refraction, or bending, of light at the water surface. Refraction in the atmosphere creates lakes in the desert, elevated islands, or castles in the air—the mirages. In mountainous country, water often appears to run uphill.

Artificial Illusions. These have been developed in great variety. The most familiar is a photograph, the two-dimensional representation of a three-dimensional scene on a flat surface, which appears to the observer as three dimensional. A picture of a totally unfamiliar situation probably would not be seen to have depth, but through experience the observer interprets the perspective relations and various color values in a painting or photograph as representing different distances from him.

OPTICAL ILLUSIONS

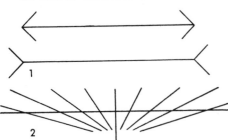

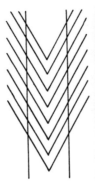

(1) The lines are of equal length. (2) The horizontal line is a straight line. (3) The vertical lines are parallel. Illusions to the contrary arise when the mind, interpreting what the eyes see, subconsciously follows the attention-directing angles.

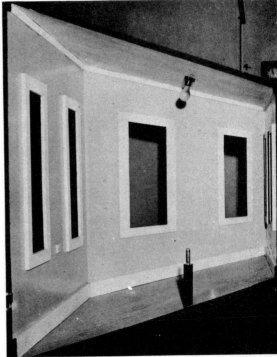

The distorted room (above) used in perception research is constructed with the angle and distance of every feature from a fixed focal point carefully calculated to reproduce the illusion of normal perspective. An observer at the focal point sees it as a normal room. Photographed from this point (left) the windows appear to be the same size although the head of the man at the right (in the smaller window) looks much larger than the head of the man at the left. (BROOKLYN COLLEGE)

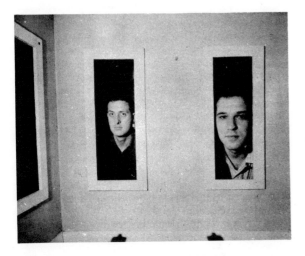

The three-dimensional illusion is enhanced by use of the stereoscope. The conventionality of such perception was demonstrated in World War II, when it was found that bomb craters in aerial photographs appeared as mounds if shadows in the pictures pointed away from the observer.

Motion pictures and television involve both the space illusion of a still picture and the additional illusion of continuous movement while viewing a rapid series of pictures. The motion illusion depends upon persistence of vision, familiar to every child who has waved a glowing stick or sparkler. The sensation produced by a flash of light does not die out immediately. If another flash follows within perhaps 1/20th of a second, the two blend into continuous impression.

Some illusions result from retinal fatigue. If one looks momentarily at the sun or other bright light, he will then see a gradually fading dark spot where the light was focused in the eye. The spot on the retina that was exposed to the intense light is temporarily less sensitive than the remainder of the retina. To demonstrate this effect, stare fixedly at a black spot on a sheet of white paper for about 20 seconds, then look toward a moderately light surface or the sky at dusk. The spot will appear light against a darker background.

P

PAIN, sensation causing distress or suffering. Nerves carry messages of various sensations, including touch, pressure, position, temperature, and pain, to the spinal cord. They travel to the brain where they are sorted and interpreted and action decided upon.

How Pain Travels. Unlike the nerves, which carry other sensations, pain nerves are naked fibers which begin as loops. Each fiber joins with many others to form trunks. The spinal cord is the main trunk and carries thousands of these fibers. Each fiber carries its individual message from a particular region of the body. As the message travels to the upper spinal cord it enters a nerve network, called the reticular formation, where it begins to enter consciousness. An actual feeling of pain does not take place until the message travels to the great receiving area of the brain, called the thalamus. Here the source of pain is recognized and the message is switched to an appropriate part of the cerebral cortex for interpretation, processing, and reaction. Now the full message of pain is realized and the person is fully aware of his pain and its location. The reaction to an individual pain message varies as it is compared automatically with stored memories of other sensations and reactions, and as learned emotional responses are drawn forth. All the data are gathered to interpret the pain's intensity. Then reactions are decided upon. The stoic may decide to disregard his pain, the highly sensitive individual will scream in anguish.

Where Pain Arises. Caused by many types of stimuli, pain is the symptom which most often leads patients to the doctor, who searches for its source. Superficial pain, as on the skin, is easily pinpointed. Pain originating within the body in hollow organs or joints may be accurately localized, but such pain is often "referred" to other areas, because information about the pain's source is misinterpreted at the reticular formation or thalamic level. For example, the pain of early appendicitis may be referred to the middle of the upper abdomen, rather than felt in the right lower abdomen. A diseased upper molar may produce earache, as may some throat infections. A diseased hip is often felt as knee pain. And irritation or stimulation anywhere along the course of a pain fiber may be misinterpreted as arising at its end point. Phantom limb pain is an example of this phenomenon. After leg amputation, a patient may feel great pain apparently arising in the lost foot. Causalgia, a severe persistent pain, and the very sharp pain of neuritis, as in shingles, are other examples of pain due to injury and inflammation of the nerve fiber or trunk. Pressure on a nerve root from injury to a spinal disc causes the pain called sciatica.

Pain as Protector. Pain fibers—unlike other sensory fibers—are not selective. They respond to any type of stimulus intense enough to cause or threaten injury. The delicate ends of pain nerve loops lie by the myriad just under skin and mucosal surfaces, and in blood vessels and hollow organs, but only the capsule, or outer covering of solid organs, such as the liver and kidney, contain pain loops. If the body lacked these tiny sensitive "pain windows," we could be stabbed or burned without feeling pain at all, nor would physical ills, such as arthritis, appendicitis, or angina, cause pain. The distribution of pain fibers is not uniform. Pain loops are most numerous in body parts most sensitive to injury. The tip of the nose and palm of the hand have only 40–70 of these endings per square centimeter, but the groin has 200 per square centimeter. An identical blow to the sole of the foot, the groin, and the eye would be painless on the sole, painful in the groin, and very painful to the eye. The fragile eye is thus protected by possessing many more pain-sensitive nerve endings.

It is now obvious that no matter how unpleasant, pain is an extremely important sensation which the body uses to protect itself from injury and illness. The pain of angina tells the patient with heart disease he has exercised enough, or eaten or worried too much, and must stop for a rest. Pain is the symptom that often reveals underlying diseases which might otherwise remain concealed. The mechanism of the pain which arises inside our bodies is not clear. Cutting or piercing does not cause pain, but pressure, chemical irritation, stretching, and inflammation do cause pain.

Pain Threshold and Intensity. The reaction to a given pain stimulus, and how its intensity is interpreted, varies from individual to individual and, at different times, in the same individual.

Both the threshold and the intensity of pain may be altered in several ways. Soldiers in battle and athletes in intense competition may not feel severe or serious injuries until their attention is directed to them. Pain may be felt more acutely when one is anxious or depressed. When awareness is redirected, as in hypnosis, even surgery may be performed without anesthesia and without significant pain. Childbirth may also be made painless under hypnosis by a physician skilled in its use. Each individual's pain threshold tends to be fairly constant, but may be altered at times by awareness and anxiety. Prolonged severe pain lowers one's threshold of pain, as may excessive concern about one's state of health (hypochondriasis). Mental illness commonly raises the pain threshold by drilling perception or interpretation of pain.

How Pain Is Relieved. Relief of pain may be accomplished in a number of ways. The most important is to remove its cause, by medical or surgical means. The pain threshold can be raised by analgesics, such as aspirin, morphine, and codeine. One may temporarily block the

Pain is a warning signal that some part of the body is being injured, stretched, compressed, or in some other way being abnormally acted on. Despite the fact that pain is among the most common of human experiences, comparatively little is known about it. The nerve pathways which conduct pain impulses, the way in which pain is recognized as coming from specific tissues, and the factors affecting the experienced quality of pain, are still in doubt.

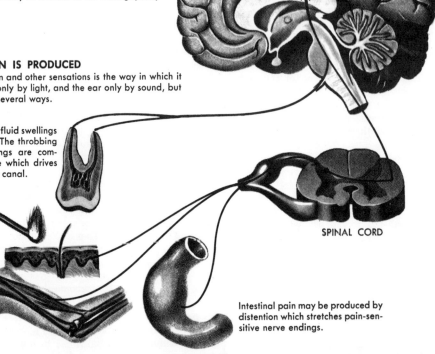

Artist: Leonard Dank

THE PERCEPTION OF PAIN

The experience of pain involves not only the recognition that a part of th body hurts, but also a feeling or emotional reaction that dominates consciousness.

The arrows indicate roughly the pain pathways in the brain. The gray arrows represent the passage of pain impulses to the higher regions of the brain (the cerebral cortex). The white arrows trace the radiation of pain to subcortical structures which may be involved in the feeling quality associated with pain.

HOW PAIN IS PRODUCED

One of the differences between pain and other sensations is the way in which it is activated. The eye is stimulated only by light, and the ear only by sound, but pain impulses can be produced in several ways.

The pain of a toothache is caused by fluid swellings within the bony canal of the tooth. The throbbing pain develops as the nerve endings are compressed by each beat of the pulse which drives blood into the inflamed and swollen canal.

Skin pain may be caused by intense heat, cold, or mechanical injury to the skin.

Muscle pain may be caused by the liberation of certain chemical substances into the tissues following vigorous exercise.

SPINAL CORD

Intestinal pain may be produced by distention which stretches pain-sensitive nerve endings.

THE PROBLEM OF PAIN IN THE WRONG PLACES—"REFERRED" PAIN

In a number of disorders involving the deep tissues, pain appears some distance from the actual source of irritation. This phenomenon, known as "referred" pain, is important in medical diagnosis.

SOME EXAMPLES OF "REFERRED" PAIN

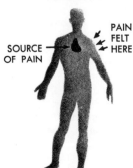

SOURCE OF PAIN

PAIN FELT HERE

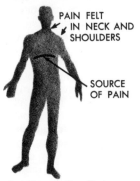

PAIN FELT IN NECK AND SHOULDERS

SOURCE OF PAIN

In certain heart conditions pain is felt in the left arm.

In disorders of the diaphragm pain may be experienced in the neck and shoulders.

SOME PROPOSED EXPLANATIONS

TO BRAIN

FROM SHOULDER

FROM DIAPHRAGM

SPINAL NERVE CELLS

SPINAL CORD

In the diagram above, it can be seen that nerve impulses from the shoulder and diaphragm enter the spinal cord at the same level. It is believed that impulses from the diaphragm may then proceed to the brain along the pathways for shoulder pain. A second possibility is that the impulses from the diaphragm and shoulder share common nerve pathways in the brain and spinal cord. In this case the brain would interpret pain impulses from the diaphragm as coming from the shoulder, since pain from this region is more common.

nerve fibor's ability to carry messages with a local anesthetic, for instance, by local, temporary freezing, when suturing or in dental work. A spinal anesthetic temporarily "freezes" the whole spinal cord at the desired level. Attention may be redirected with the use of counterirritants, such as mustard plaster or oil of wintergreen, or by hypnosis. Considerable research has been done on effective types of distraction, such as music, and static noise, sounds called white sound, and visual stimuli, to reduce pain sensation. Pain conduction can also be reduced or stopped by surgical or chemical destruction of the main nerve trunk. Rarely, pain fibers are cut at the point where they enter the spinal cord in a very delicate operation called a rhizotomy. Of more academic interest than practical importance is leukotomy, surgical severing of nerve fibers leading to the cortex of the brain. After such surgery, pain is felt but no longer bothers the patient. Leukotomy severs association traits, so that past experiences, interpretations, responses, and emotional reactions no longer aid in the interpretation and reaction to pain. *See also* NERVOUS SYSTEM.

PARANOIA [păr-ə-noi′ə], a mental disorder characterized by the gradual development of firm delusions which become the center of the individual's life. It develops in persons usually in their late forties who are sometimes described as "paranoid" personality types, being suspicious, rigid, resentful, and socially unhappy individuals who lack understanding of their own problems. Comparatively few paranoid personalities actually develop true paranoia. While pure paranoia is rare, paranoid symptoms may appear as aspects of other mental disorders, such as schizophrenia. The illness generally takes four forms:

Delusions of Persecution. The patient may feel that his life is in danger from organized plots against him. Such beliefs tend to isolate the individual from the community, causing him to lead a fear-ridden existence.

Delusions of Grandeur. This may be viewed as another aspect of ideas of persecution. The paranoiac reasons: "If I am persecuted then I must be someone of importance." He has an exalted idea of his abilities and may even identify himself with famous persons.

Litigious Type. The patient often reaches the psychiatrist via a long path of lawyers whom he has enlisted to argue his case against those he believes to have wronged him. In such cases, the paranoid person may consider himself to be persecuted by former employers, the local government, or various organizations.

Erotic Type. Such an individual believes that he or she is the object of someone's affections. Frequently a prominent member of the community or a movie star is chosen.

There is no known cure for paranoia. Most patients are permanently hospitalized.

PARAPSYCHOLOGY [păr-ə-sī-kŏl′ə-jē] is a division of psychology dealing with those psychical effects which appear not to fall within the scope of what is at present recognized law. (This definition comes from the glossary used by the *Journal of Parapsychology*.) A synonymous term is "psychical, or psychic, research." Other terms associated with aspects of this field are "clairvoyance," "telepathy," "extrasensory perception," and "psychokinesis."

Throughout history human activities have been described which appear to involve knowledge of distant or future events or unexplained modes of contact with the minds of other persons. Likewise, events suggesting the unexplained influence of mental activity upon physical processes have often been reported. Such reports are usually associated with beliefs that there may be commerce with unseen beings, whether deceased human beings or benign or malignant spirits. Systematic investigation of such matters began in the 19th century. In 1882 the Society for Psychical Research was founded in London. This was followed by the establishment of similar organizations in the United States and in many Continental countries. University scholars played an important part in the new movement, and an increasing use of systematic laboratory experimentation has characterized recent decades.

Spontaneous and Experimental Telepathy. The first great task of the Society for Psychical Research was to gather and assess a large number of narratives relating to apparent contact with distant events, especially accidents and deaths. The society also attempted both to rule out coincidence as an explanation and to make psychological sense in terms of such factors as motivation and freedom of the mind to make contact despite the distraction of immediate surroundings. A number of studies were published, and ambitious attempts were made to create a systematic psychology of apparitions, telepathic interchanges, and precognitive experiences, both in sleeping and in waking conditions.

During the 1880's and 1890's the Society for Psychical Research, followed by French and German investigators, set up experiments involving the telepathic transmission of drawings and other visual material, playing cards, numbers, and the like, to persons nearby and to persons at a distance. This was done under conditions permitting the assessment of the likelihood of achieving by chance alone a certain number of correct "hits" on the material selected. Telepathy was defined by one of the investigators, F. W. H. Myers, as "the communication of impressions of any kind from one mind to another, independently of the recognized channels of sense." Such experiments, usually of short duration and not ideally controlled, made relatively little impact but added to hypotheses regarding the role of relaxation, semisleeping conditions, and the part played by strong motivation for contact. In 1921 three psychologists at the University of Groningen, the Netherlands, reported telepathic transmission from experimenters to a subject in another room. The subject was rigidly controlled and the experimenters relied upon a method of randomization of target material and statistical assessment of hits covering a series of trials to produce a well-defined experimental result.

Extrasensory Perception. At Duke University in 1934 J. B. Rhine reported a long series of experiments. Rhine's primary method was to ask subjects to guess cards. Instead of a deck of 52 playing cards, he used a deck containing five cards bearing circles, five with crosses, five with squares, five with stars, and five with wavy lines. Any given guess would tend, on a purely statistical basis, to be right one-fifth of the time. Much mathematical analysis and many control series have shown that this tendency ordinarily to guess five out of 25 correctly is a fact that establishes control conditions. If a subject maintains an average of 6 or of 5.5, rather than 5.0, for a long time, we can establish by a standard mathematics of probability what likelihood there would be of achieving such a result on the basis of chance alone. In one series an experimenter is reported to have successfully conveyed knowledge of shuffled cards to a subject in another building on the Duke University campus at a scoring level that would not occur by chance alone once in many billions of such tests.

In Rhine's approach, and in the *Journal of Parapsychology* which he founded in 1937, short, informal, crudely controlled experiments were often followed by those in which one or another of three types of control were used: (1) opaque envelopes to contain the target cards, (2) wooden screens to prevent the subject's observing either the experimenter or the card material, and (3) long-distance conditions. Some of the experiments were concerned with telepathy, but there were many in which the experimenter never looked at the cards. If the subject succeeded, this was an example of what Rhine called clairvoyance (a term already familiar to parapsychologists). Telepathy and clairvoyance together constituted extrasensory perception (ESP).

This research at Duke University was followed rapidly by attempts to reproduce the experiments at many other universities. A few were successful, a few unsuccessful, and a number evoked general skepticism and an argument that could never be resolved in the absence of a clear-cut replication (reproduction of the experiments with essentials unchanged). It was charged, and agreed, that many preliminary tests were poorly controlled. It was at first charged that the statistics were faulty, but after long and full debate this point has lapsed. Charges of fraud and gross incompetence are still sometimes heard. No complete replication of any of the newer methods has been published. While a considerable number of psychologists are interested in the phenomena and many laboratories are investigating the topic, the absence of full replication causes many psychologists to withhold judgment on the question. Two surveys of the opinions of psychologists suggest that about 3% regard extrasensory perception as established, about 12% as a likely possibility, and about 30% as a remote possibility, while many regard it as impossible or simply as an unknown. Philosophical difficulties having to do with a mode of conceptualizing the action of mind upon mind, of mind upon material events, or the action of material events upon mind, are clearly of great weight. Among those who believe there is a real problem here for investigation, the interest lies mainly in finding out what kind of phenomena are involved and how they can be brought under control.

The Psychology of Extrasensory Processes. Variables that have been used in experimental studies in the attempt to get control of the phenomena include motivation; fatigue, drugs, and stimulants; suggestion and hypnosis; freedom from blocking; and relaxation, drowsiness, and sleep. In addition, other factors are various types of interpersonal attitudes, such as the attitude of the subject toward the task, toward other participating subjects, and toward the experimenter.

Outstanding among such studies are those of G. R. Schmeidler. In a series of 14 large experimental attacks on the problem since 1942 he usually found that the scoring level of subjects who believe in the reality of extra-

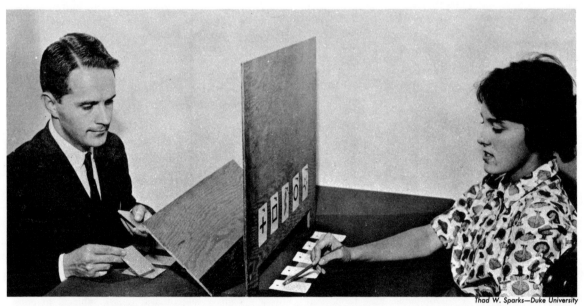

A girl being tested for extrasensory perception. She is pointing to one of five cards in an attempt to match the card in the right hand of the tester. The boards make it possible for the tester to see the girl's choice without the girl seeing the cards held by the tester or his reaction to her answers.

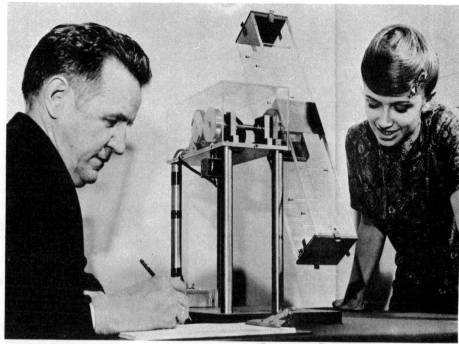

Conducting an experiment in psychokinesis. The girl is attempting to will the dice in the transparent container to land with a previously predicted face up.

Thad W. Sparks—Duke University

sensory perception is significantly higher than that of subjects who disbelieve in its reality. Schmeidler offered evidence likewise that personality factors add to or interact with this factor of attitude. There is also some evidence from experiments in which teachers test their classes in extrasensory perception. Favorable attitudes of teachers toward children and of children toward teachers lead to significantly higher levels of success than are achieved when either teachers or children are neutral or hostile. Many attempts at replication are in progress; the issue is still open.

Precognition. By the same methods of randomly preparing target materials such as cards or numbers, it should be possible to test the hypothesis that one can at times properly identify target orders (order of items to be picked) that have not as yet come into existence. That is, one may prepare the target order (pick cards, for example) after the subject has made his calls or guesses. There is some evidence of successful precognition of this sort. Rejection of precognition on philosophical grounds appears to be even more vigorous than rejection of extrasensory perception, although in some instances the controls are comparable.

Psychokinesis. In the world-wide history of the subject, reports of unexplained movements of objects, especially in the presence of certain psychically disposed individuals (mediums, for example), have been numerous. Such phenomena are covered by the term "psychokinesis" (PK). In 1943 Rhine began to report on the effects of wishing upon dice tumbled onto a prepared surface, or down a chute containing baffles, or whirled about in cages permitting no normally predictable positions in which they would come to rest. Among numerous experiments done in this way, a few have made use of the appropriate control technique of having the subject

try now for sixes, now for fives, or fours, or threes, or twos, or ones, according to a prearranged schedule. Thus the known bias of dice would be uncorrelated with the wishes used on given occasions. Some positive results have been obtained. In many such experiments, moreover, it appears clear that the results are best at the beginning of a new task.

A Swedish engineer, H. Forwald, has released dice down a chute which tumbles them onto a surface divided by a central wire. The task is to wish them to come to rest to the right or to the left of this wire (making correction for the bias caused by irregularities of the table itself). Sometimes coins or other objects are used instead of dice. Individual differences have not been stressed in PK research, although in one recent study at Bonn University the outstanding subject with coins was also outstanding in influencing a roulette wheel. Regarding PK, as regarding ESP, it must of course be noted that everything depends upon the integrity and the competence of experimenters, and that independent replication of such efforts, although it occurs here and there, has not been the rule.

Evidence for Survival After Death. Among both preliterate and literate societies there has been an interest in the alleged capacity of certain individuals to act as mediums between the deceased and the living, usually while in a dissociated or trancelike state induced by such factors as fatigue, dizziness, or drugs. Messages purporting to come from the deceased are usually received through automatic speech or automatic writing, including the Ouija board and planchette. Under the impact of American spiritualism in the mid-19th century many mediums appeared. The purported communications from the deceased often took the form of statements relating to the families' inner secrets.

The London and American societies for psychical

research undertook systematic study of such communications. Especially notable were the studies of the phenomena of Mrs. L. E. Piper by Richard Hodgson and J. H. Hyslop. After the death of the classics scholar F. W. H. Myers in 1901 a number of messages began to appear through different mediums, containing intricate references to classical poetry in which the living Myers had been deeply interested. These references were of so complex a nature that Cambridge University scholars found it difficult to track the associations down. When this had been done, however, it frequently appeared that crisscrossing references through different mediums, or automatists, had been given within a span of a few months. No living person had been aware of the fact that a literary puzzle fitting together various classical components had been worked out. Thus the "Lethe" case gives an intricate system of association related to the River Lethe as contained in Ovid and Vergil.

A few years later another type of intricate evidence began to be offered by Mrs. Willett (a pseudonym). In two reports written by G. W. Balfour messages appeared that included associations characteristic of the interests of two deceased scholars, A. W. Verrall and Henry Butcher. The result is the celebrated "Ear of Dionysius" case. Opinions vary as to the value of this material. Some scholars assert that the evidence for survival is convincing; others that telepathic interchanges among the living are certainly involved but not evidence of survival from the deceased; while a third group is still reluctant to accept even the evidence for telepathy.

The Organization of Parapsychology. Research on these problems has been in progress at about 20 American and about 10 British universities in recent years, and there is a wider awareness today of the scientific issues involved than at the beginning of the 20th century. While most of the books dealing with psychical research are devoid of interest from a scientific point of view, there are several journals that maintain serious standards.

A continuous effort is being made by psychologists, philosophers, and other scholars to construct a conceptual system in which the data will appear less incredible. It is thought by some that the philosophical difficulties will be simplified by developments in physics. But while there are many systematic psychological theories about states favorable to the appearance of such phenomena—lacking only a specification of a physical basis for the phenomena—the physicists have not as yet offered coherent hypotheses. Among the dozen or so physicists who are known to be actively interested in these phenomena, some seem to feel that parapsychological phenomena may ultimately be accommodated to physics. Others believe that physics will have to accommodate itself to any strange new facts that can be authenticated.

PATHOLOGICAL LYING, habitual lying, often needless, and unexplained by self-interest. It may involve both falsification of actual events and the development of fantasies. Pathological liars have no meaningful motivation for their antisocial behavior. They appear unable to separate truth from falsehood. They seem charming and competent, but behind this facade is a complete lack of morality and social stability. Nevertheless, some pathological liars,

through their lies, achieve something in the world, and such persons have even functioned temporarily as professional men. Most impostors quickly reveal the shallow base of their promises and claims. They further increase their chances of being detected by the frequency of their lying.

If the pathological liar becomes criminal, he is most likely to engage in swindling. Except for swindling, occasionally writing bad checks, or slander, the pathological liar may have little trouble with the law. At present, the possibility of successful treatment is limited by their lack of insight into their own behavior.

See also SOCIOPATHIC PERSONALITY.

PAVLOV [päv′lôf], **IVAN PETROVICH** (1849–1936), Russian physiologist, famous for his studies of digestion and his subsequent discovery of conditioned reflexes. Pavlov received his medical degree in 1883 at St. Petersburg Military Medical Academy, where he continued as a tutor until 1888. After study in Germany he returned to the academy in 1890 to hold various positions, becoming professor of physiology in 1895. Following the Revolution of 1917, Pavlov held the distinguished post of director of the physiological laboratories of the Russian Academy of Medicine. His researches on the physiology of digestion, summarized in *The Work of the Digestive Glands* (trans., 1902), earned him the Nobel Prize of 1904.

While studying digestive responses, Pavlov found they were easily modified. Experimenting with salivation in dogs, he discovered that the animal could be trained or "conditioned" to salivate at the sound of a bell or the sight of a circle of light. These formerly neutral stimuli alone were capable of eliciting the response for food (salivation), even though no food was offered. These investigations led to a concept of the brain as a primary signal system, and the results were published in English in *Conditioned Reflexes* (1927).

Pavlov's systematic experimental studies on conditioning in dogs and other animals profoundly influenced the theory of learning, and the concept of conditioning helped shape behaviorism as a branch of psychology. He was able to create "experimental neuroses" in his animals by making a correct choice in a conditioned animal increasingly difficult, thereby insidiously confusing the animal. Pavlov's *Conditioned Reflexes and Psychiatry* (trans., 1941) sparked the experimental approach to the study and treatment of human mental disorders. However, the premise that his approach could explain thinking as a result of a secondary signal system has not been borne out.

See also CONDITIONING.

PENTOTHAL SODIUM [pĕn′tə-thôl], also sodium pentothal, a fast-acting barbiturate used to produce anesthesia, and in psychiatry to produce a relaxed state in which the patient's problems can be more easily explored (narcosynthesis). The drug may dangerously depress breathing and must be used with caution.

See also BARBITURATES.

PERSONALITY. *See* PSYCHOLOGY: *Psychology of Personality*

PERSONALITY TEST, test or technique used in the assessment of personality traits—for example: rating scales; inventories of attitudes, opinions, and values; and measures of personal adjustment to the environment. *See* PROJECTIVE TECHNIQUES; TESTING, PSYCHOLOGICAL AND EDUCATIONAL.

PERSONNEL PSYCHOLOGY. *See* PSYCHOLOGY: *Personnel and Industrial Psychology.*

PHENOBARBITAL [fē-nō-bär′bə-tôl], drug used to induce sleep, to relieve apprehension, and to control epileptic convulsions. A slowly acting barbiturate, phenobarbital exerts its depressant action on the central nervous system for six hours or longer. Repeated use may lead to habituation and addiction.
See also BARBITURATES.

PHOBIA [fō′bē-ə], neurotic disorder characterized by an irrational fear of a particular object or situation, such as closed spaces (claustrophobia), heights (acrophobia), traveling, animals, dirt, or diseases. The individual is generally aware of the unreasonableness of his fear, but is unable to control it.

Psychiatrists consider phobias to develop as a defense against anxiety. In phobia the anxiety, instead of being diffuse and "free-floating," is displaced onto a concrete object. By avoiding the phobic object the individual can reduce his anxiety, although this forces him to restrict his activities and movements. According to psychoanalytic theory, the choice of phobia is symbolically related to the underlying psychic disturbance. This view stems from Freud's analysis of "Little Hans," a five-year-old boy who feared that a horse would fall on him or bite him. Freud related this fear to the child's unconscious hostility toward his father. The falling horse represented the child's wish for his father's death; the biting horse constituted symbolic punishment for this wish. Another, somewhat simpler, theory of phobia advanced by psychologists describes it as resulting from associations of the phobic objects or situations with painful experiences.

Phobias commonly tend to extend, including more objects and situations and imposing successively greater restrictions on the activity of the patient. Phobias are treated through psychotherapy.

PHRENOLOGY [frĭ-nŏl′ə-jē], study of the relationship between skull contours and personality characteristics. Phrenology is rooted in the notion that the mind can be analyzed into a number of discrete faculties, such as cautiousness and spirituality, and that each faculty is located in a specific part of the brain. Bumps and depressions on the skull, according to this theory, represent the degree of development of various faculties. Using these signs, the phrenologist believes he can determine the subject's personality and abilities. The practice of looking at the form of the skull to determine personal character was known in ancient cultures. It was brought to life again in the 19th century by two German scholars. F. J. Gall and J. G. Spurzheim. Their writings and teaching drew attention to specific areas of the brain associated with specific kinds of mental activities. Phrenology's principles have been largely refuted by modern anatomy and physi-

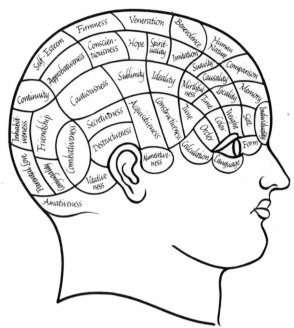

Chart indicating the seat of 42 human faculties, according to the theories of 18th- and 19th-century phrenologists. Modern studies of physiology and brain functioning show that such mapping of the brain is invalid.

ology, but they were important in provoking more intensive and detailed study of the brain. Such studies led to the discovery of specific brain areas for vision and hearing and to the development of neurophysiology.
See also FACULTY PSYCHOLOGY.

PIAGET [pyȧ-zhě′], **JEAN** (1896–   ), Swiss psychologist known for his studies of the fundamentals of child development. Piaget was a precocious student with interests in biology who published his first article at age 10. He received his doctorate in the natural sciences in 1918 from the University of Neuchatel, with a dissertation on mollusks. His interest in the philosophy of science led him to study the development of knowledge and thought in children, to probe the relation between logic and thought, as well as questions of epistemology, the means of knowing.

Piaget's methods of investigation are unique in the history of psychology. First he simply followed small children, including his own, through their daily activities, carefully observing and recording. Later he developed techniques of directly questioning children and methods of presenting little experiments in physics, without soliciting contrived answers from his young subjects. Observations of his own children's earliest encounters with various objects, and the most casual movements of their eyes, arms, and legs enabled him to describe in detail the world of the child.

Piaget construes the developing child as an organizer of reflex actions and sensory perceptions, in dynamic equilibrium with his environment. This dynamic interaction is established by assimilation of sensory material and accommodation of reflexive behavior. During development different stages of such equilibria are fixed in order of increasing complexity. Piaget's early work was devoted to elucidation of the progressively complex levels of intellective behavior, which he characterized in definite, though overlapping, stages of development corresponding roughly to age levels. In his later work he used symbolic logic to describe the abstractions of thought, much as the physicist uses mathematics to describe the objective world.

Piaget became director of studies at the Institut J. J. Rousseau in Geneva in 1921, then director of the Bureau International d'Education, which later became affiliated with the International Office of Education and UNESCO. In 1955, with the help of the Rockefeller Foundation, he established the Centre International d'Epistémologie Génétique in Geneva.

See also CHILD DEVELOPMENT; PSYCHOLOGY: *Developmental Psychology.*

PINEL [pē-nĕl′], **PHILIPPE** (1745–1826), French psychiatrist known for his reforms in the treatment of the mentally ill. As chief physician at two French hospitals he removed the chains from patients, some of whom had been bound for over 30 years. Pinel turned to psychiatry as a result of the tragic experience of a friend who became mentally ill. He heralded a new enlightenment in the attitude toward mental patients by stressing that the demented were ill. In his *Traité médico-philosophique sur l'aliénation mentale* (2d ed., 1809) he advanced the concept that mental disorders stemmed from diseased brain tissue.

PROJECTION, in psychology, the attribution of one's own traits, attitudes, or acts to other persons or things. Projection is often an escape mechanism, an attempt to reduce the tension caused by anxiety or guilt. It can take several forms. In assimilative projection, a person assumes that others think or act as he does. For example, a chronic liar may be convinced that everyone is dishonest. In disowning projection, a person denies responsibility for some attitude, misdeed, or inadequacy by putting all the blame on other persons or objects. Examples are the workman who blames his tools or the insecure person who joins in discrimination against, or persecution of, minority groups. In both cases the function of projection seems to be to protect the self or ego.

Assimilative projection may be observed in a more general, less clearly defensive, form. Children commonly seem to assume that adults feel and think as they do, and some grownups treat children as if they were small adults. This form of projection is related to an apparent tendency for people to judge things outside them in accordance with their own attitudes and emotions. Because of this tendency, projective techniques are widely used to study personality.

See also PROJECTIVE TECHNIQUES.

PROJECTIVE TECHNIQUES. The term "projective techniques" covers a number of devices psychologists and psychiatrists use to study personality. Common to these methods is the fact that they present semistructured or unstructured material—such as inkblots, pictures, or beginnings of sentences—to an individual who is encouraged to tell what he sees in the inkblot, to relate a story about the picture, or to complete the unfinished sentence. Since there is no "correct" response, the subject, in reacting to such stimuli, must answer in his own individual way. This free situation provokes from the person reactions that reveal inner needs, fears, strivings, and conflicts of which he himself may not be aware. Projective methods are in sharp contrast to the so-called "objective" methods, like the standard intelligence and achievement tests, on which the response is scored either "right" or "wrong." They also differ from the standard paper-and-pencil personality tests on which the response to an item like "Do you worry over possible misfortunes?" is restricted to one of several choices—"Yes," "No," "Sometimes," or "?".

Theories Underlying the Use of Projective Techniques. The general assumptions underlying projective devices may be summarized as follows: (1) When an individual is confronted with ambiguous stimuli and he cannot rely on previous learning to produce an answer, the meanings he attributes to these stimuli are considered to be peculiar to him and the way he sees the world. (2) In the process of creating a response, an individual identifies himself with a person actually pictured or projected in the situation by his own fantasy. (3) The individual's sample of behavior in this situation is assumed to be representative of the way he is likely to behave in other unfamiliar situations. It is believed that he projects his own characteristics into the blot or picture before him.

Although the term "test" is often used to refer to these procedures and responses to them are compared to norms (responses given by large numbers of subjects), they are more properly described as "techniques" or "devices," since the information obtained is primarily qualitative and diagnostic rather than quantitative. Parenthetically, it should be mentioned that most of the projective devices were developed initially for individual administration. Some, however, have been adapted for group administration.

The Rorschach and Other Widely Used Techniques. The best-known and most widely used projective technique is the Rorschach inkblot device, which was created by Hermann Rorschach, a Swiss psychiatrist, in 1921. The technique employs 10 inkblots, 5 achromatic and 5 colored, each on a card. The blots are presented in sequence to the subject, who may give as many or as few responses as he wishes. These responses are recorded and scored in terms of content, that is, what is actually seen; the area of the blot described; how well the concept fits the areas; how often and in what way the subject used the shape, the color, or shading qualities of the blot; what kind of movement is projected; and whether the responses are popular (commonly given) or original. Although suitable for subjects of all ages, the technique is more successful with adults and with children over 10.

An interpretation follows, based on an analysis of the quantitative scores on all the 10 cards as well as a qualitative evaluation of all the responses. Information pertaining to the individual's ability to cope with stressful situations, to attend to reality, to control his impulses, to relate to other people, as well as his feelings about himself and the way he might handle intellectual problems—these are among the facets of personality that may be uncovered.

The Thematic Apperception Test, otherwise known as the TAT, is often used along with the Rorschach. The former supplements the Rorschach findings and provides information more specifically concerned with (1) the person's relationships with significant people in his life and (2) his feelings about achievement and about intellectual and emotional involvement. The test consists of 19 pictures and 1 blank card. The subject is directed to tell a story about each picture, including in the story what has led up to the situation depicted, what the people are thinking about, and what might happen at the end. A modification of the TAT, devised for young children, is called the CAT (Children's Apperception Test) and differs from the TAT in that the pictures (10 in number) are of animal figures only.

The Figure Drawing Technique and some of its modifications, like the House, Tree, Person Test, may be used for subjects of all ages. In the Figure Drawing Test, the subject is first asked to draw a person, and then to draw another person of the opposite sex. Sometimes the subject is asked to tell about the people he drew. The drawings often reveal the acceptance of or confusion about a sexual role, the capacity for contact with others, the presence of anxiety, and generally the subject's feelings about himself. Drawings have also been used as a means to estimate intelligence for children up to 12 years of age. The House, Tree, Person drawings are handled similarly. The information obtainable from these devices depends greatly upon the clinical experience and skill of the examiner.

The Sentence Completion Test and Word Association Test are best considered together. The two methods may be so structured as to evoke from the person various kinds of reactions: feelings toward authority figures (parents, teacher, boss), siblings, or himself; and attitudes toward school, sex, or almost anything else. Typical beginnings of sentences are "There is no one . . ." or "Fathers are . . ." or "I envy . . ." or "My worst mistake . . ." The word association technique uses words that may or may not be emotionally charged, such as "woman," "dark," "ocean," "sour." Words on which the subject blocks (gives no response) or on which uncommon associations are given are particularly significant.

A projective device less often employed is the Make-A-Picture-Story Test (MAPS), in which the subject makes use of male, female, child, or animal cutout figures against a stage background. He then proceeds to tell a story for the setting he has constructed. Another is the Bender Gestalt, a test requiring the subject to copy nine geometric designs and then to reproduce them from memory. Accuracy of reproduction, additions to the original designs, and combinations of parts from different designs are some of the items observed. This technique is often used to evaluate brain damage. Among other projective devices occasionally employed are the Szondi, the Picture Frustration Test, and the Mosaic Test.

Uses of Projective Techniques. For the assessment of something as complex as personality, a single method cannot be expected to provide the necessary information. Psychologists, therefore, often use more than one method to throw light on various aspects of the personality and for corroboration of one set of results. In the hands of a well-trained psychologist who has also had wide clinical experience, these devices serve many useful purposes.

The most important reason for using a projective technique is to gain understanding of why an individual behaves the way he does. Psychologists and psychiatrists working in child-guidance clinics or in mental and penal institutions, as well as those in private practice, have come to rely on these methods for making a diagnosis and deciding upon treatment. It may be desirable for legal purposes to ascertain whether a person should be classified as neurotic, psychotic, suffering from brain damage, or normal. A diagnosis on the basis of an expert's experience, supported by the findings from projective techniques, has more validity than either one alone. These devices are also used effectively in vocational guidance, in educational planning, and in marriage and family counseling.

Projective techniques are utilized in business, industry, and the armed forces for the selection and placement of personnel. High-level positions are often filled only after a comprehensive examination of the candidate which includes a number of projective devices. They may also be used for prediction of success on specific jobs. Anthropologists have employed projective methods to aid in the understanding of the relationship between culture and personality. Therapists use them for evaluating success of psychotherapy or drug therapy. Research psychologists use them to lend insight into the developmental problems of thinking, perception, and learning.

PSYCHIATRY [sī-kī′ə-trē], that branch of medicine which deals with mental illness and emotional disorders.

History

Though psychological insights occurred throughout philosophy and literature, there was no formal practice of psychiatry until the 18th century, when medical personnel began to supervise the mentally ill. Prior to that time mental patients were maintained in monastic shelters or prisons.

The modern mental hospital may be said to have originated in revolutionary France under the guidance of Philippe Pinel (1745–1826), an enlightened and humane administrator who freed mental patients of their chains. Pinel abolished other coarse methods of treatment and introduced the practice of accurately recording case histories. Later Pinel's successor, Jean Esquirol, persuaded the French government to build a number of hospitals for the mentally ill. By the middle of the 19th century psychiatry was established as a discipline centered about the care of hospitalized patients. Disturbed individuals outside of institutions were usually treated by general practitioners, when they were treated at all.

The great classifier of mental disease was the German psychiatrist Emil Kraepelin (1856–1926). His textbook *Psychiatrie*, published in 1883, described and distinguished a number of disorders (dementia praecox, manic-depressive, psychosis, paranoia), introducing order into what had previously been a mass of unsystematized observations. Kraepelin's emphasis on the organic basis of disease was balanced by the approach of Adolf Meyer (1866–1950), a Swiss-born American psychiatrist, who believed that life experiences played a major role in causing mental illness.

Psychoanalysis and Psychiatry

Sigmund Freud (1856–1939) developed a systematic theoretical scheme for interpreting and treating emotional disorders. This system, called psychoanalysis, was revolutionary in a number of respects: (1) it offered an over-all explanation of normal as well as abnormal behavior; (2) it dealt with emotional disorders in individuals outside the mental hospital; (3) it conceived of the basis of mental illness as lying in childhood experiences; and (4) it offered a system of therapy based on an interpersonal relationship between patient and therapist.

Psychoanalysis spread from Vienna throughout Europe and to America and became a central technique in psychiatric practice. Splinter groups, differing in various points from the orthodox Freudian position, developed quickly, as Freud's early disciples, notably Carl Jung and Alfred Adler, set up schools of their own. Later, psychoanalysis became one of many techniques of psychotherapy, some of them based upon theories of human behavior greatly differing from Freud's original concept (*see* PSYCHOANALYSIS).

The Scope of Practice

Psychiatrists generally distinguish between two major groups of conditions: the organic diseases and the so-called functional disorders.

Organic Diseases. These involve physical changes in the tissues, such as might be caused by disease or injury to the brain and nervous system. In arteriosclerosis, or hardening of the arteries, narrowing of the arteries in the brain may diminish the blood supply to the brain, causing a decline in memory and mental alertness. Alcoholism may indirectly cause brain damage resulting from vitamin deficiencies. Many hereditary degenerative diseases of the nervous system cause psychiatric symptoms.

Functional Disorders. These include conditions in which there are disturbances in mental function without demonstrable tissue changes. Although these disorders are generally thought to originate from psychological stress, some authorities feel that they may really be caused by abnormalities in body chemistry. This point is still controversial.

This group of disorders may be subdivided into the psychoses, the neuroses, and the so-called character disorders. In the former, the individual suffers from distortions of reality in the form of hallucinations and delusions; extreme cases of psychosis usually require hospitalization. In the neuroses the individual is troubled by rigid, repetitive behavior which he is powerless to control. The aim of neurotic behavior is believed to be the control of anxiety. The neurosis may take the form of a phobia: an irrational dread of heights, closed places, or of any number of objects or situations. Neurosis may also appear as compulsive behavior (for example, repeated hand washing), or obsessive, nightmarish thoughts, such as the idea of burning one's house.

Persons with character disorders are essentially normal persons who are troubled by patterns of behavior which cause them difficulty in dealing with people. An example can be seen in the passive-aggressive personality who is unable to show open hostility, but may express his anger indirectly to those who do not deserve it. The passive-dependent person may become depressed when his slightest wish or need is not fulfilled.

Among the most difficult and perplexing patients seen by the psychiatrist are the psychopathic personalities, or sociopaths, who lie or cheat or abuse their friends and loved ones without apparent remorse or anxiety.

Diagnosing and Treating Disorders

The principal diagnostic procedure is the psychiatric interview, during which the patient's feelings and attitudes are explored by the psychiatrist and viewed in relation to his background and life history. The psychiatrist may call upon the psychologist to assess the patient's intelligence or to administer Rorschach (ink-blot) tests or other instruments for evaluating the central problems of the patient.

The psychiatrist makes use of two broad categories of treatment: the biological and the psychotherapeutic.

Biological Techniques. The biological approach makes use of drugs, surgery, and electrical stimulation.

Insulin coma therapy, introduced in Vienna by Manfred Sakel in 1932, was one of the earliest of these techniques. In this technique patients are given doses of insulin, a hormone which lowers the concentration of blood sugar. Since the brain depends upon sugar exclusively as an energy source, the individual lapses into a coma as the blood-sugar concentration falls. In some manner, as yet unknown, this "shock" to the nervous system produces improvement in some cases of early schizophrenia. Insulin shock treatment is no longer as popular as it once was.

Electroshock therapy is now widely used in mental hospitals. In this procedure an electric current is quickly passed through the brain, producing convulsions. The treatment is often effective in cases of depression and manias, and in some cases of schizophrenia. From 6 to 20 treatments are necessary to produce improvement.

Psychosurgery involves severing the fibers which link the frontal lobes with the rest of the brain. This is considered a drastic procedure and is used as a last resort when other forms of therapy fail. The operation apparently reduces anxiety and enables the patient to withstand frustration. In some cases, distressing personality changes, such as apathy, loss of drive, and a loss of a sense of social propriety, have resulted from the operation.

Psychopharmacology. A fairly recent and promising development in the treatment of the psychiatric disorders is the introduction of the tranquilizing drugs. Unlike the earlier barbiturates and other sedatives which calmed the patient by inducing drowsiness, the tranquilizers have the remarkable property of relieving depression and quieting excited patients without reducing mental alertness. Many of these compounds apparently affect the quality of the individual's emotional experience. Tranquilizers have quieted the wards of many mental hospitals and have significantly diminished the return rate in state hospitals.

Psychotherapy and Psychoanalysis. Psychoanalysis is the most intensive and prolonged form of psychotherapy, and is applied most often to the neuroses and character disorders. The analyst employs the technique of free association, in which the patient is expected to voice all thoughts which come to mind without attempting to censor those which he might feel to be embarrassing or irrelevant. The object of therapy is to give the patient an understanding of the history and nature of his disturbances so that he may act upon them. Treatment is given four or five times a week over a period of two to eight years, depending upon the individual case.

Other forms of psychotherapy are usually less intensive and ordinarily do not attempt to probe as deeply into the origins of the patient's problem. These shorter-term therapies may be applied to some psychotic patients as well as to neurotics and those suffering from character disorders.

Directive therapy differs from psychoanalysis and other types of psychotherapy in that the therapist attempts to suggest a course of action and attitude to be adopted by the patient. Directive therapy may make use of hypnosis or may rely solely on the strength and authority of the therapist.

Are Patients Cured? The word "cure" cannot be applied in its strictest sense to these modes of treatment. Although a single episode of depression may be interrupted or a patient freed of a delusion or an anxiety state relieved, these patterns of behavior tend to recur. If the recurrence is mild or temporary and does not disrupt adaptation or function, the patient may be said to be cured. Many patients, especially schizophrenics, may have to be treated continuously.

Biological Versus Nonbiological Psychiatrists. Psychiatrists tend to be divided into those who rely heavily on organic forms of treatment and those who are oriented to psychotherapy. The first group uses more electric shock, insulin shock, and drugs. They consider psychotherapy to be an adjunct to these forms of treatment. The second group relies heavily on psychoanalysis, seeking to understand the roots of the patient's disorder. The division is not, of course, hard and fast, as many psychiatrists use both approaches, modifying them to the case at hand.

Training. The psychiatrist's training consists of four years of medical school and one year of general internship, followed by a minimum of three years in residence in his specialty. During his residency the psychiatrist treats mentally ill patients under the supervision of trained practitioners. After his resident training, he must practice or work in a hospital for two or more years before he is eligible for certification by the specialty board. He may continue his training to specialize in a sub-field, such as child psychiatry, or enter a psychoanalytic institute to train as a psychoanalyst. Once he is fully trained, the psychiatrist may elect to remain in hospital work or he may enter research or private practice.

See also MENTAL ILLNESS; NEUROSIS; PSYCHOANALYSIS; PSYCHOTHERAPY.

PSYCHICAL RESEARCH. *See* PARAPSYCHOLOGY.

PSYCHOANALYSIS, also called "depth psychology," both a theory of human behavior and a method of treatment for some mental disorders. Psychoanalysis as a system was introduced by Sigmund Freud and later elaborated and modified by himself and others, including his daughter Anna Freud.

History. Psychoanalysis originated with *Studies in Hysteria* (1895), in which Joseph Breuer and Freud contended that the abnormal behavior of hysterical patients could be explained in terms of forgotten important events (*see* HYSTERIA). This observation formed the basis for the first important tenets of psychoanalysis. Psychological events are determined, not accidental, and there is meaningful continuity in mental life. Current psychological events, even those that seem strange or absurd, are part of an ongoing stream which is meaningful in its entirety. This continuity may not be apparent to rational awareness nor manifest in acts of will, for a large part of the mental stream is unconscious. The workings of the unconscious have been most clearly illustrated in Freud's dream research, in which he shows that even the most absurd dream may relate to desires of the dreamer and events of preceding days.

These two basic tenets provide the framework for the third: all mental activity is goal-directed. It is always intended to satisfy a drive, even though the drive and the intention may be unconscious. At this point Breuer and Freud parted ways, because Breuer could not attribute purposeful action to the unconscious. He considered unconscious processes an outcome of disruption of conscious purposiveness under stress.

Freud extended this third hypothesis further by asserting that the basic drives are simple and few in number. The list varied as the theory developed, but the instincts of sex and self-preservation were always prominent. Limiting the number of basic drives is important in psychoanalysis as well as in most other psychological theories, for it commits the theorist to try to understand the varieties of mental processes as numerous elaborations on a few simple themes.

Freud continued to build his theory, at first alone, later with an ever-increasing number of doctors, the famous Vienna Psycho-Analytical Society. The theory reached completion with its fourth basic tenet, that the experiences of early childhood predominate in shaping the personality, an idea that was hardly new. Freud's innovation was his emphasis on the unconscious character of early influences, especially those pertaining to sex. His doctrine of childhood sexuality outraged many of his contemporaries and drove away some of his followers, notably Jung.

Psychoanalytic Theory. According to Freud, the mind consists of three basic structures in constant interaction: the primitive, pleasure-seeking id; the superego, which guards morality and sets the standards for ideal behavior; and the practical ego, which has the responsibility of satisfying the id without affronting the superego, always within the limits imposed by the real world.

The energy to drive the mind is derived from instinctual urges that activate us unconsciously, so that we usually have no awareness of our basic motives. When the urges of the unconscious id are managed by the ego to the satisfaction of the superego, all is well. However, when the ego is overpowered by impulses from the id or restraints of the superego, anxiety may appear as a sign of dysfunction. This anxiety must be alleviated by means of defense mechanisms; or mental disorder, neurosis, and even psychosis may result.

The Freudian scheme of behavior may be best understood by considering the structures of the mind, the en-

MODEL OF THE MIND

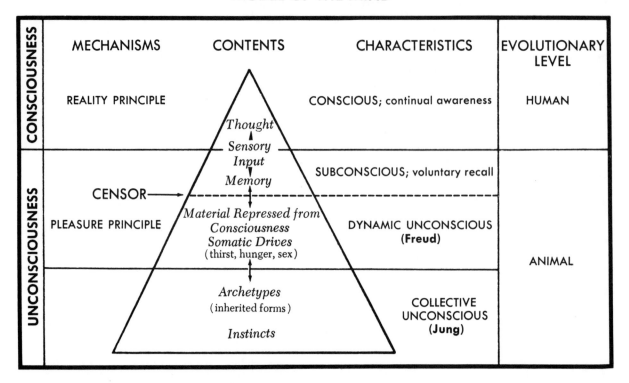

	MECHANISMS	CONTENTS	CHARACTERISTICS	EVOLUTIONARY LEVEL
CONSCIOUSNESS	REALITY PRINCIPLE	*Thought*	CONSCIOUS; continual awareness	HUMAN
UNCONSCIOUSNESS	CENSOR→	*Sensory Input Memory*	SUBCONSCIOUS; voluntary recall	
	PLEASURE PRINCIPLE	*Material Repressed from Consciousness Somatic Drives* (thirst, hunger, sex)	DYNAMIC UNCONSCIOUS (**Freud**)	ANIMAL
		Archetypes (inherited forms) *Instincts*	COLLECTIVE UNCONSCIOUS (**Jung**)	

ergy and instincts which move it, and the anxiety which plagues it.

Structures of the Mind

The id is the only part of the mind present from birth and is described by Freud as a "cauldron of seething excitement." It consists of instinctual needs seeking immediate gratification. Urges such as the impulse to urinate or defecate arise in the id and create tension, normally relieved by reflex activities that accomplish the desired act. In satisfying itself, the id obeys the pleasure principle of immediate gratification. To achieve this the id uses the primary process, the direct release of tension through body activity. The primary process cannot always act in this way, however, as in the case of hunger. Since no reflex can satisfy hunger, the id attempts to conjure up, or hallucinate, past memories of food, an obviously ineffective form of satisfaction. Because of the inadequacies of the primary process and because of the pressures of the real world, the id, which constitutes the whole mind in early infancy, eventually disconnects a part of itself to form the ego.

The ego is the mind's managing director, forming the seat of consciousness and developing as a mediator between the id's primitive desires and the realities of life. The id demands gratification, the ego decides if, when, where, and how the id desire can be satisfied. Freud compared this id-ego relationship to that of a horse and its rider, with the id the horse and the ego, the rider. The ego obeys the reality principle, which seeks to postpone gratification until conditions in the outside world are suitable.

The ego follows the reality principle through the use of the secondary process, the application of thought and judgment to decide how the id can best be satisfied. Once the ego has decided what is to be done, it puts the proposed solution into action and notes the outcome. This is known as reality testing.

The superego is the seat of conscience and morality and the last structure of the mind to develop. The final form of this structure depends upon a great crisis in the life of the child, resolution of the Oedipus complex. For a boy this complex describes his desire for his mother and consequent jealous antagonism toward his father. Since the boy cannot successfully compete with his father, a serious conflict arises which is normally solved by the boy by identifying with his father, figuratively taking him into his mind, to form the superego. The corresponding superego formation in the female stems from the Electra complex. Codes of conduct, concepts of morality, and ideals of society are now represented in this "parent-in-the mind," or superego.

When the child lives up to the superego's standards (the ego ideal), he is rewarded by feelings of pride. When he transgresses, he is punished by that part of the superego which may be called the conscience and which floods the ego with guilt.

Instincts and Mental Energy

Flow of Energy in the Mind. Mental energy is generated by biological drives such as thirst, hunger, and sex. Originally this primitive energy is found in the id and is discharged by reflex action (primary process) as quickly as it is formed. Later, with the development of the ego and the reality principle, the energy can no longer be quickly dissipated but is invested in memory, thought, and other ego activities (secondary process).

Instincts. Prior to 1920 Freud recognized two types of instincts, the ego instincts, concerned with the preservation of life, and the sexual instincts, concerned with the propagation of life. Later, to account for love, Freud merged the ego and sexual instincts into the life instinct, Eros. The death instinct, Thanatos, in opposition to Eros, accounts for aggressive and destructive impulses.

The manifestation of Eros is called libido and originally embodied only the sexual instinct. But when sex and ego instincts were merged into the life instinct, the term libido lost its exclusively sexual character, and came to refer to the general life force, comparable to Henri Bergson's *élan vital*.

The sexual instincts undergo a well-defined sequence of development. In the earliest stage, the oral phase, pleasure is obtained by sucking, biting, and other activities employing the mouth. Next comes the anal phase, wherein pleasure is associated with excretory activity, and later the phallic stage emerges, in which pleasure stems from genital stimulation. The child then passes into a latent stage which terminates at puberty, when the various phases merge into the adult sexual patterns. This sequence of development gives rise to such concepts as "oral" and "anal" personalities to describe individuals in whom traits associated with certain phases of development predominate.

Thanatos is manifested by aggression. The role of this self-destructive instinct has been little elaborated in psychoanalytic theory, and aggression has never been shown to be as necessary for an organism as the sexual drive or self-preservation.

The concept of sublimation is usually associated with the sexual instincts and describes the channeling of instinctual energy into socially productive activities. Freud believed that civilization is made possible by the sublimation of sexual energy into love for humanity and intellectual creativity.

Anxiety and Mental Disorder

Originally Freud conceived of anxiety as the outcome of id frustration. When a powerful id impulse is prevented from entering the ego, so the dammed up id energy is converted into anixety. In 1926 Freud revised this theory to stress the roles of anxiety and defense mechanisms in the handling of instinctual demands by the ego. The symptoms of mental disorder are explained as the ego's defective adaptation to inadequate integration of the instincts into the personality. The cure must therefore lie in treatment of the underlying, typically unconscious dynamics and not in the external symptoms.

The prototype of anxiety is birth, at which time the psyche is overwhelmed with stimulation. In infancy early anxiety-producing experiences involve a flooding of the immature ego with strong id desires, with which it is powerless to deal. For example, the id demands satisfaction of hunger, which cannot be obtained without the mother. Anxiety results if the mother is absent and the ego cannot bring her back by crying. Eventually the mother's absence alone may be sufficient to produce anxiety, since it signals the possibility of recurrence of the earlier situation to the ego. Adult anxiety occurs in two ways, when the ego is overwhelmed with stimulation and when it perceives the danger of being so overwhelmed.

The ego can be threatened from three directions, the id, the superego, and the real world. Id, or neurotic, anxiety stems from powerful drives, such as sex and hunger. Moral anxiety concerns the superego and occurs when the ego becomes aware of urges to violate the moral code. Realistic, or objective, anxiety emerges when the ego perceives a source of danger in the real world.

In self-protection against anxiety, the ego may employ defense mechanisms. Mental illness develops either when these mechanisms dominate and distort behavior or when too much energy is consumed by the ego's efforts to avoid anxiety. The individual may experience anxiety directly as nervousness, sweating, palpitations, and sleeplessness. More often the symptoms are indirect and give no obvious clue to their cause. In such cases a form of psychotherapy, including psychoanalysis, is indicated as treatment.

Psychoanalytic treatment is a form of psychotherapy that preceded the formulation of psychoanalysis as a general psychological theory. The technique started when Freud replaced hypnosis with the method of free association in the cathartic therapy of hysteria. Freud's own definition of psychoanalytic treatment can be summed up in his admonition, "where id was, shall ego be," that is, the patient should be helped to achieve awareness of the major contents of his unconscious.

The patient is asked to lie in a relaxed position and speak out whatever thoughts come into his mind, no matter how trivial or shocking they may seem to him. This technique is intended to reach unconscious material with as little interference as possible from the controlling defenses of the ego. Another method to probe the unconscious is the interpretation of dreams, which Freud labelled the "royal road" to understanding personality. Small lapses of normal speech and small anomalies in ordinary behavior also reveal the unconscious problems and processes described by Freud in his *Psychopathology of Everyday Life* (1904).

The unconscious material elicited with these methods is commented upon and interpreted by the analyst, an intimate procedure made possible by the peculiar relationship that evolves between patient and therapist called transference. Transference refers to the simultaneous affectionate and hostile relations that the patient develops with the therapist. These emotional responses are not based on actual situations with the therapist, but on the patient's former relations with his parents, such as the Oedipus complex. The therapist must "work through" these relationships with the patient to disentangle them, restructuring the patient's reactions to his childhood education and experiences.

Later Developments in Psychoanalysis. The above discussion is based primarily on Freud's own concepts and theories. Subsequent modifications introduced to the theory and practice of psychoanalysis have produced an overwhelming literature. The viewpoints of contemporary investigators change as knowledge increases.

The expanders of psychoanalytic theory who have remained essentially faithful to Freud's points of view are members of the "committee" formed in 1913. They include Ernest Jones, Sandor Ferenczi, Karl Abraham, Hans Sachs, Otto Rank, and later M. Eitington. Important contributors after the thirties were Anna Freud and Melanie Klein (child analysis), Franz Alexander (psychosomatic medicine), Géza Roheim and Abram Kardiner (anthropology and sociology).

Early dissenters among Freud's erstwhile followers were Adler, Stekel, and Jung, who broke with him before World War I. Adler founded what is known as *individual psychology*, stressing the aggressive reactions of the ego to a basic feeling of inferiority. His accent thus lies on the child's method of dealing with environmental conditions, especially the attitude he adopts toward his defects.

Jung based his *analytic psychology* more closely on the findings of psychoanalysis. He rejected, however, the primarily sexual meaning of libido, added a collective unconscious, and postulated a futuristic determinant in the behavior of the individual.

Later dissenters include Karen Horney, Eric Fromm, and Harry Stack Sullivan, who all place greater emphasis on individual adaptation to life situations, mainly of an interpersonal and social nature. Like Adler they emphasize environmental influence and try to incorporate it into their theories.

Status of Psychoanalysis. A compelling feature of psychoanalysis is its attempt to encompass both normal and abnormal behavior in a single system. Freud's theory has succeeded in explaining something about human behavior that has value in understanding human actions. Psychoanalysis, however, cannot account for the full range of psychological phenomena, nor can any other single theory of psychology.

Psychoanalysis is essentially a theory attributing psychological meaning to personal experience. Therefore, it may be considered only a psychology of meaningful connections (Jaspers) and thus may never account for causal relationships as it purports to do. Its greatest value lies in attempts to discover and describe the meaning of past events in terms of the patient's present life. This does not mean that therapeutic success can be expected only after adequate analysis of childhood memories, a position generally held until the thirties, because a patient may benefit even if ego cannot completely replace id.

Through psychoanalysis it has become generally accepted that the mind has unconscious, continuous, goal-seeking, and developmental aspects. It also represses thoughts or wishes, and mental disorder may relate to fixation of such repressed material or to regression of the psyche to prior developmental stages. Psychoanalysis has caused a shift in psychiatry from interest in symptoms to an analysis of the content.

Dissenters from classical psychoanalysis have partly revealed its shortcomings and restrictiveness, and currently under scrutiny by proponents as well as opponents of the theory are infantile sexuality and the drive structure. Both these concepts have been based on adult patients' statements rather than on their daily lives. The psychoanalytic literature lacks observational evidence in normal infants that sexuality really appears in satisfaction derived from

oral and anal pleasure zones and that the libido activates such areas.

Newer developments in child psychology (*see* CHILD DEVELOPMENT) question the relationships between normal infantile behavior and the appearance of specific characteristics in adults such as sexual perversions. Recent research in psychology and ethology is clarifying the role of different drives in the formation of behavior. A self-destructive instinct opposing a life instinct seems to be based more on the psychology of individual patients than the general behavior of human and animal societies.

See also:

DEFENSE MECHANISMS	OEDIPUS COMPLEX
DREAMS	PSYCHIATRY
FREUD, SIGMUND	PSYCHOTHERAPY
JUNG, CARL GUSTAV	SUBCONSCIOUS AND UN-
NEUROSIS	CONSCIOUS

PSYCHOKINESIS. *See* PARAPSYCHOLOGY.

PSYCHOLOGICAL WARFARE, the application of psychology to the conduct of war in an effort to win victories without force. Though psychological warfare embraces the use of unorthodox military techniques or unfamiliar instruments of war to panic, unnerve, or depress the enemy, the term has generally come to mean the use of propaganda, which has been defined as "organized persuasion by non-violent means." The object is to change the minds of the enemy. In the broadest sense, psychological warfare synchronizes political, propaganda, subversive, and military efforts with modern psychology to attain specified goals. The term "psychological warfare" is a recent one, but the actual practice of psychological warfare, which calls for a sure human touch, an inventive mind, and forcefulness in speech or writing, is as old as man.

Psychological warfare is directed against troops and civilians. It seeks to subvert beliefs and ideals; to promote treason; to cultivate resentment, cowardice, distrust, and prejudice; to divert public opinion; to depress morale; and to facilitate social disorganization and, ultimately, surrender. Strategic psychological warfare or propaganda wages a sustained campaign in an effort to achieve gradual, long-range influence. Tactical psychological warfare, or propaganda, seeks to accomplish immediate short-range results, usually in a local combat situation.

"White" propaganda, information issued from an acknowledged source, is overt psychological warfare. "Gray" propaganda does not clearly identify a source. "Black" propaganda, which purports to emanate from a source other than the true one, is covert or illicit psychological warfare. All are used.

Psychological warfare may employ truth or deception in the battle for men's minds. The means used include posters, loudspeakers, pamphlets, leaflets, radio broadcasts, news releases, and agents spreading rumors. In World War I and II and in the Korean War, leaflet printing became an adjunct to field operations. "Surrender passes" bearing promises of safety and good treatment were printed to entice enemy soldiers to give themselves up and were distributed by artillery shells and airplanes.

The British in World War I waged a superb propaganda

campaign among neutral nations. In comparison, the Germans were amateurish. The American psychological warfare effort in that war was the work of the Creel Committee, which distributed printed and filmed material and also provided speakers. In France the American Expeditionary Force (AEF) used morale and surrender leaflets effectively.

Propaganda, or psychological warfare, was later developed into a highly potent weapon, particularly by such dictators as Benito Mussolini, Adolf Hitler, and Joseph Stalin. During World War II American psychological warfare was under the direction of the Office of War Information and the Office of Strategic Services.

Brainwashing, a subtle technique allied to psychological warfare, first won attention during the notorious Soviet purge trials of the 1930's, when high officials made spectacular and implausible confessions. Use of drugs or hypnosis is sometimes suspected in brainwashing, but the technique is generally believed to be derived from social psychology. Once the individual is isolated from the group and his sense of social cohesiveness has been destroyed, he becomes susceptible to suggestion and conversion to a particular point of view or ideology. Some American and allied prisoners of war were brainwashed in Korea by the Chinese Communists.

PSYCHOLOGY [sī-kŏl'ō jĭ]. As a science, psychology may be defined as the systematic study of the processes whereby the individual human being—or animal—interacts with the environment. As a profession, it may be defined as the attempt to apply the knowledge and methods of psychology to the solution of problems of human welfare.

Psychology as a Science

The definition of psychology as a science includes an emphasis on *systematic study of processes* in order to set scientific psychology apart from prescientific, or "common sense," psychology. This latter sort of psychology is likely to be casual and one-shot rather than systematic or cumulative and is likely to be more concerned with immediate prediction than with the formation of a complete picture of the processes involved as the organism lives its life. Many psychologists would prefer to substitute the term *behavior* for the term *processes* in the definition, for objectively observable behavior is the bedrock subject matter of the science. In fact, psychology is frequently described as a behavioral science. The general term *processes*, however, does not exclude *conscious* processes from the proper province of psychology. For purposes of definition it does not matter that the conscious processes of one individual can be studied by another individual only through observation of what that individual says and does.

The term *individual* is included in the definition to draw a distinction between psychology and those disciplines—such as sociology, cultural anthropology, and political science—that tend to focus their interest on groups, institutions, or cultures rather than on individuals. Actually, social psychology, a field on the border between psychology and sociology, often does concern itself with groups, but even in that borderline specialty there remains an emphasis on the individual as he behaves in a group or social setting. The definition also uses the general term *organism* rather than the more specific term *human organism* to indicate that psychologists, though primarily concerned with human beings, are interested in all organisms, or in the living organism in general, and seek the basic general laws of organismic interaction with the environment. Hence the frequent use of subhuman organisms in experimental research. The phrase *interacts with* is used instead of the frequently encountered *adjusts to* to emphasize the active and dynamic nature of behavior. Psychology does not regard living as a matter of relatively fixed and relatively passive responses to environmental events.

Beginnings of Psychology. In a general sense the history of psychology is as long as the history of the human race. Since the dawning of human self-consciousness man has had a curiosity about himself and has tried, often in strange and wonderful ways, to understand and predict his own behavior. Scientific psychology, however, cannot be said to have begun until the second half of the 19th century. A frequently cited year of birth is 1879, the year of the founding of Wilhelm Wundt's Psychological Laboratory at Leipzig, Germany. Previously, however, there had been a good deal of research and writing which, at least in retrospect, appears psychological in character. Wundt himself had already produced his monumental book *Outlines of Physiological Psychology* (1873–74), and philosophers, physiologists, and others had turned concentrated attention to psychological matters.

More than two centuries before Wundt, René Descartes had written about reflex action, had speculated about the role of the nervous system in behavior, and had formulated a theory of mind-body interaction. Thomas Hobbes in his *Leviathan* (1651) had written about the social nature of man and had evolved a theory of motivation and of the association of ideas. John Locke, George Berkeley, and John Stuart Mill in England, David Hume in Scotland, and J. F. Herbart in Germany had written extensively about the processes whereby the individual interacts with his environment.

In Germany the physiologist E. H. Weber had conducted his experiments in the physiology of the senses and had become interested in sensation. Gustav Fechner had turned from physics to philosophy and to experiments on the systematic relationship between sensation on the one hand and physical stimuli on the other. Hermann von Helmholtz had conducted his studies of nerve conduction and had published his *Physiological Optics* (1856). In France, Philippe Pinel and others had begun early in the 19th century the enlightened psychological interpretation of insanity. In England, Charles Darwin had published *Origin of Species* (1859), a book that was to have as enormous an influence on psychology as on other disciplines. The versatile Sir Francis Galton had begun his studies of individual differences and had evolved his ingenious techniques of measurement.

Wundt's laboratory, however, was the first research establishment given an explicit psychological label. Wundt was the first man deliberately to undertake the creation, through the experimental approach, of a systematic, scientific body of knowledge about the interaction of the organism with its environment.

Psychology in America. By the start of the 20th century, psychology had come to the United States to stay. Since then, except for the influence of psychoanalysis, originated by the Viennese physician Sigmund Freud, and the contribution of the German Gestalt psychologists Max Wertheimer, Kurt Koffka, and Wolfgang Köhler, all of whom eventually moved to the United States, the young science has been primarily an American science in both location and flavor.

William James, G. Stanley Hall, and E. B. Titchener were, in point both of time and of influence, pioneers in American psychology. James, an eminent philosopher, psychologist, and physiologist, was conducting psychological experiments at Harvard as early as 1875 and soon thereafter began work on his classic *Principles of Psychology*, published, after 12 years of work, in 1890. Hall, a Massachusetts farm boy, early decided to go to Germany to study with Wundt but landed instead at Harvard where he worked with James, taking his doctoral degree in psychology in 1878. He then went to Germany for a period. Returning to the United States and to the new Johns Hopkins University, he established in 1883 what is regarded as the first psychological research laboratory in America. In 1888 he became the first president of Clark University and helped make Clark a leading center of psychological research. Titchener, an Englishman who studied with Wundt at Leipzig, moved to Cornell University in 1892 and took charge of the newly established psychological laboratory, which he directed for the next 35 years. Although working in America, he continued to represent the Germanic tradition in psychology.

Among the other leading psychologists in the early history of the discipline in America was J. McKeen Cattell, who studied with Wundt at Leipzig and with Hall at Johns Hopkins, founded the psychological laboratory at the University of Pennsylvania in 1888, and went on to Columbia University in 1891. He remained there for 26 years, doing pioneer research in a wide variety of fields, including that of the measurement of individual differences. The list of American pioneers also included John Dewey, philosopher and educator, who worked with Hall at Johns Hopkins, G. T. Ladd, J. M. Baldwin, Joseph Jastrow, E. C. Sanford, James Rowland Angell, and Harvey A. Carr.

Schools of Psychology

The early American history of the new discipline may be described as an era of schools of psychology. A school of psychology can be defined in terms of its basic conception of the proper subject matter of psychology and of the proper approach to its study. The historically definable schools include (1) structuralism, (2) functionalism, (3) behaviorism, (4) Gestalt psychology, and (5) psychoanalysis.

Structuralism, with Wundt and Titchener its most eminent proponents, concerned itself with the "structure of mind." According to this school the basic problems of psychology are (1) the analysis of mental phenomena into their elements by means of introspection and (2) the discovery, also through introspection, of the ways in which the elements are connected. The structuralists, therefore, studied sensations, images, feelings, perceptions, and ideas and sought to understand the basic regularities and laws of mental life. Introspection implies "looking into" oneself and attempting to report what goes on.

The functionalists, with Dewey, Angell, and James in the forefront, had no patience with the neat introspective approach of the structuralists. They wished not so much to understand the structure of mind but rather the function of mind as the organism goes about its business of interacting with its environment. They were more akin to Darwin in emphasis on the adjusting organism than to Wundt in his emphasis on the conscious organism. Also, the functionalists inclined more toward the objective observation of behavior than to the introspective observation of awarenesses.

Behaviorism, historically associated with the name of John B. Watson, grew up around the time of World War I. Like functionalism, it arose as a protest against the introspective approach and against the sterility of a concentration on the study of consciousness. Watson maintained that the true subject matter of psychology is behavior and that its aim, as in other natural sciences, is prediction and control—in this instance, of behavior. He further maintained that its method is the objective observation of actual behavior—the doings and sayings of people—rather than the introspective study of conscious states, which Watson did not believe could be established as scientifically nutritious phenomena.

Gestalt psychology grew up in Germany shortly after the turn of the century under the initial leadership of Max Wertheimer and his two illustrious students, Kurt Koffka and Wolfgang Köhler. Gestalt may be translated "pattern," "organization," or "configuration." The adherents of this school rejected what they considered a fruitless concentration on elements in both the structuralistic and the behavioristic approaches. They felt that both the Titchenerian elements of mind and the Watsonian elements of behavior represented artificial entities produced by the methods of the researchers and that all experience and all behavior are, in psychological reality, organized. Behavior is not to be viewed in terms of specific responses to specific stimuli, but in terms of patterns of behavior in a complex psychological field. Similarly, conscious life is a life of organized perceptions and meanings rather than a life built up through the bundling together of separate elements of mind.

The psychoanalytic school, if it can be called that, originated with Sigmund Freud in Vienna. It had historical roots in the philosophy of Herbart and Franz Brentano and in the ideas of Jean Charcot and Pierre Janet about the nature of mental aberrations. Psychoanalysis developed outside the pale of what was, in the first decade of the 20th century, traditional psychology. It dealt with motives and personality, concepts then foreign to psychology. Freud, facing a wealth of data on the strange inner lives of disturbed individuals, created a dynamic theory of personality in an attempt to account for the behavior he observed. His view of personality, as modified somewhat by himself and his followers, still influences the way psychologists and psychiatrists conceive of personality.

In a broad sense, psychoanalytic psychology is but one facet of what may be termed dynamic psychology—psychology that emphasizes, as does present-day common-sense psychology, the role of the individual's motives in producing observable behavior. In this sense Freud and William McDougall, the later studying the role of what used to be called instincts in human behavior, belong in the same category. These two, with others, can be viewed as the fathers of that segment of modern psychology concerning itself with human motivation and with other aspects of the dynamics of personality.

Modern Psychology

Modern psychology is a many-branched product of its history. Its journals and books show diversified flowerings of each of its historical roots. No one approach, no one theory, no one school has come to dominate the field. After World War II even the definable schools of psychology had become indistinct. Each had made an impression, each a contribution. E. G. Boring, psychology's leading historian, observed that each of the schools had died of success. Each made its point and each influenced many psychologists, but without winning actual converts. Modern psychology is not characterized by schoolishness but by tremendously varied specialization. The specialization is determined not by philosophic slant, or by method, or by loyalty to a gifted master. It is determined, rather, by the curiosity of the individual psychologist as it is focused on one aspect or another, and at one level of analysis or another, of the process whereby the individual organism interacts with its environment.

The diversity of approach and of content in psychology is shown in the various classification systems of its branches, which are used to classify books and articles relating to psychology. A system that has often been followed is the one that appeared in the 1960's in the *Psychological Abstracts*, an American journal carrying summaries of published materials judged to be of interest to psychologists. The branches of psychology can be described and classified in various ways. For example, industrial psychology (or, as it is often called, personnel psychology) may be treated as a field by itself rather than being grouped with military psychology. The two fields are closely related, since many of the same personnel problems are found in industry and in military services. It is neither possible nor desirable to make complete distinctions between branches of psychology. This point is further illustrated below in the discussion of psychology as a profession. For example, tests and measuring devices —although sometimes regarded as belonging in a separate field—are used in the measurement of personality, of abilities, of educational achievement, and in other areas. Clinical psychologists, the largest professional group, draw information from the categories "Therapy, Guidance, and Mental Health," "Abnormal Psychology," and others.

Psychology as a Profession

Psychology as science had not long existed when it became apparent that scientific psychological knowledge had relevance for man's practical affairs. It became clear also that the methods evolved by scientific psychologists to increase their knowledge could be employed in gathering data bearing directly on problems of no direct concern to scientists but having considerable significance for improving individual adjustment and for various purposes of business, industry, education, and government. Applied psychology grew out of purely scientific psychology, and psychology as a profession evolved from psychology as a science. By the 1970's more than half the 26,000 psychologists in the country were employed outside the academic setting. They were engaged either in research in applied psychology or in rendering professional services of a psychological character.

Growth of the Profession. World War I saw the first large-scale application of psychological knowledge to the solution of practical problems. A pressing wartime problem was selecting personnel for military service and assigning individuals to duties that matched their intellectual abilities. Under the leadership of Robert M. Yerkes, psychologists organized themselves, first as volunteering civilians and later as an official military group, to adapt existing tests of intelligence for use on large groups of people and then to test and classify millions of citizen soldiers. During the generation after World War I there was continued progress in applying psychology to the solution of practical problems.

World War II brought on a truly major effort to turn psychology's resources to practical affairs. Psychological tests—of intelligence, of abilities and aptitudes, and of personality—were used on an unprecedented scale to select and to classify military personnel. Psychologists also worked extensively on other problems, such as effective training methods, the design of equipment for most efficient human use, morale, organization, and leadership, and on clinical problems involving the diagnosis and treatment of emotional disturbances.

After World War II and the wartime demonstration of psychology's practical usefulness, psychology became firmly established as an applied science and psychology as a profession became a reality. Of the various professional specialities, clinical psychology showed the most rapid growth, with approximately 40% of all psychologists classifying themselves as clinical. Large numbers of clinicians were employed in mental hospitals, mental health clinics, and other settings where they were concerned with the diagnosis and treatment of various kinds of emotional troubles of individuals.

Also after the war there was a significant increase in the numbers of industrial, counseling, school, engineering, and other kinds of applied psychologists. Under the last six of the eleven headings in the classification of psychological literature can be found a listing of the major problems of an applied or professional nature with which psychologists concern themselves. The term "consulting psychology" is often applied to work in these fields. The distinctive feature of consulting psychology is that the psychologist is in private practice and serves on a fee basis rather than being on the staff of a school, clinic, hospital, or other organization. Firms of consulting psychologists have been organized and offer counseling to individuals and organizations. The postwar increase in the number of applied psychologists was accompanied by an approximately proportional increase in the number of psychologists devoting themselves to research and teaching in academic settings.

Standards for Professional Practice. By the 1960's psychology had become firmly established and organized as a profession. The American Psychological Association (APA) had formulated and adopted a code of professional ethics and had established procedures for dealing with unethical conduct on the part of its members. It had also established a number of boards and committees to deal, on a national level, with purely professional matters. The American Board of Examiners in Professional Psychology had been independently established as a specialty board equipped to issue diplomas to those clinical, industrial, and counseling psychologists judged to meet high standards of professional competence. Many states had enacted legislation providing for the issuance of certificates or licenses to psychologists who met explicit standards of competence for professional practice.

Moreover, the qualifications of the professional psychologist had been specified. At the highest level, he was defined as an individual who had received the Ph.D. degree or its equivalent from a recognized institution of higher learning, who had had five or more years approved experience in a psychological specialty, and who had satisfactorily passed the relevant examinations of the American Board of Examiners in Professional Psychology.

At a lower level, a professional psychologist was defined as an individual who had received some graduate training in psychology from a recognized institution of higher learning, was gainfully employed in rendering psychological services, and had been certified by a state or other agency as competent to perform psychological services.

Where there are no state or other agencies for certifying the professional competence of psychologists, it becomes difficult for a prospective client to know whether a person who calls himself a psychologist has a legitimate right to do so. Most reputable psychologists in the United States, whether they are performing professional services or are engaged in research and teaching in academic settings, are members of the APA. The purpose of this major national organization of psychologists is "to advance psychology as a science, as a profession, and as a means of promoting human welfare."

To become an associate of the APA an individual must have completed two years of graduate study of psychology in a recognized graduate school and must be devoting full time to work or graduate study that is psychological in nature. Alternatively, he must have obtained a master's degree in psychology from a recognized graduate school, have completed one year of experience in psychological work, and be employed in work of a psychological nature. One may become a full member of the APA upon the completion of the doctoral degree in psychology from a recognized graduate school. Fellows of the association must have the Ph.D. degree, have five years of experience beyond the degree, and show evidence of an outstanding contribution to the field of psychology.

Psychology in Canada. In Canada the national professional organization is the Canadian Psychological Association. Just as the American body has affiliated groups in the states, the Canadian organization has affiliated associations in the provinces. Canadian psychologists, like their colleagues in the United States, have for years been aware of the need to set standards for the practice of psychology. One notable step was the Ontario Psychologists Registration Act of 1960. This law empowered a board of examiners to register as psychologists those who met qualifiations for a professional title.

PSYCHOLOGY, ABNORMAL

Abnormal psychology is devoted to the study of emotional and mental disorder. Like psychiatry, the medical specialty concerned with such disorders, abnormal psychology studies recurring patterns of behavior desturbances. Unlike psychiatry, however, it concentrates exclusively on research into the cause, description, and classification of these abnormalities, rather than on their treatment. Along with experimental and physiological psychology, abnormal psychology was recognized as a distinct field of study around 1900. It provides much of the theoretical and empirical basis for psychiatry and clinical psychology and has gradually become closely connected with these fields. Presently there is much cooperation among the practitioners of all three. The results and methods of experimental and physiological psychology are also proving relevant to the study of abnormal behavior, as exemplified by the effects of conditioning and drugs on behavior and emotional states.
See also MENTAL HEALTH; PSYCHIATRY.

PSYCHOLOGY, CLINICAL

Clinical psychology is a branch of psychology dealing with diagnosis and treatment of problems in behavior. Originally concerned with the evaluation of mental abilities through intelligence tests, clinical psychology is now much expanded. It includes assessment of personality, and diagnosis and treatment of mental disorders. The psychiatrist, seeking to find out the kind of disorder and the recommended treatment for a patient, might refer him to a clinical psychologist for special testing or interviews.

The clinical psychologist is a Ph.D. who has received clinical training, enabling him to act as a psychotherapist. His practice partly overlaps that of the psychiatrist. But, while both are trained in the treatment of mental disorders, the psychiatrist possesses a medical degree, which permits him to prescribe such medical treatment as drug and shock therapy. The clinical psychologist may be part of a mental health team in a psychiatric hospital or outpatient treatment center. He may work in a mental health clinic or have a private practice. Often, he is engaged in research on mental disorders. Both abnormal psychology and clinical psychology are involved in studying mental disorders, but clinical psychology tends to emphasize the evaluation of practical procedures for dealing with behavior problems. In the 1960's clinical psychologists also became involved in community mental health activities, to design programs for preventing mental disorders.
See also COMMUNITY PSYCHIATRY; MENTAL HEALTH; PSYCHIATRY.

PSYCHOLOGY, COMPARATIVE

Comparative psychology, sometimes called animal psychology, deals with similarities and differences in the behavior of animals as related to similarities and differences in bodily structure. Animals of all degrees of complexity, from protozoans to primates, are studied. The researcher assesses their sensory and motor capacities, their needs and preferences, their emotional reactions, and their learning and problem solving. These studies are made, not only in the native habitats of the animals, but also in the laboratory, where the conditions of observation are more easily controlled and where more precise measurements of behavior are possible. Zoologists as well as psychologists study animal behavior. Zoologists are interested for the most part in the instinctive activities of animals drawn from the lower end of the evolutionary scale, since in them the mechanisms underlying behavior seem particularly accessible. Comparative psychologists are interested for the most part in the intellectual capabilities of animals closer to man in the scale, since man is their principal concern.

The first textbook of comparative psychology, *Animal Intelligence* (1881), by G. J. Romanes, was based largely on anecdotal materials—tales told by hunters, pet lovers, zoo keepers, and other casual observers. This book greatly exaggerated the animals' achievements and the kinship of these with human achievements. An important figure in the turn-of-the-century transition from anecdotalism to the modern, experimental movement was C. Lloyd Morgan, an English psychologist. He emphasized the need for systematic and sustained investigation and for cautious interpretation. In compensation for the common tendency to humanize animals, Morgan suggested the following rule: Do not attribute to the action of higher processes any behavior that can be interpreted as well in terms of the action of lower processes.

If one person can be said to have ushered in the modern period, it is Edward L. Thorndike, an American psychologist, who devised ingenious techniques for the study of learning in animals. His work with chickens, cats, dogs, and monkeys led him to a bold new theory, published in *Animal Intelligence* (1911). All animals, said Thorndike, may be regarded as systems of connections between sensory and motor mechanisms. Some systems are inherited, and some are acquired in the course of experience. Intellectual differences among animals reduce to differences in the speed with which they form connections and in the number of connections they are capable of forming. There is no qualitative difference, Thorndike asserted, between the intelligence of man and that of the lower animals. It is only because "he learns fast and learns much, in the animal way" that man may seem to function in a manner of his own.

Observing a variety of animals in a variety of experimental situations patterned after those of Thorndike, the early comparative psychologists were more impressed by the similarities in behavior than by differences. Although skeptical at first, they quickly succumbed to the Thorndikian view. As a result (since specialization has obvious advantages), the scope of research narrowed sharply. Attention gradually became fixed on a small number of mammalian forms—primarily the rat—which were chosen largely for reasons of convenience and were treated as representative of animals in general. It was not until the

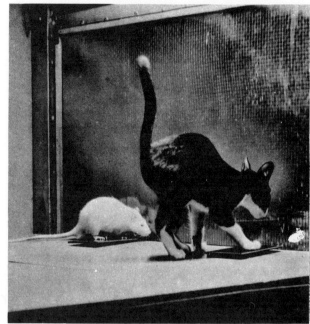

Wide World

The rat and cat in a comparative psychology experiment have learned to co-operate in pushing floor buttons to reach food.

second half of the 20th century that the Thorndikian hypothesis began once more to come under critical scrutiny and the foundations of a systematic comparative psychology began to be laid.

See also CONDITIONING; INSTINCT; LEARNING.

PSYCHOLOGY, DEVELOPMENTAL

Developmental psychology is a branch of psychology devoted to the study of the behavior of children. Historically, emphasis has been placed on the search for those elements of behavior in the child which are thought to be prerequisite for complex adult behavior. Theories have been developed which attempt to account for the constantly shifting patterns of these elementary processes as they mature and combine throughout childhood.

In the 19th century the young child was thought to be no different from the adult except in size. As knowledge of the function of the nervous system increased, biologically and psychologically oriented theories of growth and development evolved. Prominent is the psychoanalytic concept of child psychological development. In this concept, Freud's insight into the crucial nature of early experiences in the formation of adult personality patterns is worked out. The work of Arnold L. Gesell in the United States and Jean Piaget in Switzerland have also greatly influenced our views on child behavior. In the 1960's developmental psychologists were called upon to lend their best efforts towards ameliorating the problems of underprivileged children. It was felt that application of already well-established child development theories could correct growing problems in the education of the poor.

See also ADOLESCENCE; CHILD DEVELOPMENT.

PSYCHOLOGY, EDUCATIONAL

Educational psychologists are concerned with broad applications of the principles of psychology to problems of education, both in and out of the classroom. Since students and teachers are people, consideration of the psychology of their behavior could be as broad as the psychology of people anywhere. In other words, the study of educational psychology could be identical with the study of total psychology itself. In view of the fact, however, that educational psychologists often place special emphasis on the activities of the teacher and learner centered around the school situation, three basic problems of educational psychology can be categorized: (1) the preparation of the teacher for engaging in the teaching process, (2) the application of psychological laws to the teaching process itself, and (3) the psychological evaluation of the success of the educative process.

Preparation of the Teacher

The teacher must know how and what kind of information to gather regarding the student he is to teach. Each child brings with him to the classroom a unique biological and cultural background. Children are differently endowed with intellectual gifts and handicaps and have had various types of upbringing and early experiences. These differences seem to be among the important reasons why students tend to stand at different points between the two extremes, the earnest learner and the passive slacker.

If the teacher is to bring out the best efforts of his students, he must be able to gather information about their levels of intellectual, social, emotional, and physical maturing. The varieties of home life and child-parent relationships of his students and the extent to which the individual student has the ability to put himself in another person's place will be important. The educational psychologist is concerned with these aspects of the student-learner and can supply the teacher with much useful information concerning the relationship of learning ability of students to their personality characteristics.

The teacher should also be acquainted with the vast literature dealing with the judicious and effective use of rewards and punishments and their effects on the speed and efficiency of learning. Since each child is different from every other child, not all rewards and punishments are equally effective in the learning situation for all children. Part of the preparation of the teacher, therefore, consists of familiarizing himself with what psychology has to say about this very important motivational aspect of the learning situation.

The teacher must also achieve a reasonably accurate psychological picture of himself. Even though a teacher may have studied the psychology of people in general, he may not know how he as a person stands in relation to others. He may thus make many needless mistakes as a teacher. With a reasonable amount of self-insight, he may not fall so readily into the trap of projecting his own faults and strong points onto his students. The clinically oriented educational psychologist can be of service in helping the teacher to acquire such necessary self-knowledge.

Application of Psychology to Teaching

The teaching process is concerned not only with the teaching and learning of academic material, but also is extended by some educational psychologists to include the teaching of such things as the rules of good conduct, good citizenship, and emotional maturity. Learning, no matter where it takes place—in the laboratory, in the classroom, or in less formalized life outside the school—is possibly governed by the same basic laws that govern learning in the classroom. A similar statement can be made in regard to motivation, thinking, and problem solving. For this reason, these topics will be discussed briefly as they apply to the academic situation.

Learning in the Classroom. According to some theories, learning is motivated by a condition of learned or biologically determined need. Because of this need, the person may become active. It is not necessary that he be conscious of the reasons for his activity. During the course of such activity he may, by purpose or by chance, behave in such a way that his need will be reduced. Such a response, which thus has eventuated in the need reduction, will be learned and will become more probable in the future, if such a need arises again in comparable circumstances. Such learning, often referred to as instrumental or operant learning, is said by many leading learning theorists to be the reason for the development of much important human behavior. It should be noted, however, that some learning theorists explain all learned behavior on the basis of a second type of learning to be considered later in this discussion.

The duty of the teacher, then, might be to arrange situations in the classroom so that students will feel a need—experience a "felt discomfiture"—when faced with a problem which they are supposed to solve. As a result of this felt need, it is hoped that the student will engage in appropriate activities such as reading, discuss material that could be involved in the eventual solution of the problem, or in some other way gather information that may bear on the solution. As a result of such activities, he may discover the solution to the problem, or the teacher may help to guide him to its solution. If such a discovery of a solution is satisfying to the student, he will be more likely, in future problem situations, to behave similarly and discover solutions to other and perhaps increasingly difficult problems. The good teacher sees to it that all of the students are faced with a procession of problems requiring solutions; that occasional success accompanies reasonable effort on the part of the student; and that his successes are followed by circumstances interpreted by him as pleasurable.

Coupled with the learning of solutions to felt problems as described above is perhaps a second kind of learning. When a stimulus, object, person, or even a situation that an individual neither likes nor dislikes is paired with a stimulus, object, person, or situation that an individual does like or dislike, the result may be as follows: The neutral stimulus takes on some of the nonneutrality of the second stimulus with which it has been paired. This previously neutral stimulus, onto which the nonneutral stimulus has "rubbed off," can now become one which the individual will work to get or to avoid. For example, when gold stars are continually paired with praise from the teacher, classmates, or parents, gold stars tend to take on reward value of their own, and students may work to obtain them.

It is a prime task of any teacher to know which rewards

or punishments are important motivators for the students in his class. These are the rewards that will help to maintain the learning activities of his class. If there are few rewards common to many members of the class, the wise teacher will develop more. He will do so by pairing such potential rewards with situations that are thought of as pleasurable by most of the students in the class. Good grades, a smile of approval, the granting of extra privileges, or the mere pointing out of the general usefulness of knowledge may become rewarding enough to motivate all sorts of productive work on the part of the student.

Methods of Motivation in the Classroom. What has been said about learning theory indicates that motivating students to think and learn is a prime problem of the classroom teacher and the educational psychologist. They must be on a constant search for reasonable goals toward which reasonable students will strive.

A few students will engage in all sorts of learning and thinking activities when their only apparent satisfaction is that of knowing that they have added new information, techniques, or understanding to their already considerable knowledge. Other students work most diligently for the approval of their teachers, parents, or classmates. Others are sparked to their greatest activity by grades or degrees. Still others find great rewards in their ability to apply newly learned knowledge to such things as a conversation with a friend, a summer job, or the study of another academic discipline. The educational psychologist is searching for answers to such questions as why students differ in their choice of goals and what rewards are most effective for motivating desirable activity. Something is known in these areas, but much needs to be discovered.

The educational psychologist can make many suggestions to the teacher about such topics as the following: the possible temporary effect of punishment; the desirability of easily graded steps of presentation of the subject matter to the student; the possibility that much less is forgotten by the student than is usually believed; the fact that the biological inheritance and background of experience in previous learning affect the learner's ability to perceive; the fact that the ability of children to think and learn is affected by their differing physical ages and receptor sensitivities; and that all learners differ, both quantitatively and qualitatively, in their patterns of basic and learned needs, drives, and tensions.

Thinking in the Classroom. Thinking, particularly the process of creative problem solving, is another area with which the teacher should be concerned. It is an area to which the psychologist and educational psychologist also have something to contribute. Here again, as in the field of learning, the student will often have to be made conscious that problems exist and are in need of solution. The educational psychologist can point out to the schoolroom teacher that a person involved in the creative thinking process typically follows certain steps toward the solution of problems. Correct solutions are most often reached by those possessing the most knowledge of how others have reached solutions to roughly similar problems. The teacher should know that by careful organization of material he can make for more meaningful and rapid solutions of problems and that the mental "set" or prejudices of a student may impede or enhance his ability to solve problems.

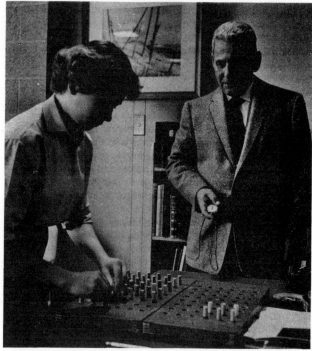

Hays—Monkmeyer

A high school guidance counselor gives a student a manual dexterity test. Trained in personnel psychology, the counselor uses test results to advise the student on choice of occupation and studies.

Evaluating the Educative Process

Evaluating any program, particularly an all-embracing educational program, is a task any reasonable person will approach with humility. The educational psychologist can aid the teacher in his quest for better and more accurate measuring techniques and instruments. To evaluate any educational program, it is necessary to be familiar with the student at the start of the program and to be able to measure the student at the end of the process of formal education or at the end of a stage in the process. How such an educated student compares with people of the same age who have had less education is a necessary third ingredient for measuring the success (or lack of success) of any educational program.

In order to obtain such information it has been necessary for the psychologist and the educational psychologist to develop, revise, discard, and redevelop countless measuring devices: intelligence tests, tests of attitudes, and of social, emotional, mental, and intellectual maturity, to name but a few. Such tests, together with those that attempt to measure biological differences in the developing individual, differences in ability to respond to learned motivators and be goaded to activity, and differences in goals toward which students strive, are major interests of the educational psychologist.

It is apparent that the educational psychologist must lean heavily on psychologists working in all fields. In the future he may lean particularly heavily on the physiological psychologist, whose work is destined to probe the mysteries of the physiology of such processes as learning and memory. The "conquest of the student" is, in many ways, identical to the conquest of man himself. It is probably true that the laws that govern the learning process in the school are the same laws that govern the learning of man in less formalized learning situations.

See also CONDITIONING; LEARNING; TESTING, PSYCHOLOGICAL AND EDUCATIONAL; THINKING.

PSYCHOLOGY, EXPERIMENTAL

Experimental psychology studies behavior by means of experiments, usually in a laboratory. This kind of investigation may apply the most sophisticated and complex methods, such as computer-controlled programs for the teaching of reflex actions. Nevertheless, experimental psychology is limited to those areas of behavior which can be studied in an experimental situation. Experiments are best suited to study such events as the number of trials needed to learn something or to solve a problem. Problems are often reduced to their simplest forms, such as having a rat press a bar for food. The variables which influence the process are then studied systematically, and from the data laws are deduced to be applied to behavior in general.

Psychophysics, a branch of experimental psychology, is concerned with human perception, such as reaction time, as it is affected by different conditions and stimuli. Another branch, originated by the Russian physiologist Ivan Pavlov, is the study of conditioning. Pavlov studied automatic physiological reflexes, such as the flow of saliva after presentation of food, and the ways in which such responses could become associated with other conditions.

Pavlov's work led to the operant-conditioning techniques of B. F. Skinner and others, in which animals can be conditioned to respond to a stimulus with a complex

St. Louis Post-Dispatch—Black Star

The cat in a discrimination test has learned to choose the black bowl, concealing liver bits, and to ignore the empty white bowl.

materialize, and the great stress and risk involved in some peacetime and many wartime situations.

A large number of basic psychological techniques have either been originated or vastly improved as a result of their application in military environments. The first successful group intelligence testing was done in World War I by U.S. Army psychologists, who developed tests for assessing the trainability of both literate and illiterate recruits. The personnel testing program that grew up in action, for example by pressing a bar for food. Gradually, experimental psychologists incorporated the ideas of Gestalt psychology and began to investigate the ways in which animals respond to a whole situation, as well as to its separate parts. Most recently, under the influence of ethological findings, they have begun to study types of learning, such as imprinting, which are not the result of conditioning. Practical applications of experimental psychology have included new approaches to education, most recently the introduction of teaching machines and programmed learning.

See also CONDITIONING; ETHOLOGY; PAVLOV, I. P.; REACTION TIME; REFLEX.

PSYCHOLOGY, MILITARY

Military psychology is the application of fundamental psychological principles and techniques to military problems. Many problems of the military psychologist are similar to those encountered in the civilian culture. However, the military situation differs from the usual civilian environment because of factors such as the following: the very large number of people deliberately organized along somewhat authoritarian lines, the great complexity and technicality of military equipment, the difficulty of preparing and training for action which hopefully will never industry between 1920 and 1940 was based on this early military effort. World War II marked a great resurgence and expansion of military psychology. Each of the military services established vigorous programs. The largest programs were concerned with the screening, selection, and placement of enlisted and cadet personnel. For example, all Army Air Force pilots, navigators, and bombardiers were selected for training as the result of an extensive series of paper-and-pencil tests as well as muscular coordination tests. The services also established large research projects which investigated special training problems and studied the difficult sensory and perceptual discriminations required in using radar, sonar equipment, and gun-laying apparatus.

Since World War II there has been a great increase in the application of knowledge in engineering psychology. This is particularly important in military weapon systems such as high-speed airplanes and missiles, and in large, computer-based command and control systems. Psychologists help design these systems so that they can be used easily by military operators.

Since in peacetime there is no chance to train against a real enemy, military psychologists have devised elaborate training programs to simulate war situations. One of the best known is the System Training Program developed for the U.S. Air Defense Command. With this program all the individual radar operators, interceptor pilots, and commanders, and the staffs of higher headquarters can be

Fried—Pix

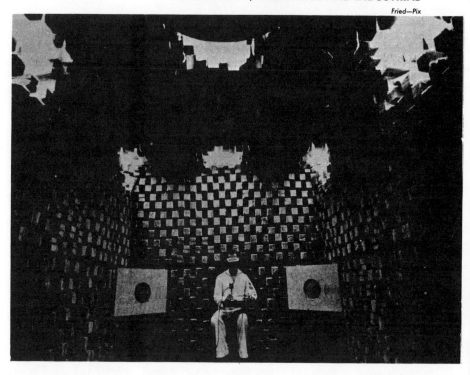

A subject takes a sound-direction test in an echo-proof chamber at the nuclear submarine school of the U.S. Naval Submarine Base, Groton, Conn. Test data are used by designers to help improve nuclear submarine sonar equipment.

simultaneously exercised by simulating as far as possible the problems that they would face if a major attack had been launched on the country. Through such exercises various defensive tactics, communications and control procedures, and rules to guide decision making can be developed and learned.

In the Army special psychological studies have been made of the difference between fighters and nonfighters. It has been estimated that in an infantry attack as many as 75% of the men in the action do not fire their guns. During the Korean War, Army psychologists identified a number of men who were known to have been good fighters and a number who were known to be poor fighters—for example, men who had thrown down their guns or panicked. Both groups of men were studied intensively, and it was found that the fighters, in contrast to the nonfighters, were more intelligent, more masculine, more socially mature, were "doers," and were preferred by their peers. They also had greater emotional stability, more leadership potential, better health and vitality, and a more stable home life. The fighters were the kind of men needed for all demanding activities, whether in front-line combat or elsewhere.

Military commanders were disturbed by the behavior of men who had been "brainwashed" while prisoners of the Communists in Korea. Psychologists have studied this problem through sensory-isolation experiments. Soldier volunteers were confined to small cubicles in each of which there were a bed, food, and chemical toilet but no light, sound, or other sensory stimulation. Although not subjected to threats or painful stimuli, over one-third of the men asked to be let out before the scheduled four-day period was completed. Typical complaints were "I can't take it" and "The darkness is getting me." These men lost

time orientation and found it difficult to distinguish between wakefulness and dreaming sleep. Such experiments help the services devise ways to train men to resist brainwashing.

PSYCHOLOGY, PERSONNEL AND INDUSTRIAL

The terms "personnel psychology" and "industrial psychology" are used individually or together to cover a number of applications of psychology. The applications of psychology in industry has been largely to personnel problems such as placing and training men and women. Since World War II, however, other areas have been taken in. Personnel psychology has many uses in military service and in civilian government as well as in business and industry. In fact, it is used in virtually all organizations with large numbers of people.

Selecting and Placing Personnel. The first and most frequent application of personnel psychology has been in occupational selection and placement. There have been many cases, especially in the largest organizations, where careful assessment of the man and the job has resulted in more efficiency and more satisfaction on the part of employees. Satisfied employees stay longer on a job.

Personnel psychology, especially through the work of Carroll L. Shartle and associates in the U.S. Employment Service, has made great progress in methods of determining aptitudes for various occupations. The U.S. Employment Service has developed a general aptitude test battery, a reliable and valid series of measures of the factors that have been found to underlie intellectual and motor aptitudes for occupational performance. The 10 areas measured by the test battery are intelligence; verbal, numerical, and spatial aptitudes; form perception; clerical percep-

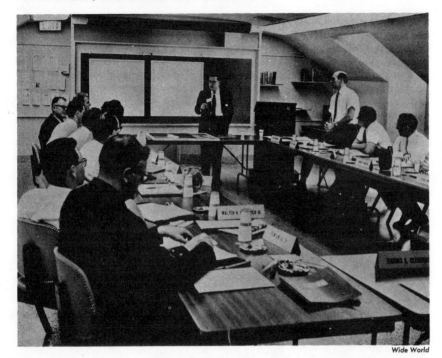

Industrial executives attend a special psychology seminar at the Menninger Foundation in Topeka, Kansas. They hope to understand better, and solve, some of the personnel mental health problems engendered by the conditions of modern industry.

Wide World

tion; aiming; motor speed; finger dexterity; and manual dexterity. The tests for these aptitudes are combined in varying ways to predict how well prospective employees will do in numerous occupations. Though many large companies have developed similar tests for their own use, others may and do use, at no direct cost to themselves, the services of state employment offices. These employment offices have available the measures used by the U.S. Employment Service.

The measurement of interest has also been a major concern in personnel psychology. Here the Strong Vocational Interest Blank has been the most thoroughly studied over a longer period of time, although the Kuder Preference Record has become more popular because of its ease of scoring. The Strong Interest Blank measures the extent to which one's interests correspond to those of people who have made a living for a minimum of two years in one of several fields, chiefly business and professional. Findings from this Interest Blank have been found to correlate more with job turnover than with any criterion of productivity. The implication is that interests are more closely related to staying with a job than to working hard at the job. The Blank has been uniquely valid in predicting the productivity, as well as the job turnover, of life insurance salesmen, regardless of their experience, age, or education.

Personnel Training. There have been substantial applications of psychology to the training of employees. Work in this area started with the training of rank and file employees, but during and after World War II there was considerable activity in attempts to train supervisors. The central research problem here, as in research on selection and placement, has been the quest for an adequate criterion of vocational success. The lack of such a criterion with managers has impeded any demonstration of the effectiveness of management training. Nevertheless, by the 1960's industry was spending millions of dollars each year on this type of training. The largest companies conduct their own courses. In addition, industry sends men to universities for courses in management development.

The lack of an accepted criterion of success appears to be due in large part to the situational nature of the manager's job. Managerial success depends, to a certain extent, on what an executive's boss, associates, and subordinates anticipate and what their perceptions are. What others expect of a manager and how they feel toward him are conditions that vary with time, location, industry, and company.

Training Methods. The major need in management training has been thought to be understanding people. Most frequently training is by the conference method. One way of giving practice with supervisory problems is through role playing. Two or more participants are assigned parts to study—perhaps one takes the part of a department head, another the role of an employee whose work is unsatisfactory. Each one's view of the situation is kept secret from the other participant or participants so that the play simulates actual personnel problems. Usually the other members of the training group serve as observers. Following the play they discuss the behavior of the role players and attempt to analyze their feelings and thoughts. The aim is to develop empathy, or the ability to understand the feelings of others.

What is called "sensitivity training" has been introduced into a few industrial companies in an attempt to increase the extent to which managers alter job performances as a result of training. The need for this has become evident in studies such as one of a group of foremen. They were found to be less considerate six months after returning to their jobs than they had been prior to attending a training course, although immediately after the course they had been more considerate. The foremen evidently found the autocratic example of their bosses more power-

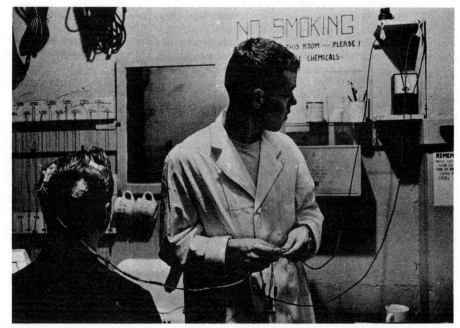

An example of research in physiological psychology. Human brain activity during dreams is studied in the "sleep lab" of the department of psychology at the University of Chicago. The electrodes attached to the subject's head will be connected to an electroencephalograph to record patterns of brain activity after the subject has gone to sleep. (FLORES—PIX)

ful than the theory of the classroom in shaping their behavior.

Both education and industry have made increasing use of teaching machines. While the term "teaching machine" may refer to mechanical devices, it is essentially a procedure involving careful programming of what is to be learned, active response by the learner, and immediate feedback of information so as to reinforce correct responses. Teaching machines have been used to teach employees an assembly process and are being used to teach accounting and other subjects useful in industry.

Other Problems for Industrial Psychology. The application of psychology to the design of industrial equipment grew out of somewhat similar applications in World War II. In fact, human engineering, the careful consideration of the capacities and limitations of the human organism as a guide to design, remains primarily a military rather than an industrial concern.

Social psychology has had some application in industrial research in showing the importance of understanding human behavior in informal situations as well as in formal groups. These findings have been incorporated into some training programs for managers.

The principles of clinical psychology have been applied in industry by large companies that have used a clinical approach to the selection, placement, and guidance of executives. For example, some concerns make an intensive study of the personalities of men who are being considered for posts in management. More rarely, clinical psychologists are assigned to help with the personal problems of maladjusted rank and file employees.

Labor unions have been studied by a few psychologists, but in the view of some critics this area has been inadequately studied because psychologists have been the "servants of power." The argument is that since they are almost always employed by management, they must please management in order to be hired and retained.

The application of the principles of psychology to industry is being carried on by hundreds of psychologists. They are employed either by single industrial companies, by consulting firms to serve more than one company, or by universities from which they serve as consultants to industrial companies. The majority of them are members of the American Psychological Association's Division of Industrial and Business Psychology. Their work tends to interweave with that of consulting psychologists to the extent that the latter are engaged by industry and business. *See also* TESTING, PSYCHOLOGICAL AND EDUCATIONAL.

PSYCHOLOGY, PHYSIOLOGICAL

This branch of psychology studies the relation of bodily processes to behavior. While contemporary emphasis is on the central nervous system, the subject includes description of the part played by sensory, muscular, glandular, digestive, and other physiological systems in determining behavior. Starting in the early 19th century, major advances were achieved. Vision and hearing were analyzed. Separate nerves controlling sensory and motor functions were identified. The dependence of the quality of sensation on the nervous system was discovered. Sensory and motor areas in the brain were localized. The nerve cell, or neuron, was identified as the structural unit of the nervous system. The early years of the present century were dominated by research on brain mechanisms in learning and memory.

Around 1950 physiological psychology entered a period of rapid development. Advances in electronics made it possible to amplify and to measure the minute electric currents generated by nerves. Techniques were devised for placing electrodes in the brains of laboratory animals. It became possible to map brain functions. Experimental findings led to changes in basic concepts of how the nervous system functions. One conclusion is that the activity of the brain is a complex pattern of facilitation and inhibition of the passage of impulses along the nerves. Although separate areas of the brain are related to different functions, each area interacts with all other areas.

The most influential research finding of the post-World War II period concerned a hitherto undetected manner of control of the integrative activities of the brain. It has been demonstrated that sensory stimulation leads to two types of central nervous system activity. The first, known for a very long time, is the transmission of excitation along relatively insulated nerve tracts to specific loci in the brain. By this means detailed information about the sights, sounds, tastes, and smells of our environment is carried to the brain. But the same sensory stimulation also results in transmission to a pooled system receiving excitation from all sense organs active at any time, with this system transmitting relatively generalized stimulation to wide areas of the brain.

This latter consequence of sensory stimulation, called activation, is crucial for normal behavior. Without the activation the brain is unable to deal with specific messages from sense organs. Absent or very low levels of activation are characteristic of sleep. High states of excitement, motivation, and emotion are accompanied by very high levels of activation. The activation system also has properties of inhibiting activity, not only within itself but in other brain areas as well.

There are good reasons for believing that the subtle and complicated processes of awareness, attention, and memory will be illuminated by continuing research on this activating system of the brain.

Of almost equal psychological importance is the discovery that animals with electrodes implanted in certain areas of the brain learn a variety of complex habits solely for the reward of small pulses of electric stimulation of the areas of the brain under the electrodes. This indicates that the "pleasurable," or rewarding, consequences of action may depend on activity in definite brain locations. Stimulation by electrodes in other areas leads animals to learn to avoid further stimulation, indicating the possibility of "punishment," or pain, centers as well. Coupled with a growing knowledge of brain regions crucial to hunger, thirst, temperature and respiratory control, and sexual behavior, these studies give hope for an understanding of the physiological basis for human behavior.

See also Brain; Emotion; Nervous System; Sleep.

PSYCHOLOGY, SOCIAL

This branch of the social sciences is primarily concerned with the socially influenced behaviors, attitudes, and beliefs of human beings. It is also concerned with the social behaviors of lower animals as a source of insights into human activities. Social psychology overlaps traditional psychology and sociology, which are its intellectual ancestors. Because a substantial number of the concepts, techniques, and problems of social psychology are shared with psychology and sociology, social psychology is known as a bridging discipline. It combines findings and insights of the two parent branches of learning in much the same fashion that biochemistry unites certain phases of the biological and chemical sciences.

Although psychologists and sociologists have always been concerned with somewhat similar subject matter, they have not usually achieved very close working arrangements with one another. Psychologists have been concerned with the investigation of the behaviors and internal processes of the single individual, while sociologists have almost always taken the group, or society, as their unit of investigation. Each of these approaches to the study of man is legitimate, and each has been highly productive. But rigid adherence to either approach inevitably overlooks the whole class of relationships which link the individual and the group. These relationships are studied by the social psychologist.

Origins of Social Psychology. The field is both very old and very new. Its philosophical origins can be traced back almost to the beginning of written literature. For civilized man seems always to have been self-conscious about his relationships with his fellow men. Early religious documents speculated about the psychological bonds that hold men together in societies and about the rules of individual conduct that are conducive to cohesion within the group. From Plato and Aristotle to Hobbes and Locke, writers attempted to describe the instincts, gregarious motives, and social contracts that unite human beings into social organizations.

During the 19th century and the early part of the 20th century many writers, impressed by the dramatic excesses of crowd behavior, described the motives and processes that might transform a self-sufficient individual into a mere puppet of the masses. These discussions featured quasi-scientific arguments about concepts bearing such labels as "herd instinct," imitation, suggestion, sympathy, hypnosis, the id, and prepotent drives. It is now recognized that these concepts do not adequately explain crowd behavior, but the arguments they generated years ago served to stimulate interest in the more careful study of man's complex social behavior.

Contemporary Social Psychology. Modern social psychology began during the 1930's. The previous decade had brought an increasing concern for the use of empirical and scientific methods in the investigation of interpersonal behavior. It was not until the Great Depression and World War II, however, that a concerted attempt was made to test the social psychological speculations and theories generated during earlier centuries. Stimulated by the widespread breakdown of social institutions and the need to develop new means of social control, scholars in many disciplines gave renewed attention to problems of an interpersonal nature. A very significant aspect of this endeavor was the effort to understand people's attitudes toward one another, toward authority figures, and toward their jobs, religion, government, and family. New and more reliable means of measuring attitudes were developed, and scientific techniques for selecting representative samples of peoples were devised.

With these methodological improvements came a growing awareness that attitudes are strongly influenced by social factors and have very important social consequences. There was a rapid accumulation of evidence indicating that an individual's political, economic, or social attitudes tend to reflect the influence of other people with whom that individual has satisfying or dissatisfying relationships. It became equally clear that an individual's attitudes tend to influence his behavior in a wide variety of situations. The morale of an army, the productivity of a factory, or the stability of a family cannot be fully understood unless psychological factors are considered. But traditional psychology had relatively little to say about people's relationships to one another. It was a branch of learning devoted to the study of the sensory, motor, emotional, and learning behavior of the individual.

Field and Laboratory Studies of Attitudes. Most of the early investigations of attitudes and related social psychological phenomena were field studies. Investigators observed people in their everyday environments and noted the effects of social and situational factors. It was often difficult, however, to find exactly the kind of natural situation the social psychologist wanted to study. Even when the appropriate situation could be found, inability to control the speed or extent of natural processes made it difficult for the investigator to reach definite conclusions. Led primarily by Kurt Lewin, social psychologists gradually turned to the study of people in contrived, or created, situations. Just as the chemist creates the special circumstances in which he can observe the reactions of chemical substances, social psychologists since the 1930's have been devising their own social microcosms in which to witness the reactions of human beings. Two or more individuals are brought together for a period of time, from a few minutes to several days, while many circumstances are kept constant and only a few are permitted to vary. Sometimes the people studied are selected because they have the same or different attitudes, knowledge, personalities, professions, or jobs. Some sort of problem is created for the experimental group. Sometimes members are led to believe that an especially important event has occurred—perhaps that the building in which they are meeting has caught fire. In such contrived situations it has been possible to study many factors. These include the effects of group size and composition on how members feel about the group and how much the group accomplishes, the effects of social roles on attitudes and performance, the impact of the group on how the individual views himself and how much he hopes to achieve, and the influence of numerous personal and situational factors on how well the group holds together and works together.

Laboratory investigations of people in contrived situations have not replaced field studies. The laboratory study permits the experimenter to exercise more control than is possible in field studies and to reach confident conclusions about the events that have occurred in the contrived situation. It is by no means certain, however, that these conclusions apply to natural situations outside the laboratory until they have been substantiated by field studies. Laboratory studies are valuable in that they permit the investigator to examine rapidly a large number of alternative hypotheses. The most promising of these can then be subjected to test under field conditions.

Interpersonal Relations and Perceptions. In addition to the intensive study of attitudes and of social influences on the behaviors of interacting individuals, social psychologists are vitally concerned with problems of interpersonal perception. Humans often respond to their own impressions of other people, rather than to the actual qualities of other people. For example, a man may have a general impression of "boss" or "foreigner" or "teen-ager" which distorts his view of actual employers, tourists, or high school students. Consequently an adequate understanding of individuals' reactions to one another must take account of complex processes involved in how one perceives others. Social psychologists have shown that a leader's perceptions of his coworkers are related to the group's productivity. As an everyday example, when sales are high the sales manager is likely to have a high opinion of the personal and business qualities of his men. Changes in interpersonal perceptions have been shown to produce changes in the likes and dislikes among group members. Self-perceptions are often related to perceptions of other persons. For example, the man who feels he is a capable leader may see capabilities in those he is leading. The uncertain leader may tend to see more weaknesses. On the other hand, the leader's perception of himself is influenced by the attitudes of his followers. The social psychologist's interest in the study of self-perceptions and interpersonal perceptions is shared by personality theorists, who have tended to emphasize the effects of the perceiver's personality upon his perceptions.

Although the problems cited above are the kind that concern scholars in many disciplines, they are approached by the social psychologist from a particular point of view. He alone among the interested scholars deliberately attempts to treat interacting individuals as psychological beings who are, at the same time, parts of a larger unit: the group or organization. In this manner he attempts to employ the insights and techniques of the psychologist and of the sociologist, and to unite the relevant portions of both disciplines into a more meaningful body of knowledge.

Applied Social Psychology. Practical applications of social psychology are numerous. In business organizations social psychologists deal with problems of worker morale, leadership, and productivity. In military settings they are concerned with problems of brainwashing, psychological warfare, and propaganda analysis. They assist in planning political campaigns, sales drives, and labor union activities. They conduct opinion surveys, and they sample consumer preferences. They work with organizations attempting to bring about social change or to prevent such change. They also co-operate with clinical psychologists, psychiatrists, and social workers in the investigation and treatment of mentally disturbed individuals, criminals, and juvenile delinquents. But their most basic function is to discover new knowledge about the individual as a participant in collective action.

See also SOCIOLOGY.

PSYCHOLOGY OF ADOLESCENCE. *See* ADOLESCENCE.

PSYCHOLOGY OF CHILDREN. *See* CHILD DEVELOPMENT.

PSYCHOLOGY OF LEARNING. *See* LEARNING; PSYCHOLOGY: *Educational Psychology.*

PSYCHOLOGY OF PERSONALITY

One characteristic of human behavior evident even in casual observation is that it tends to remain consistent at different times and in different situations. A salesman who approaches his customers in an aggressive manner is likely to be aggressive in his dealings with people away from his job. Although notable exceptions to this rule can be offered—such as the changes in behavior that occur as the child develops into adulthood or the special times when a person acts "out of character"—still the thread of sameness in an individual's actions cannot be denied. Personality is the name given to this pattern of samenesses characterizing each person. There is disagreement about how personality shall be defined and the way that personality develops. Most experts agree, however, that when we talk about an individual's personality we are talking about what are consistent behaviors for him.

Theories of What Personality Is

Why has there not been better agreement about the nature of personality and the manner in which it develops? One reason is the basic disagreement among theorists as to whether an individual's personality should be considered an inner system that actually exists—much as the nervous or gastrointestinal system resides within the human body—or whether personality is simply a convenient name for the regularities of behavior observed to characterize the person. The argument is rooted historically in the revolt of John B. Watson against the philosophical and physiological origins of psychology. His principles, outlined in *Behaviorism* (1930), stress the importance for psychology of dealing only with behavior that can be observed and not with speculations about what goes on within the human body. The latter he felt a more fitting province for such sciences as biology and physiology. Behaviorism, Watson's school of psychology, remains only as a historical marker, but its profound influence upon personality theorists has been transmitted by learning theorists such as Clark Hull and Kenneth Spence.

Personality Conceived as an Inner System. The most influential concept of personality emphasizing inner systems and forces is the psychoanalytic formulation of Sigmund Freud, described in *A General Introduction to Psychoanalysis*. He conceived of the personality as being made up of three aspects. One part, the id, exists without our being aware of its presence and includes the uncivilized urges and wishes society would condemn and punish if they erupted without being toned down in some manner. The second part, the ego, is that part of our personality that is in direct contact with the world about us and has the difficult assignment of forcing back the id's uncivilized urges or of disguising them in such a way as to make them socially acceptable. The ego is the rational, "common sense" part of personality, which deals with the id and with the real world.

The third aspect of personality, according to Freud, is the superego, or the conscience of the person, which he absorbs from his parents. The superego provides the sense of right and wrong which keeps the ego from straying far from the path of socially acceptable behavior. The emphasis on inner forces is clearly evident in Freud's view, with the surging id forces and critical superego battalions persistently attacking the rational ego to gain control of the person's behavior. The learned behaviors by which the person satisfies these demands from within, as well as the requirements of social group living, provide the consistencies in thought and action that we call personality. Freud's contention that the early experiences of the child were very important in determining how personality will be shaped pioneered a point of view that has been universally accepted by psychologists and may represent his most important contribution.

Personality Defined as Observable Behavior. The opposite view, which holds that inner structure and function are unobservable and should not be considered in defining personality, has not been associated with any one person as much as it has been tied to the behavioristic philosophy. An example of this view would be David McClelland's definition of personality (1951) as the most extensive picture of a person's behavior that a scientist can give at a moment of time. Thus one's personality consists of all that an observing scientist can see and not of the inner structure of the human being.

One difficulty with thinking about personality only in terms of what can be seen by outsiders is that this approach merges into two popular but misused versions of the term. Personality is sometimes used to refer to the degree of social impact a person has upon other people. "He has a wonderful personality" or "If he had more personality, he would have gotten the job" are two examples. Although it is true that others may be either favorably or unfavorably impressed by the manner in which a person behaves toward them, the unimpressive person has no less personality than the social charmer. He merely has a different personality.

The second misuse of the term "personality" is as a substitute for "reputation" and often involves a moral judgment. The best illustration of this is found in psychiatry, where the term "psychopathic personality" is used to describe a person whose behavior consistently runs counter to social rules and who, in this sense, is a "bad person." However, when individuals who are called psychopathic personalities are more closely examined, it is found that, aside from the common attribute of nonconformity to society's rules, their personal traits vary considerably. It is even more misleading to depend upon popular reputation to describe personality, since this adds the element of rumor and individual moral biases to confuse the picture.

Theories About the Important Elements in Personality

The question of whether personality should be conceived as something that exists within the person and provides the direction and force for his acts or as a convenient label for his characteristic and observable behaviors is only one of the issues that have bothered psychologists. Another major difference in viewpoint is the question of which elements should be considered the most important part of personality. Among the more famous theories of personality are those of Sigmund Freud, Carl Jung, and Harry Stack Sullivan. Each of these thinkers placed a unique emphasis upon different aspects of human behavior and the forces that determine it.

Freud's Theory. Freud, in addition to the structural elements of personality as discussed above, placed great emphasis upon two wellsprings of behavior. Positive and affectionate tendencies, he believed, are based upon energies that are primarily sexual in nature, whereas negative and destructive tendencies stem from other energies, unnamed by Freud. It would be an oversimplification to say that he considered the personality of an individual to be determined by these two opposing energy systems. However, the manner in which the person comes to control the energies and the direction in which the energies become mobilized are certainly basic. For example, Freud might consider the choice of physician as a profession to be a result of personality development in which the sexual energies have been channeled into helping others and the destructive energies directed toward the extinction of disease. If nothing more, Freud brought sex out from its mid-Victorian cloak and forced psychology and Western culture to consider its vast importance in everyday behavior.

Jung's Theory. Carl Jung, who was initially closely aligned with Freud's ideas regarding personality, broke away because he could not accept the heavy emphasis on sex. Jung also viewed the personality as based upon an energy system and the person as molded by the manner in which the energies are directed. One of the distinguishing features of Jung's theory was the importance he placed upon the positive, striving nature of man. He felt that man in particular, and man in general, is seeking a completeness in himself so that all aspects of his personality will be in harmony. There was also a heavy emphasis upon the inherited nature of personality, since he assumed that we all share a storehouse of experiences passed down from countless generations of primitive human and animal ancestors. Thus we all are born with a tendency to act in a certain way toward mothers, since human beings have always had mothers. One feature of Jung's concept of personality that has been more popularized is his notion that attitudes of "extroversion" and "introversion" are present in each person, one usually being stronger than the other. By extroversion he meant an orientation toward the real world about a person, whereas introversion referred to an inward interest in one's own personal experiences.

Perhaps one reason why Jung's view of personality never commanded the attention accorded to Freud is its mystical quality. Scientific psychology has been critical both of his contention that man's destiny is guided by events which have yet to occur rather than by his past experiences, as well as of his proposal of common inheritance of psychological tendencies from our ancestors. Neither, it is felt, can be evaluated by scientific test.

Sullivan's Theory. In contrast to Freud and Jung, who were products of European psychology with its stress upon instinctive forces, American-born Harry Stack Sullivan focused his thinking upon the social experiences which from birth mold the individual's personality. The personality for Sullivan is a system of energy and has the reduction of tension as its major purpose. Tension in man stems from physical needs such as hunger and thirst, and from anxiety, which results from feelings of insecurity in human relationships. Sullivan sketched stages in the development of the human being, much like Freud, suggesting at each stage the characteristic ways in which anxiety is experienced and the methods by which it is reduced. Like the other theorists, Sullivan attempts to explain the way personalities of all men develop, but he does so in such a way as to highlight the demands made by society and the efforts of the individual to live more comfortably as a social animal.

Summary. It is difficult to escape the conclusion that all attempts to explain the nature of personality encountered in psychology to this point are only steppingstones toward a more vital explanation that will some day emerge. Steadily increasing evidence points toward a concept of personality that must include a variety of elements. Our characteristic modes of behavior seem to depend in part upon inherited qualities, and physical factors within our bodies set limits on what we can be and do. But more than anything else our behavior patterns depend upon the way we learn to deal with our fellow men and with the demands of social living. This is a hopeful theory, since it suggests that personality is only in part an unchangeable thing and in the main is alterable through further learning experiences.

See also BODY TYPES; CULTURE AND PERSONALITY; EMOTION; INTROVERSION-EXTROVERSION; PSYCHOANALYSIS.

PSYCHOMETRICS, term used to mean (1) psychological measurement or the study of such testing and (2) the branch of psychology that applies mathematical procedures to the problems of psychology. See TESTING, PSYCHOLOGICAL AND EDUCATIONAL.

PSYCHOPATHIC PERSONALITY, a term describing one of the most perplexing disorders known to psychiatry. Superficially the psychopath appears charming and competent. His intelligence is often above average, and he is capable of mastering the most subtle occupational skills. This façade conceals a complete lack of morality and positive human feeling in all his personal relationships and an absence of normal occupational and social goals. Despite his excellent personal and intellectual equipment, the psychopath consistently fails in all endeavors. He repeatedly abandons his job and family in pursuit of the most casual impulse. His sexual life is shallow, impersonal, and promiscuous. He may cheat, steal, or even kill, showing no remorse. He is incapable of understanding his own behavior or profiting from his experience. It is important to distinguish psychopaths from psychotics and psychoneurotics. The psychopath neither has any bizarre notions concerning the world nor does he suffer from anxiety. An early writer, in describing this condition, marked the distinction between psychopaths and overtly deranged persons by designating the former as "morally insane."

Centuries of speculation have not clarified the nature of the disorder. Some have attributed it to a "constitutional inferiority," while others have cited family relationships and childhood experiences. Psychiatrists recognize in these persons the most difficult and fruitless subjects for treatment.

See also PSYCHIATRY.

PSYCHOPHARMACOLOGY [sī-kō-fär-mə-kŏl'ə-jē], the study of the effect of drugs on the mind. Drugs that produce mental effects have long been used in medical practice. These include opium, alcohol, cocaine, and more recently the barbiturates, which are widely used as sleeping pills. The subject has received special attention since the introduction of newer drugs, such as the tranquilizers, which calm excited psychotic patients, and the discovery of substances, such as lysergic acid diethylamide (LSD), which produce hallucinations and changes in mood. The psychopharmacological agents may be considered in three categories: the tranquilizers, the hallucinogens, and the stimulants.

Tranquilizers reduce anxiety and agitation in psychologically disturbed individuals. They differ from sedatives, such as the barbiturates, in that they quiet the patient without producing drowsiness. The best-known tranquilizers are reserpine and chlorpromazine (Thorazine).

Hallucinogens produce mood changes and hallucinations of sight, space, and time. At times they cause irrational behavior and speech similar to that seen in certain mental disorders. Although drugs such as alcohol and marihuana also produce mental changes, the hallucinogens are distinguished by their high potency, being effective in small dosages.

The Indians of the southwestern United States have used a hallucinogenic drug (mescaline, obtained from the mescal cactus) for centuries as part of religious rituals. The hallucinogenic effects of lysergic acid diethylamide (LSD) were accidentally discovered in 1943 by a Swiss chemist, who developed peculiar visual disturbances while working with this compound. He correctly surmised that his symptoms resulted from swallowing traces of the material he was handling. This drug has been of considerable interest to psychiatrists in producing experimental symptoms similare to those seen in mental disorders (psychoses).

Stimulant Drugs. In contrast to the tranquilizers, which calm, quiet, or even depress the patient, the central nervous system stimulants (or psychomotor stimulants) alert the patient and relieve depression. Members of the group include the familiar amphetamine (benzedrine), which has been available for many years, and newer drugs, such as iproniazid, methylphenidate, pipradol, and imipramine.

How Psychopharmacological Drugs Work

The dramatic effects on behavior produced by tranquilizers, hallucinogens, and stimulants have aroused much interest in the chemistry of the brain. There is some evidence that these compounds may not act directly on the nervous system but rather through their effect on a number of special substances long known to exert profound effects on the functioning of nervous tissue. These substances (epinephrine, acetylcholine, norepinephrine, and serotonin) are normally present in the brain and other parts of the body and are intimately involved in the transmission of nerve impulses and in the action of the heart, glands, viscera, and blood vessels. It has been found that whereas some tranquilizers, such as reserpine, reduce the amounts of serotonin in the brain, LSD has the reverse effect. It is also possible that some stimulant drugs work in an even more indirect way, inhibiting the action of an enzyme (monoamine oxidase) which, in turn, increases the quantity of serotonin (and possibly other compounds) in the brain. These mechanisms remain speculative since they deal with one of the most poorly understood aspects of physiology—the functioning of the nervous system.

See also NARCOTICS; TRANQUILIZERS.

PSYCHOSIS [sĭ-kō′sĭs], term given to a category of mental disorders in which the individual suffers from hallucinations, delusions, or other distortions of reality. This may take the form of a complete severance from the real world,

as seen in certain trancelike states in schizophrenia, or a partial distortion of reality such as occurs in the paranoid, who is normal save for his belief that malevolent persons are "after him." Psychosis is a more serious disorder than neurosis; in the latter, the individual is aware of the real world but is the victim of persistent and troublesome patterns of behavior which he may be powerless to control.
See also MENTAL ILLNESS; NEUROSIS; PARANOIA; PSYCHIATRY; SCHIZOPHRENIA.

PSYCHOSOMATIC [sĭ-kō-sō-măt′ĭk] **MEDICINE,** branch of psychiatry which deals with physical illnesses that result in part from emotional conflicts. The basic principle of psychosomatic illness is the spilling over of anxiety, fear, resentment, and other forms of psychological tension into the nervous and hormonal channels which normally regulate the activities of the internal organs.

The focus of the conversion of psychological stress into physiological activity lies in certain portions of the brain involved in internal control. These areas control internal activity by means of the autonomic nervous system and through control of the endocrine glands. The autonomic, or visceral, nervous system is a vast network of fibers which co-ordinates the action of the heart, digestive system, and glands. The complex effects of emotions on the body are produced through the fibers of this system and by means of endocrine secretions (hormones) traveling in the blood stream. Fear, for example, may blanch the stomach lining, squeeze blood from the skin and intestines, quicken the heartbeat, and raise the blood pressure. Repeated or prolonged episodes of fear, tension, or anxiety may eventually cause permanent tissue damage. One concept of the mechanism of such tissue destruction was advanced by the physiologist Hans Selye, who stated that prolonged stress might produce body damage through the release of excessive amounts of certain hormones from the adrenal glands.

Disorders in which psychological factors are believed to be important include heart ailments, migraine headaches, peptic ulcers, asthma, skin eruptions, and hyperthyroidism. Menstrual difficulties and sexual problems often have a psychosomatic basis. Not all of the psychosomatic ailments involve actual tissue damage (for example, headaches may be caused by temporary constriction of the blood vessels of the head).

An intriguing question is why a specific organ should be affected in one individual but not another. Much of the theorizing in the field of psychosomatic medicine has been an attempt to answer this question. Some theorists have suggested that an inherited weakness of particular organs may be responsible: thus there would be "stomach types," "heart types," and so forth.

The psychiatrist Helen Flanders Dunbar proposed that particular personality types were susceptible to specific psychosomatic ailments. Franz Alexander stressed the nature of the emotional problem as a selecting factor: thus individuals with a strong desire to be dependent on others would develop peptic ulcer and asthma, whereas those with aggressive emotional patterns might develop migraine and high blood pressure. The bulk of the evidence to date favors a nonspecific theory, according to which sustained tension will "break through" at a point of least resistance. The psychosomatic ailments are treated both medically and psychiatrically.

PSYCHOTECHNOLOGY. *See* PSYCHOLOGY: *Personnel and Industrial Psychology.*

PSYCHOTHERAPY [sī-kō-thĕr'ə-pē]. In one sense psychotherapy may be said to have been practiced whenever one person attempted to console another, or when the influence of the philosopher, priest, or medicine man was directed at relieving mental distress. However, as a systematic method of therapy based upon a theory of human behavior, it began with the work of Sigmund Freud of Vienna. Freud's work was the starting point in a development that has led to the various schools of psychotherapy.

Freud's Approach

Freud became interested in a case being treated by his colleague Josef Breuer. The patient was a young woman who suffered from paralysis of the right arm and leg, impaired vision, and a number of other serious and puzzling disturbances. The symptoms could not be traced to any underlying organic disturbances. Such cases of profound disturbances in the absence of pathology had been known since the time of the ancient Greeks (who had ascribed it to a wandering of the womb through the body, hence the term "hysteria," from the Greek *hystera*, "womb"). While ordinarily physicians felt themselves powerless to deal with ailments of this kind, Breuer was led by certain chance observations to attempt a treatment. He had noted that the girl repeated several words to herself while in a trancelike state of altered consciousness. He hypnotized the patient and repeated these words to her. This led to the recall of memories concerning phantasies of the patient at the bedside of her ailing father. Following these sessions the patient's symptoms would disappear for a period of a few days or sometimes weeks. Eventually Breuer was able to alleviate some of the symptoms by the technique of reviving memories which the patient could not recall while fully conscious.

Breuer and Freud both believed that the girl suffered from a splitting of the psyche. Where in the normal personality thoughts and feelings were well integrated in the mind, in hysteria certain unacceptable thoughts wandered about the unconscious creating difficulties, like a splinter or other foreign body in the flesh produces an inflammation.

While Breuer and Freud agreed as to this point, they developed different views as to the nature of the split. They stated their ideas in separate chapters of their book, *Studies on Hysteria*. Breuer thought that some constitutional weakness might be responsible, whereas Freud offered an entirely new, purely psychological theory which he later called "psycho-analysis."

Basically the new theory held that:

(a) *The cause of the "neurotic" disturbance is an emotional conflict between two or more incompatible needs or desires*—for example, a girl is in love with her friend's husband.

(b) *The conflict becomes submerged in the unconscious*

—instead of shifting her affection from this man to another, the girl may try to escape the painful conflict by pushing all thoughts and feelings relating to him out of her awareness, that is, she *represses* them.

(c) *The repressed conflict produces neurotic symptoms* —these thoughts and feelings thus excluded from consciousness continue to exert an influence on her, returning into consciousness in an indirect form no longer recognized by her as having anything to do with the original feelings. She may now develop a cough similar to that of the wife. The symptom symbolically expresses her desires toward the man—by imitating one feature of the friend and rival, she expresses the now unconscious wish of wanting to be in her place. Thus the symptom can be understood as an unsuccessful attempt at resolving an intolerable conflict in which the individual can escape the psychological tension only at the price of a more or less painful symptom.

Making the Unconscious Conscious. These insights suggested to Freud the direction the cure would have to take: the patient would have to be made to readmit to consciousness the conflict-laden thoughts and feelings. But how could this be accomplished? How could something unconscious be made conscious again?

At first Freud used hypnosis to help the patient recover memories of experiences and thoughts which he could not recall spontaneously because they were related to underlying conflicts. Freud abandoned hypnosis when he found that he could not hypnotize all of his patients. He also noted that in those who could be hypnotized relief of symptoms was usually only temporary. In place of hypnosis he substituted "free association"—a procedure in which the patient was encouraged to relax and allow his thoughts to wander without any preconceived goal of his own or direction by the therapist. The basis for this technique was Freud's assumption that the repressed ideas affect not only the symptoms but also influence the patient's conscious thoughts. By connecting the apparently unrelated musings of the patient, the therapist hoped to make the patient recognize what he had previously pushed out of his mind.

Accepting the Unconscious. Free association brought into focus another difficulty. If the conflict which gave rise to the symptom was so painful that it could not be tolerated, would not the patient resist having to experience it all over again in therapy? This "resistance" proved to be one of the crucial problems of psychoanalytic therapy and was partially overcome with the aid of "transference"— the emotional attachment which the patient develops toward the therapist. This enables him to face what he had not been able to face earlier. Thus the therapist was drawn into the interplay of the psychological forces operating within the patient. It is the importance of this support gained from the transference which makes psychoanalysts feel that self-analysis is well-nigh impossible.

Resolving the Conflict. Presuming that the patient can be made to confront his conflicts, what reason is there to believe that he can resolve them? Clearly the theory of unconscious conflict alone did not fully explain why people can be made to give up their symptoms through therapy. The completion of the psychoanalytic explanation of therapy was achieved by locating the origins of the conflict in childhood experiences. This might explain why conflicts could be resolved in therapy since (a) the conflicts arise in childhood, (b) they cannot be adequately dealt with by the immature child mentality, but (c) they can be better handled by the mature adult mind provided they are brought to consciousness later in life.

The theory of childhood origins of neurosis also made it possible to account for the difference between normal and neurotic reactions on the basis of differences in childhood experiences. These experiences centered around the child's basic needs and the child's dependency upon his parents for their gratification. Freud described the stages of psychosexual development in the child and saw in them a fertile area for the development of conflicts beyond the capacity of the child to resolve.

To summarize the principal points underlying the psychoanalytic approach to therapy:

(a) The basis for neurotic patterns of behavior occurs in childhood (genetic principle of explanation).

(b) Thoughts, ideas, and desires which would conflict with accepted attitudes or norms are then prevented from entering consciousness by the mechanisms of defense, for example, repression (dynamic principle of explanation).

(c) Buried in the unconscious, they generate painful neurotic symptoms (structural, or topological, principle of explanation).

The therapy itself proceeds on the assumptions that:

(a) The nature of the unconscious conflicts can be discovered by the method of free association and the analysis of dreams and other symbolic materials.

(b) Resistance can be overcome and the patient can be made to face the unpleasant ideas emerging from the unconscious through the agency of the therapist and the emotional power of the transference relationship.

(c) The patient can then resolve as an adult the problems which he was incapable of handling as a child.

Divergent Schools

Not long after Freud introduced his basic ideas, divergences of opinion arose among his followers which led to changes in the methods of therapy. C. G. Jung and Alfred Adler, who belonged to Freud's original circle of adherents, ultimately established schools of their own. They retained the concept of unconscious mental processes and conflicts but gave it a somewhat different meaning.

Adlerian "Individual" Psychology. Adler was the first to break away from Freud by citing actual or imagined weaknesses or deficiencies (inferiorities) of the person as the central cause of emotional disturbances instead of psychosexual problems as emphasized by Freud. According to Adler, the attempt at "overcompensation" for these inferiorities results from a striving for dominance or power over others—a pattern which might interfere with interpersonal relationships. Adler was particularly concerned with such asocial tendencies and in his therapy attempted to remove the obstacles to social adjustment.

Jung's "Analytic" Psychology. Jung concentrated on the study of what he called the "collective unconscious," the deepest layers of the mind containing the ancient thought patterns of the race as they manifested themselves in myths, legends, customs, and rituals. Jung saw in the similarities in the myths of distant peoples evidence of a common psychic heritage. For example, myths of the sun

as a "god-hero" who is born every day and makes a perilous "night journey" during the dark hours are common to many distant cultures. He interpreted these legends as the prototypes of problems facing humanity everywhere. Thus the god-hero myth is an expression of the need to admire a superior person or being.

Like Adler, Jung discounted Freud's emphasis on infantile sexuality as the source of neurosis. To him emotional problems appeared to be more a reflection of the eternal problems of the human race—how to become a person, how to find meaning in life, one's relation to the significant people in one's life, and so forth. He believed that loneliness, hopelessness, and despair as to life's meaning could be overcome by developing an awareness of the connection between the forces working within the collective unconscious and the personal unconscious. That is, one could find the link between the personal life of the individual and that of the entire human race. The goal of therapy was thus to help people find meaning in life and for this reason was thought by Jung to be an answer to the therapeutic needs of the older person. He continued to recommend Freudian psychoanalysis for younger people because its emphasis on instinctual urges seemed to him more suited to their needs.

Although they started out in opposite directions, both Jung and Adler arrived at a similar therapeutic objective —overcoming the sense of isolation of the individual. The methods differ. Adler aims at a re-education of habits and attitudes and the development of a "social sense"; Jung seeks to develop a personal philosophy of life. These goals differ from the "classical" psychoanalytic objective of resolving neurotic conflicts, but they are by no means incompatible with it. The fact that Jung and Adler took psychoanalysis as a point of departure and what they have in common with psychoanalysis (for example, the concept of unconscious mental processes) justifies their being considered as belonging to the psychoanalytic school of thought. It is what they disregarded or abandoned (specifically, the theory of psychosexual development) that marks them as distinct from the Freudian school.

Rank's Approach. After World War I, Otto Rank, one of Freud's younger disciples, developed a variation of psychoanalysis which was initially based on a different interpretation of the therapeutic process. Rank believed with Freud that the essential element of therapy lay in the transference relationship—the emotional attitudes developed by the patient toward the therapist which could be understood as a re-enactment of unconscious attitudes toward parents and other significant people in his childhood. But he held that the re-experiencing of an intense personal relationship and the working through of the feelings of separation at the termination of therapy had a unique significance. The reason for this lay in Rank's concept of neurosis as stemming from the act of being born— the birth trauma experienced by the infant as it leaves the all-protective environment of the womb. The patient-therapist relationship is then the re-creation of this situation, and the act of separation from the therapist is intended to allow the patient to assert his striving for independence and to conquer the anxiety which surrounded these strivings. Clearly this notion places the interpersonal relationship of the therapist and the patient in the center of the therapeutic process and concentrates their work on the specific experience of separation, thus limiting the scope of the exploration of the unconscious.

Influence of Various Approaches. The divergent movements described above did not seriously rival Freudian analysis as the principal therapeutic approach, but they did exert a considerable influence on the thinking of workers in the field generally and on the public at large. Jung's philosophical orientation was well received in Europe, while the concepts of Adler and Rank appealed to many in the United States. They have also provided models for certain trends and shifts in emphasis regarding either theory or technique. For example, Adler's emphasis on the social aspects of personality development is reflected in certain ideas of Karen Horney, Erich Fromm, Abram Kardiner, and others. Jung has served as the prototype for those movements which seek to relate psychoanalysis to various philosophies of life. Among these are the "existential" analysts who attempt to relate the anxiety of neurosis to the uneasiness of persons who are troubled by philosophical questions as to the meaning of life.

Nonpsychoanalytic Therapies. There are a number of schools of psychotherapy which may be said to ignore completely theory and interpretation of the patient's past or current behavior. One of the better known is the Carl Rogers school of "nondirective" therapy, in which the task of the therapist is to provide a warm, positive atmosphere in which the patient can explore his attitudes and feelings. This differs from the role of the counselor who attempts to advise and direct the individual. Such forms of therapy differ from psychoanalytic therapies in that they do not seek to explore the unconscious or to alter the patient's personality on the basis of a theory of human behavior. They generally seek to encourage the patient's exploration of his attitudes, and to support him in his attempts to think and act in a more fruitful manner.

Significance of Differences

The fact that wide differences of theory and method exist has raised the question as to the validity of psychotherapy in general. With regard to psychoanalytic theory, analysts point out that no scientific body of knowledge or theory is ever complete and forever closed to revisions. The more ambitious the theory in its attempt to explain a large number of facts, the more likely it is to require revision. Also, the newer a theory, the more it is open to misunderstanding or misinterpretation. Frequently differences of opinion among experts are more a difference of language or emphasis than of substance. Psychoanalysts consider the deviations within their own group as having contributed to elaborations of psychoanalytic theory. This does not mean that they consider everyone to be equally right, but that seen in historical perspective the differences are less irreconcilable than they may have originally appeared. Psychoanalysis has, of course, never claimed to be the only feasible method of therapy. At most its adherents have claimed it to be the only theory of human behavior sufficiently comprehensive to provide an explanation of the therapeutic effect of various approaches.

Despite theoretical differences, however, most forms of psychotherapy have important elements in common. These are that a personal relationship is established for the specific purpose of helping a person to deal with his psychological problem, and that the therapeutic situation thus created is "permissive"—meaning that the patient realizes he may speak freely without fear of being judged, scorned, or condemned by the therapist. Finally, the resolution of the difficulty is expected to come about through a searching exploration of the nature of the difficulty on the part of the patient, leading to some new understanding of his problems.

Some therapists would argue that these common elements allow the conclusion that all approaches are of equal value and that the underlying theories have no practical significance. Others would maintain that the common elements constitute what might be called the minimum requiremnts for therapeutic help. In some instances such minimum help will be sufficient to produce improvement; in other cases it is only an initial step. It may be that even a brief period of therapy satisfying these minimal conditions can be of great importance in the life of a person suffering from an acute emotional difficulty. But it is one thing to come to someone's help in an emergency and another to help a person with a long-standing set of symptoms which make his life seem hardly worth living or which endanger his family.

Theory also influences the course that therapy will take. If the therapist believes that a full resolution of the difficulty in question cannot be achieved without exploring childhood conflicts, he will obviously proceed differently than if he believes that the problems are not related to them. If two therapists holding such divergent views were dealing with the same type of problem, not only would the therapy have a different character, but it would also lead to different results. The differences of opinion are modified somewhat by the considerable overlapping of theories held by any given therapist (for example, an Adlerian therapist may accept certain Freudian concepts and vice versa). Furthermore, there is often a gap between what therapists do and what they think they do. This may be because they proceed intuitively or because their own personality plays a more important role in their effectiveness than they realize. Another factor minimizing differences between therapists is that in many instances differences of opinion do not become relevant because they apply only to certain kinds of problems.

Paradoxically, the possibility exists that a therapist might be quite successful in helping people even though he bases his therapy on a faulty theory. This may be analogous to the supernatural explanations given by primitive peoples to the action of certain herbs—the herbs worked in spite of, not because of, the explanations given.

Over and above all these considerations, it must be kept in mind that even the most comprehensive and systematized theory can do no more than establish general principles and guide-lines for the therapist. The enormous variety and complexities of the problems which beset human beings and which the therapist is called upon to deal with present a continuous challenge to his ingenuity and resourcefulness. His ability to "think on his feet" may often contribute more to the therapist's success than some fine points of theory. For this reason the notion that psychotherapy is more an art than a science may contain a kernel of truth.

The form psychotherapy takes in any given case will also be determined by the therapeutic goal which the therapist and patient set for themselves. Some patients might be satisfied just to be freed from a particular symptom while others would want to be sure that it does not return. The latter might require a modification of the personality structure which underlies and gives rise to the symptom.

It must be realized that these goals cannot always be set at will by either patient or therapist. The nature of the disturbance also sets limits as to what can be accomplished, since not all forms of emotional disturbances are equally amenable to psychotherapy. Most readily susceptible to treatment are neurotic reactions, such as anxieties, phobias (irrational fear of animals, heights, places, and so forth), compulsive thoughts or actions (repeated hand washing even when the hands are clean), and various bodily disturbances which have no organic cause. Also susceptible to treatment are the so-called "character neuroses," which involve dominant and troublesome personality characteristics (such as being too inhibited or too rigid). Addictions, perversions, and psychoses are far more difficult to treat by psychotherapy alone.

Practical considerations also influence the kind of therapy given in a particular case. The cost may be considerable in forms of therapy requiring regular sessions ranging from one to five times a week over periods of months and years. Often the goals of therapy may have to remain limited for purely economic reasons.

Other Forms of Psychotherapy

Earlier, we noted differences between schools of psychotherapy based upon varying theories. Adlerian and Jungian therapy acted upon different concepts of the basic problems, and nondirective therapy rejected the theory upon which the psychoanalytic types of therapy were based. This by no means exhausts the bewildering variety of labels which have been attached to various forms of psychotherapy. Among these variants can be found differences based on theory (what is wrong), on goals (what shall be done about it), and on techniques (how should or can it be done). In terms of goals, "short-term" therapy attempts to relieve only particular neurotic symptoms, while "long-term" therapies seek to alter the basic personality structure.

"Supportive" therapy also aims at treating certain symptoms (for example, anxiety) and, as the word implies, involves reassurances, encouragements, and warmth on the part of the therapist to help the patient deal with his problems. In terms of technique, many specialized forms of therapy are used. "Hypnotherapy" utilizes hypnosis to help overcome the patient's inability to communicate. "Environmental" psychotherapy is directed at changing the circumstances which contribute to the emotional difficulty. This may require taking a child out of one class in school and putting him in another or removing an emotionally disturbed soldier from the combat zone. "Psychodrama" is another specialized technique of psychotherapy in which the individual spontaneously acts out a particular role suggested by the therapist in a dramatic setting with others. In the dramatic situation he may find freer expression of unconscious attitudes than he would otherwise be capable of.

Group Therapy. In this procedure the members of a group discuss their personal problems under the leadership of a therapist. The therapy is more or less modeled along the lines of individual therapy sessions but is to varying degrees modified by the interaction of the members of the group. An interesting variant of this approach is Alcoholics Anonymous—an informal association of former alcoholics who help themselves and others to overcome their addiction through mutual support and encouragement.

Family Therapy. This focuses on the entire family as the object of therapy. The family is considered to be all those who live under one roof. The therapist conducts his sessions with the family and attempts to diagnose the lines of cleavage and dissension and to reduce the psychological tensions existing between its members.

Play Therapy. This is used with children. The therapist may use the symbolic significance of the play activity as a clue to understanding the child's unconscious conflicts.

Training of the Therapist

The fact that the therapist's personality is one of his major professional tools affects both the selection and training of candidates. For this reason students are selected on the basis of personality characteristics for which it is difficult to establish an objective system of evaluation, such as grades for scholastic achievement. Also, the therapist is required to submit himself to therapy, both to understand more thoroughly the process and to gain insight into aspects of his own personality which might interfere with his professional functioning.

The highly personal and subjective nature of the therapist's training is difficult to fit into the more formal requirements of general academic institutions, and consequently most therapists receive their training in private institutes. Even so, more and more medical schools and graduate psychology departments have introduced theoretical and clinical programs designed to formalize the training of psychotherapists.

The distinction between medical and nonmedical therapists refers to their academic training, not to any difference in theoretical persuasion. Psychotherapists may have an M.D. or a Ph.D. degree. The term "psychiatrist" designates a physician who specializes in mental disorders. He may practice psychotherapy or may use drugs, shock therapy, and other medical procedures. A nonmedical therapist does not use the latter means.

Criticisms of Psychotherapy and Some Open Questions

The enthusiastic acceptance of psychotherapy in some quarters has been matched by an equally vigorous criticism in others. The critics have demanded "objective" proof of its value—of the same order as that obtainable in the physical sciences. Some studies have been made, claiming that psychotherapy produces no greater improvement than would normally occur with the passage of time. The protagonists of psychotherapy have, in turn, criticized such studies as being too superficial. They cite the difficulty of defining what a "cure" or even "improvement" is in objective terms. What seems incontestable is that "test-tube" proof of the effectiveness or ineffectiveness of psychotherapy is not applicable to this problem.

This is not felt to be a problem of great urgency or importance by the therapists because they see the changes which they effect in patients right before their eyes as a continuous process—and so do patients. As a matter of fact, most of the theory is based on the systematic observation of these changes in patients.

Aside from uncritical overestimation or rejection of psychotherapy and the practical limitations to its applicability—time, money, personnel—psychotherapy raises many problems concerning ethics, responsibility, and values. For example, is a soldier who develops certain inappropriate reactions a willful malingerer or is he "sick"— should he be punished or treated? To what extent can an individual be held responsible for an antisocial act if it is true that he is acting under the influence of internal pressures over which he has no more control than over a headache? Will therapy change a person's values and lead him to reject previously held beliefs, such as religious convictions? Also, if it is granted that the therapist influences his patient in some ways, to what extent is his philosophy of life transmitted to the patient, even though this is consciously avoided?

Perhaps the most profound implication of psychotherapy has to do with the rearing of children and their education. If the theories are correct in tracing the majority of adult neurotic problems to childhood experiences and events, then the clear possibility exists of adjusting child rearing to the psychological needs of the child. If this can be done, then an "ounce of prevention" may indeed be worth more than a "pound of cure."

See also PSYCHIATRY; PSYCHOANALYSIS; PSYCHOLOGY.

PYROMANIA, literally fire-madness, an irresistible desire to commit acts of arson which have no obvious purpose. The reasons for this behavior may be neurotic or psychopathic. The neurotic may wish to draw attention to himself, or his pyromania may indicate an emotional disorder. If pyromania is a sociopathic personality disturbance, it reveals two characteristics of the psychopathic personality in extreme form, lack of motivation in committing antisocial acts and lack of neurotic anxiety concerning those acts. Individual antisocial acts are, in most cases, attributed to personal motives, such as hate or jealousy. The pyromaniac sets his fires without apparent motive. For most people, the thought of violent and antisocial acts is accompanied by feelings which range from uneasiness to outright anxiety. The psychopath feels no anxiety and, even after committing the crime, does not seem to have a guilty conscience. The pleasure derived from seeing something burn has been attributed to destructive instincts or aggression. But it is also understandable as resentment of society. During times of social breakdown, such as wars and riots, the destructive impulses that otherwise show only in sick individuals may be released simultaneously in many members of a group.

R

RANK [*rängk*], **OTTO** (1884–1939), Austrian psychoanalyst and early associate of Sigmund Freud. Rank split with Freud, developing his own concept of the birth experience as the central factor in neurosis. He practiced psychoanalysis in Paris from 1926 to 1935 and then in New York until his death.

RATIONALIZATION [*răsh-ən-əl-ə-zā'shən*], in psychology, a mental device by which an individual invents acceptable explanations for his own behavior. For example, the public official who accepts a bribe "rationalizes" that he is underpaid and overworked and thus converts an unethical act into an acceptable one. According to many psychologists and psychoanalysts, rationalization is one of the defense mechanisms which protect the individual from anxiety by avoiding the necessity of recognizing one's less palatable motives.
See also NEUROSIS; PSYCHOANALYSIS.

RAUWOLFIA [*rou-wŏŏl'fē-ə*], powdered whole root of *Rauwolfia serpentina*, a climbing shrub found mainly in India, Ceylon, and Burma. Used for centuries in the tropics for a number of disorders, rauwolfia came to medical attention in the 1930's when a number of its active ingredients (reserpine, deserpidine, alseroxylon) were isolated. Although knowledge of its action is incomplete, evidence indicates that reserpine affects the circulatory and nervous systems by its action upon certain hormones (serotonin, norepinephrine) which are important in nervous function. Reserpine and rauwolfia have been used as tranquilizers in psychiatric patients, but their use in this respect has been curtailed by a tendency to produce serious depressions. The drugs are of value in reducing high blood pressure.
See also PSYCHOPHARMACOLOGY; TRANQUILIZERS.

REACTION TIME, the interval between presentation of a stimulus, such as a buzz, and the response to that stimulus, such as pressing a button. Interest in this field was first aroused by the German astronomer F. W. Bessell. In 1830 Bessell noted consistent personal differences among various astronomers in recording the time of passage of a star across the field of their telescopes. He attributed these differences to individual variations in the time interval between the physical occurrence of the star's passage and the perception of this passage as determined by the actuation of a stopwatch.

In 1880 the German physiologist Hermann Helmholtz attempted to use the phenomenon of reaction time to measure the conduction speed of nerve impulses. He stimulated a subject with a weak electric shock, first on the toe and then on the thigh, and noted the time difference in the reflexive twitch from the time of stimulation. Helmholtz theorized that the time difference corresponded to the nerve conduction time between the toe and thigh.

The Dutch physiologist F. C. Donders distinguished three types of reaction time: (1) Simple reaction time, pressing a button in response to a brief flash of light. (2) Discrimination reaction time, pressing a button when a green light is flashed but not if a red one accompanies the green. (3) Choice reaction time, pressing one of several buttons associated with several lights, only one of which is correct. He found that reaction time increases with the complexity of the situation. The Danish physiologist Carl Lange refined Donder's work by demonstrating that reaction time is shorter when the subject concentrated on the response, rather than on the stimulus. Thus, an automobile driver starts faster when a stoplight turns green if he concentrates on depressing the accelerator rather than on anticipating the light change.

Recent studies of simple reaction time have shown that each individual's reaction time is fairly constant over a large number of trials, with the same stimulus intensity and duration. This fact is being widely used to measure the effects of various stimulus conditions, such as varying levels of sound, and varying subject conditions, such as different levels of fatigue or lack of sleep. These experiments are of value in the analysis and evaluation of many human skills, such as flying and driving.

REFLEX [*rē'flĕks*], automatic response to a stimulus. The simplest reflex arc is exemplified by the knee jerk. A blow on the patellar tendon just below the knee sends a message along an afferent (sensory) nerve to the spinal cord. A double message goes back, causing the extensors to contract and the flexors to relax, resulting in an involuntary kicking motion. This is one of many very simple deep tendon reflexes which are largely unaffected by the higher centers of the central nervous system. But there is always either some inhibitory effect or an enhancement of these reflexes by inflowing messages from the brain.

More complex reflexes are of considerable diagnostic help in examining premature and newborn infants. The appearance during fetal life of many reflexes helps the physician to estimate the infant's gestational age. Several primitive reflexes appear very early, and disappear at a predictable age. Failure to disappear may be the first clue to brain damage or disease. The constancy and predictability of these reflexes in infancy and childhood give an indication of overall cerebral function. In adulthood, the same predictability is useful in demonstrating functional integrity of a specific nerve arc.

Superficial reflexes elicited by lightly stroking the skin are dependent upon, or markedly modified by, connections with the brain. Thus, they are of use in diagnosing diseases higher in the central nervous system.

Emotional stimuli produce many involuntary, reflex reactions, such as blushing with embarrassment and blanching with fear. The reflexes involve the muscles found in all small arteries, causing them to dilate or contract, sometimes to the extent of altering the blood pressure. The breathing rate may be similarly affected. Lie detector testing uses these physiological changes to determine truth or falsehood, by detecting the emotional response to lying.

The great Russian physiologist Ivan P. Pavlov described a different type of reflex—the conditioned reflex. In his original work he used dogs to demonstrate a simple conditioned reflex. When a dog sights food, its salivary glands begin to flow. Pavlov always presented food in association with the ringing of a bell. The dogs learned this association and would salivate as soon as the bell rang, even in the absence of food. Much of our activity and behavior can be explained by a series of intricate conditioned responses. To an experienced motorist, most of his driving is reflex in nature. Some philosophers are convinced that most, if not all, life processes are types of reflex actions.

Knowledge of conditioned reflexes is used in some clinics for alcoholics, where patients are given a tasteless emetic in their favorite drink. The constant association of alcohol and vomiting eventually produces an aversion to alcohol alone. This type of reflex must be reinforced by repetition at intervals to remain effective. The same type of approach may be used to help people stop smoking.
See also CONDITIONING; NERVOUS SYSTEM.

REGRESSION [rĭ-grĕsh′ən], in psychiatry, a return to a more primitive and infantile mode of behavior, which occurs under conditions of stress or frustration. An example may be seen in the behavior of the adult who becomes helpless, dependent, and "childish" in trying circumstances. In psychoanalytic thinking, regression is distinguished from fixation. In the latter the individual becomes arrested at a specific stage of psychic development. The disorganization and disintegration of behavior seen in psychotic reactions is considered a form of regression.
See also MENTAL ILLNESS; PSYCHIATRY; PSYCHOANALYSIS; PSYCHOTHERAPY.

REIK [rīk], **THEODOR** (1888–1969), psychoanalyst, one of the original group associated with Sigmund Freud in Vienna. Reik also studied under Karl Abraham in Berlin and practiced in Berlin, Vienna, and the Netherlands. He went to the United States in 1938. A champion of nonmedical analysts, Reik founded the National Psychological Association for Psychoanalysis, an organization which includes both medical and lay therapists. His publications include *Listening with the Third Ear* (1948), *Masochism in Modern Man* (1949), and *The Secret Self* (1960).

REPRESSION refers to an active but unconscious mental process which makes certain mental material unavailable to conscious awareness, unless special attempts are made to recover it. These attempts may be through psychoanalysis, drugs, or hypnosis. Repression is considered the central defense mechanism of the ego, designed to control those ideas, impulses, and feelings which would create intolerable anxiety. It was first elaborated by Sigmund Freud to explain the frequent memory gaps, particularly those related to early childhood, which he observed in his patients. He came to call this childhood amnesia, a result of repressing certain unacceptable impulses and wishes which the child had been taught to reject. Since Freud's original formulations, the concept has gained wide acceptance and has found clinical support in such phenomena as "slips of the tongue" and posthypnotic amnesia. The latter follows patterns predicted by the laws of repression—that less pleasant material is most difficult to recall.

Not all "forgetting" is the result of repression. In the two large groups of memories, one has to do with neutral material, such as facts, and the other with personal history, called autobiographical memory. In the first instance forgetting follows certain laws related to time and frequency of repetition while in the second it is related to repression of material which has a more highly charged personal meaning.

There is some question as to whether repression fully explains such phenomena as childhood amnesia. Why does the unacceptable nature of some impulses serve to explain the forgetting of almost all childhood experiences? Possibly because the organization of the adult's mind no longer permits the recovery of childhood memories..

Though a normal mental mechanism, repression may become exaggerated in individuals for whom repressed material exerts a profound effect upon the total personality, leading to such disturbances as hysterical reactions and pathological amnesias. Eminently responsive to psychotherapy, these disturbances were among the first to be considered by Sigmund Freud in the development of psychoanalysis.
See also AMNESIA; HYSTERIA; PSYCHOANALYSIS.

RHINE [rīn], **JOSEPH BANKS** (1895–   ), American psychologist. A graduate of the University of Chicago (Ph.D., 1925), he joined the faculty of Duke University in 1928. In 1940 he became director of Duke's parapsychology laboratory. His extensive and careful experimental studies of such phenomena as telepathy are reported in *Extra-Sensory Perception* (1934), *New Frontiers of the Mind* (1937), *The Reach of the Mind* (1947), and *New World of the Mind* (1953).
See also PARAPSYCHOLOGY.

S

SCHIZOID [skĭt'zoid] **PERSONALITY,** prone to an emotionally rigid, secluded, and asocial way of life. It is often coupled with introversion, a preoccupation with the self. Originally Eugen Bleuler introduced the term to describe the prepsychotic personality of schizophrenic patients. However, not all schizophrenics are schizoid and many conspicuously schizoid persons never become psychotic.

The sensitive schizoid feels lonely and imperfectly understood. He is shy, self-conscious, and often paranoid. In school or college he rarely takes part in games or social activities but strives for a sense of security in a secret hobby, such as keeping a diary or by excelling in some special study. His love for literature or art often substitutes for human companionship, and he prefers abstract or philosophical subjects to concrete, objective interests. However, many schizoids lack such sensitivity. Since they also lack spontaneity, they appear emotionally dull and taciturn and are often attracted to rites and cults. Many become cold, reserved, headstrong individuals, resentful of advice or supervision. These extremes are not always applicable, and often a sensitive, tender nature is hidden beneath an aloof and unresponsive exterior.

When a schizoid personality develops a psychotic reaction, it usually resembles schizophrenia. When a schizophrenic psychosis occurs in such a personality, the process may be more severe and resistant to treatment than one arising in another personality type.
See also SCHIZOPHRENIA.

SCHIZOPHRENIA [skĭz-ō-frē'nē-ə], a major mental disease marked by a disorganization of the personality with bizarre behavior, hallucinations, incoherent speech, and detachment from the real world. It is the most common form of psychosis, accounting for approximately half of the chronic patients in state mental hospitals. The concept of schizophrenia as a single disease is questioned by some psychiatrists, and no single definition is acceptable.

Causes. Theories concerning the cause of schizophrenia are highly controversial. One group of theorists stresses the importance of psychological factors. The other searches for a physiological or biochemical cause. The first group traces the origins of the disease to an anxiety-laden early family life, beset with tension between the parents. Some even describe a "schizophrenogenic mother," an overprotective, cold, or distant person who produces the schizophrenic pattern by her inability to give herself to the child. The second group seeks an underlying organic disturbance. Several studies have attempted to demonstrate the influence of inheritance on schizophrenia. One such investigation found the greatest incidence of schizophrenia among children of schizophrenic parents.

Other investigators have examined the biochemistry of the schizophrenic in comparison with the normal and, in the words of one critic, such investigators have found the schizophrenic to be "a sorry physical specimen indeed: his liver, brain, kidney, and circulatory functions are impaired; he is deficient in practically every vitamin; his hormones are out of balance, and his enzymes are askew." This writer points out the great difficulty in determining whether such biochemical changes are the *cause* of the disease or the *result* of it. The biological school received encouragement from the fact that tranquilizing drugs were effective in calming agitated patients. It is felt that the action of these drugs may be related to the concentration of certain substances in the brain (serotonin or noradrenalin). Some investigators feel that imbalances of these substances may play a role in the disease.

Symptoms. Schizophrenia is usually a long time in developing. The individual may gradually lose interest in the world, as his personality loses its color, and he may withdraw from social contacts, preferring to sulk in his room. He may become preoccupied with mystical speculations or begin to feel that he is the target of suspicious glances. The fully developed schizophrenic episode is most common in adolescence or in early adult life. The disease involves changes in speech, thought, and behavior.

Speech peculiarities testify to the bizarre mental activity of the schizophrenic. The conversation of the patient is illogical, irrelevant, and tangential to what is under discussion. There may be an odd rhyming and punning or repetition of words (perseveration).

Thinking. The schizophrenic is unable to think abstractly, but gives a "concrete" meaning to ideas. The patient, when asked to explain a proverb such as "When the cat's away, the mice will play," merely rephrases it, saying that the mice are free to play when the cat is away. He is unable to understand "cat" and "mice" in the symbolic sense of a person of authority and individuals subordinate to that authority. Thought loses the normal logical guideposts and seems to resemble the "condensation," or lumping together of ideas, as seen in dreams. Associations are incongruous and fragmented. There may be a reckless invention of new words compounded into an incoherent jumble, or "word salad." For example, one schizophrenic produced an essay entitled *Equalitized Metabolic Demention Metabolism.*

Delusions. The patient may have delusions of persecution ("They are trying to poison me"), of grandeur ("I am Queen of Scotland, Empress of the world"), or of dissolution ("I am falling apart; I don't exist any longer"). The paranoid schizophrenic may be nihilistic ("I exist; there is no world"). The schizophrenic with delusions of persecution may have "ideas of reference," feeling that all events relate to him. He may hear a policeman's whistle and think "Cop's whistle means I can't see my girl tonight." The schizophrenic may also have delusions about his own body ("My blood is turning to stone. My back hurts, my brain is shrinking and running down my spinal cord").

Hallucinations. The commonest hallucinations are voices. Occasionally hallucinations of smell are present, particularly the odor of cooking gas or of rotting flesh.

Emotional Reaction. This is a striking aspect of the schizophrenic in which the emotional response is not appropriate to the situation. The schizophrenic may speak of the funeral of a close relative as a normal person might recite a recipe, or he may laugh at hearing of the death of a loved one. This behavior is described as a "splitting-off" of emotions from the rest of the personality. There is also a characteristic dullness and flatness to the emotional life of the schizophrenic; he lacks the "spark" of the normal person.

Loss of Identity. The schizophrenic may become deper-sonalized. He may ask, "Am I a man or am I a woman?" He may feel that he is a spectator or that he has no body. These ideas are all considered manifestations of a loss of awareness of the self as a distinct entity.

Types. There are four principal types of schizophrenia, which differ in the emphasis on the symptoms described above.

The simple type involves basically a loss of interest in people and activities, a complete inertness. Hallucinations, delusions, and disorganized thought are rarely seen. The pattern usually begins in childhood but is not recognized until late adolescence or early adulthood when the patient's lethargy, poverty of thought and emotion, and withdrawal from social contact make employment and normal living impossible. Such individuals may become vagrants or prostitutes if not cared for by some other member of the family or hospitalized.

The hebephrenic type represents extreme personality disorganization. The patient's behavior is best described as "silly." He giggles or laughs inappropriately. Speech and thought are chaotic, and hallucinations are plentiful.

The catatonic type displays extremes of withdrawal or excitement. After an initial period of agitated, purposeless overactivity, he may settle down to a stupor, refusing to move and maintaining for hours whatever position he is placed in.

The paranoid type is preoccupied with delusions, particularly delusions of persecution: people are talking about him, watching him, after him, and so on. Hallucinations are common. This type is more prevalent in older adults.

Schizophrenia in Children. Several writers have described schizophreniclike reactions in children marked by withdrawal and occasionally by hallucinations and delusions. A distinctive form is "infantile autism," occurring in children as early as the age of 2 or 3. These children avoid social interaction, remain by themselves, have a curious obsession for sameness (the furniture must always be in exactly the same position), and may not speak. Such children, although often brilliant, may seem feeble-minded.

Treatment. Treatment of schizophrenia falls into the same two groups as speculations concerning its cause: psychotherapy and physical or biological therapies. Psy-chotherapy is often used in conjunction with tranquilizing drugs which quiet the patient and make therapy possible. Other forms of treatment are insulin coma therapy, electroconvulsive therapy, and lobotomy. The tranquilizing drugs have been of great help with disturbed and agitated patients and have permitted the discharge of many who would otherwise be chronic hospital patients.

See also LOBOTOMY; MENTAL ILLNESS; PSYCHIATRY; SHOCK THERAPY.

SELYE [sĕl′yā], **HANS** (1907–), Canadian biochemist and histopathologist. Born in Vienna, Selye was an assistant in experimental pathology at the University of Prague from 1929 to 1931. He went to Johns Hopkins as a Rockefeller Research Fellow and then to McGill University under the same aegis in 1932–33. In 1945 he became professor and director of the Institute of Experimental Medicine and Surgery at the University of Montreal.

Selye performed the first experiment, clearly establishing the link between disease and the adrenal cortex. He had anticipated finding specific pathological changes in rats given a variety of drugs, poisons, and gland extracts. Instead, he noted similar responses to each substance. This led him to theorize that any life-threatening stress would elicit similar pathological findings, particularly in the adrenals. Selye named this common response the "alarm reaction." In the alarm reaction, he described a shock and countershock phase. In the latter phase, he found great enlargement and increased activity of the adrenal cortex. Lacking adrenals, the animals succumbed to shock.

Selye next studied the effects of milder but more prolonged stress, and suggested that diseases of adaptation resulted from prolonged stress. His theory gives credence to the concept that prolonged physical and emotional stress can cause specific illnesses. In man, such stress ills include arteriosclerosis, peptic ulcer, and rheumatoid arthritis. Although the relationship between stress and disease is accepted, the specific cause and effect remain imprecise.

SENILITY [si-nĭl′ə-tē], physical and mental state of old age characterized by personality changes resulting in part from the altered psychological and social situation of the elderly person and in part from actual damage to brain tissue. As his faculties begin to fail and as he finds himself increasingly alone, the aged individual may begin to feel that life has passed him by. He may become resentful of his declining influence on those around him and may feel that his experience qualifies him for a position of respect and importance in the family or even in public life. He is frequently dogmatic, inflexible, and conservative, and unable to accept or tolerate changes. Increased leisure may lead to introspection, and in reviewing his life the older person may be overcome by feelings of guilt or failure. This may culminate in a severe and sometimes pathological depression.

Whether or not such traits appear depends on the individual's earlier personality. The adverse character changes are often merely accentuations of features which were always present. For this reason it has been said that senility is a caricature of the previous personality. The social changes are less marked in smaller communities, where the aged person often retains responsibility as a respected elder, than in populous cities where the older individual becomes a neglected and anonymous citizen.

Although the exact nature of the brain changes in senility is not yet clear, they apparently involve a decrease in the blood supply to the brain and a lowered activity of brain tissue. Decline in brain function may result in memory impairment. At first the memory of recent events is vague and, later, events in the distant past are forgotten. The patient may attempt to compensate for his memory loss by fabrications. He may eventually become suspicious and feel that he is being persecuted because of the confusion resulting from his inability to recall where he has left his belongings or what he has been told. These changes may finally culminate in a psychosis (senile psychosis) characterized by confusion, agitation, depression, or exaggerated ideas of being persecuted. Hospitalization may be necessary.

One approach to the problems of senility is to keep the elderly person active and involved with people. He should be made to feel useful in a manner consistent with his physical and intellectual capacities. In cases of senile psychosis, medication and electroshock treatment for depression may be helpful.

SENSATION [sĕn-sā'shən]. All that we know of the world around us and about our own body comes from the messages started at sense receptors and carried by nerve fibers to the brain, where they are decoded and interpreted. Through this process we become aware of our environments, both external and internal. The messages are initiated by an appropriate sensory stimulus, which, by definition, is any change in energy that activates a sense organ. But all energy changes are not effective. The eye, for example, responds only to about 1/70th of the total known spectrum of different frequencies. Our eyes are not "tuned" to cosmic rays, radio, ultraviolet, infrared, and other waves. Nor can human ears hear frequencies much above 20,000 or below 20 cycles per second. All of the other senses have limits. Nevertheless, our many senses allow us to enjoy a good perfume or an opera, examine pictures, or attend to descriptions of what we have not ourselves experienced. In short, everything we do depends upon information encoded in messages from our receptors.

The Stimuli. Six classes of stimuli affect receptors: mechanical, thermal, photic, acoustic, chemical, and electrical. All of these forms of energy change serve as potential information for use by the conscious individual. Photic energy (light), for example, informs us about happenings in the three dimensions of space, as do also the acoustic and mechanical forces. Simply by looking, we preceive how high, how wide, and far away is an object. Similarly, through aural perception we learn to detect the direction and distance of the baby's cry or the kitten's meow. The chemical agents, which produce odor and taste perceptions, must reach the receptor in the nose and on the tongue before they can be effective. But since odorous gases and vapors are airborne, the nose is viewed as a distance receptor as contrasted to a contact receptor, such as the tongue. Thermal energy can work either over distance or by contact, since it is dependent upon the addition or withdrawal of heat. Electricity has the interesting property of exciting all the senses. Stimuli, then, come in a variety of forms, providing rich arrays of information during every second of the time we remain alert to them.

The Number of Senses. How many different senses respond to the six basic types of stimuli? Aristotle found only five, lumping many under "feeling." Now we know that 25 is as valid a number as 5, depending upon our system of classification. The skin possesses four, anatomically and functionally, different senses: cold, warm, pressure (touch), and pain. A given tiny spot on the skin will always respond to a warm stimulus object but never to a sharp needle prick, while an adjacent area will detect only cold, and so on. The nonauditory portion of the inner ear responds to speeding up or slowing down of

CLASSIFICATION OF THE SENSES AND THEIR RESPONSES

Sense	Normal Stimulus	Sense Organ	Receptor	Sensory Qualities
Vision	photic energy (light)	eye	rods and cones of retina	colors, discontinuities, textures, etc.
Hearing	acoustic energy	ear	hair cells of organs of Corti	tones and noises
Skin sensitivities	mechanical, thermal, and chemical energy	skin	specialized and free nerve endings	pressure, pain, heat, and cold
Smell	volatile substances	olfactory cleft high in nose	hair cells of odor epithelium	odors (minty, burnt, woody, musty, etc.)
Taste	soluble substances	tongue	taste buds of papillae	sweet, salty, sour, bitter
Kinesthesia	mechanical energy	muscles, joints and tendons	specialized and free nerve endings	pressure, pain
Labyrinthine sensitivity (statis sense and balance)	mechanical forces and gravity	nonauditory labyrinth of the inner ear	hair cells of crista and macula	none (equilibrium)
Organic sensitivity	mechanical energy	portions of alimentary tract	specialized and free nerve endings	pain, pressure

SENSATION—THE LINK BETWEEN THE BRAIN AND THE SENSE ORGANS

The brain experiences the world through the senses of sight, taste, smell, hearing, and the skin senses of touch and temperature. The nature of these sensory-brain links is still obscure: ancient Greek philosophers believed that the senses transmitted "copies" of objects to the brain; however, modern physiologists have discovered that the senses transmit only nerve impulses. Information about the world is somehow "coded" into these identical electrochemical impulses, much as a Shakespeare play or a Hindu epic could be put into the dots and dashes of the telegraph code. The problem for sense physiology is to understand how the brain deciphers the code and thus to reveal how the properties of objects are perceived by the mind.

HOW THE QUALITIES OF OBJECTS ARE RECOGNIZED

THE EYE AND COLOR

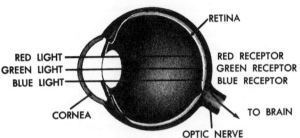

One of the most perplexing problems of sensory physiology is that of how the visual apparatus distinguishes color. Several theories of color vision are based on the idea of special color receptors in the retina — the light-sensitive membrane of the eye. According to such theories, light of specific wavelengths, or colors, would stimulate specific receptors. The best-known theory (the Helmholtz-Young hypothesis) assumes the existence of receptors for red, green, and blue light. The impulses from these receptors are presumably mixed in the brain, or the eye, or somewhere between to yield the full range of colors to which we are sensitive.

THE TONGUE AND TASTE

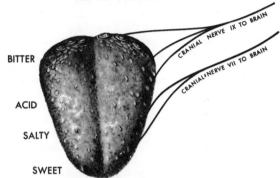

THE DISTRIBUTION OF TASTE RECEPTORS ON THE TONGUE

The sensation of taste is made possible by special sensory receptors in the tongue. Apparently the brain identifies a taste as "bitter," "sweet," "salty," or "acid," because it stimulates specific tongue receptors, giving rise to nerve impulses that travel along specific pathways to the "taste" areas of the brain.

HOW OBJECTS ARE LOCATED IN SPACE

HOW SOUNDS ARE PINPOINTED

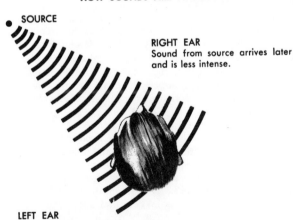

RIGHT EAR
Sound from source arrives later and is less intense.

LEFT EAR
Sound from source arrives sooner and is more intense.

Sounds are located on the basis of differences in time interval and intensity of the sounds arriving at the ears. Impulses from the two ears must thus be compared somewhere in the brain or along the nerve pathway which leads from the ear to the brain.

HOW OBJECTS ARE LOCATED ON THE SKIN

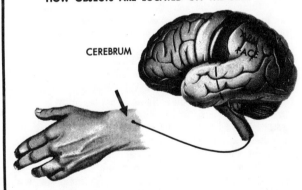

An object pressing on the skin stimulates touch receptors, giving rise to impulses that travel to a specific area of the cerebrum. In this part of the brain each section of the skin is represented by specific nerve cells, just as each section of a stretch of terrain may be represented by a corresponding area on a map. Impulses from a given part of the skin stimulate their representative cells in the skin "map" of the brain. In this way the brain locates the pressure as originating from a specific point on the skin.

bodily motion and to the differential pull of gravity. Here, the body itself is the thing perceived, and muscular adjustments are instituted to preserve or restore equilibrium. And sensory organs in the muscles "feel" the position of an arm or leg. This muscles sense, termed kinesthesia, tells us about posture and makes possible the complex motor skills involved in driving cars, flying planes, or playing golf. Without this sensitivity in the muscles, tendons, and joints, we should be forced to watch over every movement of hand or foot.

Nor are these all the senses. The organic sense located in the lining of our gastrointestinal tract makes possible reports on hunger, thirst, nausea, and a full bladder. Deeper within the body are sense systems for detecting a large variety of changes in chemical and thermal conditions. Again, all of these sensitivities do not rest logically in the single class of "feeling" advanced by Aristotle. In fact, the more we learn about each of our senses, the more we note the great variety of types of receptor mechanisms involved in knowing the world and safeguarding our lives. Not 5 nor even 25 are sufficient for the task of maintaining the complex human organism. In the interests of simplicity, only eight are illustrated in the table of classification.

Dimensions of Sensation. The sensory dimensions are quality, intensity, extension, and duration. Quality, though usually many-faceted, is the only identifying, or specifying, dimension. The other three dimensions are directed to the question of how much. In taste, a sensation may be weak or strong, disappear quickly or remain, but it must have sweetness or some other specific quality if it is to be sensed at all. Each of the other sense channels has its own special attributes, not one of which could possibly be confused with any other. Sounds may be intense or weak, large as the boom of thunder, or as small as the fife tone. They may last 2 seconds or 20 seconds. The intensity of any sensation depends upon the amount of effective energy in the stimulus, and the sensitivity of the receptor.

As noted earlier, the four dimensions—quality, intensity, extension, and duration—are inseparable characteristics of all sensations. Let any one of the four be reduced to nothing and the sensation also disappears. This does not mean that in all senses, all of the attributes are equally obvious. In vision or the skin senses, extension is more obvious than in smell or organic sensitivity, but that dimension still aids in the definition of a flavor or the degree of hunger being experienced.

Measurement of Sensation. Whatever the sense channel, a certain minimum amount of energy must impinge upon the receptor, before sensory messages can become initiated and be delivered to the brain. Senses are not infinitely acute. This minimum amount is called the absolute threshold. A statistical concept, a threshold varies from time to time, condition to condition and from person to person. Still, it expresses an important and useful relation between the physical stimulus and the psychologic response of the observer. Hence, the name given to this branch of study is psychophysics. It was founded by Ernst Heinrich Weber (1795–1878) and Gustav Theodor Fechner (1801–87). In 1834 Weber began to study the difference thresholds, or the least amount of change which can reliably be perceived as different. After investigating several departments of sense, Weber found that human judgments are relative. Lifting four, then five, postage stamps, a man may be able to discern the difference in weight, while he cannot discern the addition of a pint of water to a 50-pound bucket. In other words, the increment that can just be discriminated, or the just noticeable difference, has a constant relation to the basic intensity. The Weber fraction for lifted weights, in the middle ranges, is about $\frac{1}{50}$. For taste, it is about $\frac{1}{3}$, meaning that any taste stimulus must be increased in intensity by about $\frac{1}{3}$ before it is noticeably different. Some visual tasks have Weber fractions of $\frac{1}{60}$.

Fechner's principal contribution was a generalization relating the array of stimulus energies to the parallel sensation intensity. After creating the major methods of psychophysics, all of which are still employed, Fechner showed that as stimuli increase in geometrical progression, sensations increase in arithmetical progression. Therefore, relatively larger and larger quantities of stimulus energy are required to get corresponding sensory reactions. But both the Weber fraction and the Frechner relationship are only crude approximations.

Twentieth-century contributions to psychophysical study of the lawful interaction of stimuli and response have depended upon the newer approaches to sensed ratios, via the route of three scalar methods: fractionation, magnitude estimation, and ratio estimation. Typically, under these methods an observer functioning in highly controlled conditions observes a standard stimulus and compares a second stimulus with it as a fraction or ratio. Alternately, he may assign a number from 1 to 100 to its absolute magnitude. The reliability of such procedures has proved quite satisfactory, even when totally different senses (for example, audition and kinesthesia) are employed in the quantitative comparison.

From such procedures, which in general confirm each other, has come the power law, linking sensation magnitude to stimulus intensity. This law holds that "equal stimulus ratios tend to produce equal sensation ratios."

The Sensory Signal in the Nervous System. Though the stimulus and the sensory responses have been briefly reviewed above, little has been said of the transmission and encoding process. Nor have we described just exactly how the receptor cells turn stimulus energies into a specific signal, which, when encoded, informs the observer that he is seeing a triangle, eating a bite of banana, or grasping a sheet of sandpaper. Answers to the questions about receptor function or the process of encoding are extremely incomplete. Nevertheless, a few general stages in the total process can be enumerated.

The fact must be accepted that by various types of interaction between stimulus energy and receptor cell a signal or impulse is started along the nerve network toward the brain. Basically, the messages carried by nerve fibers are all alike. The stimulus only releases energy already in the fibers. When, and if, it responds, a nerve fiber responds completely. Because of this all-or-none response, the only way in which the message of an impulse may be coded is by its: (1) place or origin, the specific receptor stimulated; and (2) destination in the brain. Every sense system owns a particular area in the cerebral cortex where the impulse ultimately arrives, and a succession or a combination of such impulses yields additional information.

Relatively intense stimuli usually increase the number of impulses per second (the frequency of the nerve impulse), and activate more fibers at the same time. The brain somehow responds to these messages to make us aware of differences in flavor, brightness, pressure, pitch, and the like.

The unit of the nervous system is the neuron. There are three types: afferent (sensory), efferent (motor), and connector (association). Once activated, a nerve fiber is refractory (nonexcitable) for a brief interval, no matter how intense the stimulus may be. Then, during the period of recovery, a relatively intense stimulus may excite the fiber again. Thus, the greater frequency of nerve impulse is produced by a relatively more intense stimulus. As noted earlier, little yet is known about how the brain translates a sensory impulse into an immediately meaningful perception. Obviously, previous experience is important, as are attentional factors, prior levels of excitation of the sense in question, and so forth. But the means for co-operative action of the billions of brain cells involved in even a simple perception remains a mystery.

Other Experimental Approaches. Psychological studies of the effects of distorting or inverting stimuli have taught us much about seeing and hearing. Much, too, has been learned from the study of development of perception in children. And data have been gathered on the effect of one sensory experience on another. In recent years interest has been aroused in the effects of being deprived of sensory stimulation. These are a few of the areas that promise a rich potential for continuing research.

See also SENSORY DEPRIVATION.

SENSORY DEPRIVATION, also called perceptual isolation, experienced by people subjected to various kinds of isolation for extended periods of time. Different methods are used to reduce the amount and variation of sensory input. Subjects may be masked and immersed in water to exclude light, sound, and tactile impulses. Specially constructed environments are designed to control quantity and variability of sensory stimulation. In these experiments, scientists learn how much stimulation is needed for perception. They also learn how sensory experience may vary over time and observe unusual occurrences, such as hallucinations, thought disorders, disorientation in time and space, and increased irritability. These experiences resemble symptoms of mental illness, and are therefore called "artificial psychoses." Such studies are particularly important for future outer space exploration.

Physiological measurements indicate that there are also changes in the body which may underlie these changes in mental state. The connection between them is not clear, however. Studies of this type with mental patients have shown that schizophrenics are generally much less affected than normal people by sensory deprivation. This has caused some interest in the therapeutic use of decreased stimulation.

Future research with sensory deprivation will include the study of behavior under prolonged, that is, month-long, isolation of man in darkened rooms or in caves. Also, studies of isolation in groups of men are being conducted to determine the influence of diminished variability in sensory input on interactional behavior. It is clear that many social disruptions can be brought about by group isolation.

See also PSYCHOLOGY, *Physiological*.

SHOCK THERAPY, in psychiatry, a group of techniques in which comas or convulsions are induced to treat certain mental disorders.

Insulin shock therapy is based upon the injection of insulin, a pancreatic hormone that lowers the concentration of sugar in the blood. This results in the literal starvation of the cells of the brain which depend upon sugar for their energy. The parts of the brain are affected in a definite sequence. The higher brain ceases functioning before the more primitive structures succumb. The entire process takes several hours, culminating in a coma, the deepest stage of insulin shock. The patient is brought out of the coma by administering sugar (glucose) or glucagon, a pancreatic hormone which opposes the action of insulin. Treatments are usually given five or six days a week, and a series is completed after 40 to 50 treatments.

Insulin shock therapy produces considerable physical stress and is consequently not applicable to elderly patients or to those suffering from heart, liver, or kidney ailments or other chronic illnesses. Complications of treatment are seizures, respiratory difficulty, or heart failure. Usually these problems can be anticipated and can be prevented or minimized. In some cases the coma does not end in time, a condition known as "prolonged coma." This must be treated as a medical emergency.

Insulin therapy is less-frequently used today than formerly owing to the expense of its administration and the fact that similar results can be obtained more safely and economically through the use of tranquilizing drugs. Despite these drawbacks, insulin coma therapy is still valuable in the treatment of certain types of schizophrenia and is sometimes useful in the treatment of manic-depressive psychosis.

Convulsive shock therapies were introduced following observations that the symptoms of mental disease sometimes spontaneously disappeared after convulsions. In 1935 the Hungarian investigator Meduna produced convulsions by injections of camphor. Later a synthetic preparation, metrazol (in Europe "cardiazol"), came to be used in place of camphor.

The most widely used form of shock therapy is ECT, electroconvulsive therapy, which was introduced in Italy in 1937. This technique utilizes alternating current, applied through electrodes attached to the skull. The procedure is highly safe since only small amounts of current are used. Many physicians give a short-acting barbiturate to sedate the patient before the current is applied. In addition, a muscle-relaxing drug may be administered to prevent the strong muscular contractions of the convulsion from producing fractures or dislocations.

The principal side effects are temporary confusion and memory loss. ECT can be safely applied to elderly patients and pregnant women, but it is considered preferable not to treat patients who have had recent heart attacks, or those suffering from equally serious ailments.

The best success with electroconvulsive therapy has been obtained with depressed patients. A major use has been in quieting acutely agitated psychotic patients who are exhausting themselves by their activity. It is also helpful in certain types of schizophrenia. The treatment schedule varies. Most patients are treated two or three times a week, but in severely agitated cases, treatments may be given several times a day. At times maintenance treatment may be given every week, month, or at longer intervals. *See also* PSYCHIATRY.

SKINNER, BURRHUS FREDERIC (1904–), American psychologist known for his experimental work on learning. Skinner's researches employed the "Skinner box," a device in which an animal can obtain a pellet of food by pressing a lever. Skinner describes this as "instrumental learning," a situation in which the animal performs an act in order to satisfy a need. In this case the need is hunger, the instrumental act is pressing the lever, and the pellet of food is the "reward," or "reinforcement," which stamps in the learning. The Skinner box has inspired the teaching machine. Here the stimulus, or need, is the question, or problem; the instrumental act is the writing of the solution; and the reward is the confirmation of the correct answer.

SLEEP. The basic feature of sleep is a lowered level of awareness which differs from the unconsciousness of fainting or injury in that it is reversible, that is, the sleeping person can be awakened by strong stimulation such as the sound of an alarm clock. The depth of sleep is variable, being deepest during the first half of a sleep period and then becoming progressively but irregularly lighter. That sleep is not a complete loss of responsiveness is shown by the experience of dreaming and by the fairly frequent shifting of body position.

During sleep bodily processes are slowed significantly. The heartbeat becomes slower, respiration declines, the body temperature falls, urinary output lessens, glandular secretions diminish, and the muscles relax. The recuperative power of sleep can probably be attributed to this lowered general metabolism. Brain activity shares in this general decelerated pace. The pattern of rhythmic, spontaneous electrical activity becomes generally slower in frequency and higher in amplitude, indicating a lessening of spontaneous activity and an increase in synchronized "idling" of larger masses of brain cells.

Patterns of Sleep. There are two major patterns of sleep, the diphasic and the polyphasic. Man exhibits the diphasic pattern, consisting of one period of sleep in the 24-hour day. This varies somewhat in length from person to person, but averages about one-third of the total day. Other animals may have similar patterns, the duration and time of sleep varying with nocturnal or diurnal foraging habits. Infants and many animals show a polyphasic pattern, with many shorter periods of sleep and waking in any 24-hour period. The human infant gradually changes to fewer sleep periods, each of longer duration, until the adult pattern is achieved.

Theories of Sleep. Many hypotheses seeking to account

for sleep have been advanced, but few have survived experimental test. It has been speculated that sleep is caused by the accumulation of toxic substances—probably waste products of metabolism—in the blood stream. However, Siamese twins with common blood circulation can have quite different sleep patterns. Sleep has also been ascribed to a decrease in the blood supply to the brain, but evidence shows that if anything, there is an increased blood supply to the brain during sleep.

Current concepts of the problem owe much to the efforts of Nathaniel Kleitman of the University of Chicago. He suggested that possibly the real problem is *wakefulness* rather than sleep, and that the question should be: What produces wakefulness? According to this view, sleep is the natural resting state of the living system, and wakefulness the to-be-explained departure from the "normal."

Pursuing this line of thought, Kleitman then distinguishes between "wakefulness of necessity" and "wakefulness of choice." The former is responsible for polyphasic sleep patterns of primitive animals and infants, and the latter for the diphasic pattern of higher animals in their adult phase. Wakefulness of necessity is stimulated by needs such as hunger, thirst, and the avoidance of pain and yields to sleep when these needs are satisfied. Wakefulness of choice represents the gradual control of the waking mechanism by external stimulation acting on individuals who have built up habits of responding to such stimulation and have learned to conform to social customs or other environmental demands in regulating their sleep cycle. As the experience of insomnia indicates, wakefulness of necessity may also be produced by worry, excitement, or pain.

Sleep, then, starts in the young as a reflection of satisfied needs when the infant is "at peace with the world," and wakefulness is a signal of a disturbance of the balance of body needs. Thus a cue is given to the part of the brain that may be critically involved in sleep and waking. Most of the centers regulating bodily needs are located in the hypothalamus of the brain. Carefully controlled destruction of some of the anterior regions of the hypothalamus in rats or cats produces a continuously insomniac animal, and conversely, destruction of some posterior regions leads to persistent somnolescence. Thus intimately associated with or a part of brain regions mediating regulation of bodily metabolic states are areas crucially involved with sleep and waking, a fact which strongly supports Kleitman's formulation.

The "sleep center" is probably able, by its activity, to inhibit the cerebral cortex of the brain, just as the "waking center" stimulates these higher regions. External stimulation is also capable of arousing brain activity, but in the infant this source is not yet fully developed and is of minor importance. As the infant matures, he becomes more susceptible to outside stimulation and thus acquires wakefulness of choice.

Much remains to be learned about sleep. The fundamental problem of why the life of the individual is dependent on sleep still eludes solution. There is also uncertainty about the mechanism that irresistibly induces sleep following long periods of sleep deprivation. The processes responsible for the action of sleep-producing drugs need more study. Increased understanding of these matters seems possible now that we know something about the general circumstances governing sleep and waking and about where in the nervous system these basic processes may lie.

See also NERVOUS SYSTEM.

SLEEPWALKING, or somnambulism, a condition in which the individual walks during sleep. It may be considered a form of dissociation (a separation of certain mental processes from consciousness). Sleepwalking may occur nightly or at irregular intervals and is most common during childhood. During episodes the sleepwalker generally avoids obstacles, although he may injure himself. He resembles a subject in hypnotic trance, responds to suggestions, but remembers none of the experience after awakening. If awakened while walking, he is surprised at finding himself out of bed. There is no evidence that it is dangerous to awaken a somnambulist, although it should be done as calmly as possible.

Recent studies of sleep and dreams show that many psychomotor activities may occur during deep sleep, especially in children, such as talking, bed-wetting, and screaming as in a nightmare. The meaning of such dissociated activities awaits further elucidation.

SOCIOGRAM. *See* SOCIOMETRY.

SOCIOLOGY is the social science concerned with the organization or structure of social groups. It seeks to determine the kinds and causes of variation in social structure, and the processes by which social structure is kept intact or changed.

Examples of Sociological Studies

Much of the present article is devoted to discussing the parts of this definition. It will be helpful, before starting this discussion, to give a few examples of what sociologists do. Sociology, other social sciences, and the physical and biological sciences seek principles that describe or explain human behavior or other natural phenomena. Hence social scientists and other scientists often use general, abstract terms that are hard for the layman to grasp. But their theories are based on the study of particular people and facts—often thousands of them. And these studies often produce knowledge that is of immediate interest and usefulness. The concerns of sociologists can be suggested by listing some of the topics included in a survey of this social science: sociology of politics, sociology of law, sociology of education, sociology of religion, sociology of the family, sociology of science, personality and social structure, urban sociology, race and ethnic relations, sociology of occupations, social disorganization and deviant behavior, sociology of mental illness, criminology, and mass communication. Samples of work in three of these fields follow.

Occupational Sociology. The study of vocations adds to the store of information about the structure of groups. It also produces facts that are useful to vocational counselors and personnel departments. One widely quoted study, *Prestige Ratings of Occupations* (1947), by P. K. Hatt and C. C. North, attempted to find how Americans rate the prestige of occupations. A poll of a nationwide sample showed that in general professions were rated higher than other occupations. Within the professional group justice of the U.S. Supreme Court ranked 1 (of all occupations), physician 2, college professor 7, minister 14, dentist 17, lawyer 18, and public school teacher 36. The main factors determining rank were the amount of specialized training needed for a profession and the degree of responsibility called for. Although this study cannot be accepted without certain qualifications, it does suggest, for example, one reason for the difficulty of recruiting top-grade college graduates for school teaching.

Educational Sociology. Some sociologists specialize in studying teachers, students, schools as social organizations, and the role of education in society. Discussions of the aims of education often draw on the findings of sociologists. When debating the question of what the schools ought to do, one finds it useful to know what the schools are doing and what teachers, students, and others think they should do. Examples of sociological studies in this area are surveys that have been made of college and high school students in the United States. More than two-thirds of the college students polled stated that the chief purpose of higher education was to provide a basic general education or to provide vocational and professional training. Of high school students, more than one-third rated learning how to get along with other people as the first goal of high school education. Learning basic subjects rated much lower. Such findings can be useful guides to educators who are concerned, for example, with the motivation and achievement of their students. These findings can also help to build up an understanding of American society in general, since educational aims reflect beliefs about what is good for individuals and for the country.

The Sociology of Mental Illness. Another example of the work of sociologists is their studies of mental illness. Whereas psychiatrists tend to focus on individual cases, sociologists approach the problem broadly. They investigate such questions as these: How many cases of mental illness are there? Do cases tend to be concentrated in certain geographical areas or within certain groups of people? How do various cultures around the world compare with respect to amount and kind of mental illness? It has been observed, for example, that mental illness occurs in all kinds of cultures, among primitive peoples as well as in industrialized societies. Rates of incidence and causes need much more investigation. Some comparisons of incidence in different regions suggest, to some theorists, a genetic factor in mental disease. Another view is that mental illness is related to the conditions under which people live. *Mental Disorders in Urban Areas* (1960), a study of mental illness in various sections of a city by Robert E. L. Faris and H. Warren Dunham, reported that the center sections had a higher incidence of schizophrenia. These sections were characterized by rundown buildings, many rooming houses, and general social disorganization, conditions that tend to isolate people and make them vulnerable to mental illness. (It is also possible that the mentally ill tend to drift toward slum areas.) Such a study contributes material for the sociologist who is working on theories of urban group behavior and for the sociologist who is studying deviant behavior. The study also has implications for psychiatrists, social workers, architects, and city planners.

The Scope of Sociological Theory

These examples of sociological studies are background for the more theoretical discussion that follows. As the definition at the start of the article stated, sociology is concerned with social groups. Various social groups have been mentioned—city dwellers, students, and professional men. To explain the full scope of sociology it is necessary to discuss the general nature of social groups.

Social Groups. Social groups vary greatly in size, degree of permanence, and range and kinds of activity. The most comprehensive type of group is ordinarily called a society. Such a group may include millions of members, divided among many overlapping *subgroups*. It often maintains an independent existence for many generations and its activities cover all aspects of human social life. Sociologists might speak of the United States as a society or of the society of France before the Revolution. At the other extreme is the group with a membership of two. The two may interact for only a moment or for a much longer time. All social groups, large and small, distinguish between members and nonmembers, involve some communication and co-operation among members, and have some sort of organization, or structure. The members of a group are distinguishable from nonmembers in several ways: they have obligations toward one another and toward the group as a whole, and they may enjoy certain rights denied to nonmembers. The structure, or organization, of a group reflects the subgroups of which it is composed and the *roles* played by members, either in the group or in its subgroups.

A role is a cluster of group obligations or functions that one or more individuals are expected to fulfill. But not all members of a group play the same roles. As the word "structure" implies, there is differentiation. Different individuals are likely to have different functions. Each individual, furthermore, is likely to have a number of functions. Because he ordinarily belongs to many groups and subgroups, he has many social roles to play, one for each group or subgroup. A doctor, for example, may have the roles of surgeon, executive in a hospital, husband and father in a family, and member of the school board in a town. Corresponding to the functions that members of a group fulfill are the rights they enjoy as a result. Taken together those rights equal what may be called a *status*. Every position in a group has built into it status and role, that is, interacting rights and obligations. A doctor is expected to use his professional skills to treat illness. In return he is granted great prestige in American society.

Institutionalization. The more general obligations, as distinct from specific tasks, are defined by social rules, or *norms*, which may be formally or informally established. *Laws* are formally established norms, but the "rules" binding upon two friends are not. Closely linked with norms is *institutionalization*, one of the most important concepts in sociology. A norm is said to be institutionalized in a group if some or all of the group's members are expected to live according to it on appropriate occasions. Although the norm may apply only to some of the group members, other members know what it is and to whom it

pertains. They express disapproval of anyone who should, but does not, live up to it. In other words, the group supports institutionalized norms with negative sanctions —penalties for violation. The group also has positive sanctions—rewards for conforming. But because many approved actions may be rewarded even if they are not definitely expected, negative sanctions serve as better indicators of institutionalization. It should be emphasized that, in any group, institutionalization is a matter of degree. The degree depends upon several variable factors: the clarity of the norm, how many group members accept its validity, whether it applies to them or not, and the intensity of the group's disapproval of violations. Some groups—physicians, for example—have well-defined codes of professional ethics. In this case professional societies define the norm and oversee the behavior of group members.

Institutionalized rules can be general or specific about the situations in which they are supposed to serve as guides for action. Some sociologists use the term "value" for the most general rules or standards, and "norm" in a narrow sense for the more specific, more detailed rules. The U.S. Constitution, for example, defines values of American society, but norms govern the day-to-day conduct of families like the Joneses, who are part of that society. Institutionalization of social rules may take place on a number of levels. These include the level of general values, the level of norms for a particular type of subgroup or role, and the level of norms for a particular example of a particular type of subgroup or role. The various levels form a *hierarchy* of values and norms, ranging from the most general to the most detailed. Every society has such a hierarchy.

Functional Problems. The structure of a group reflects its institutionalized values and norms. A key to the concept of structure is the concept of function. Every group must fulfill certain conditions, that is, deal successfully with functional problems, if it is to survive and flourish. Structural features are functional to the extent that they help the group solve one or more of four problems. These problems are (1) goal attainment, (2) adaptation, (3) pattern maintenance, and (4) integration. They are treated below.

Goal Attainment. The maintenance of the group as a distinct social system depends on its ability to cope with changes in its environment, either by adjusting to those changes or by actively mastering them. The problem of goal attainment, in practical terms, is one of mobilizing the support of group and subgroup members and co-ordinating their activities so that relatively specific tasks are accomplished. For the society as a whole, this is a political problem.

Adaptation. This is the problem of transforming the environment in such a way as to provide the means by which the group and its subdivisions can attain their goals. For the society as a whole, this is an economic problem.

Goal attainment and adaptation may be illustrated by an example from history. Societies in ancient Mesopotamia faced the economic problem of raising food in an arid land. Irrigation provided an answer. Building irrigation systems required that individual farmers co-ordinate their work. To achieve this goal, a political organization was set up to plan irrigation canals and to direct work on them.

Pattern Maintenance. The group's life depends to a considerable extent upon its culture, including its values and norms. Pattern maintenance is the problem of preserving these and other patterns of culture: for example, science, philosophy, religion, ideology, and art. Pattern maintenance involves transmission of necessary knowledge of the group's culture and respect for that culture to the individual members of the group, above all to new members. To do this is a major aim of education in all societies, whether education be given informally by the older members of a group or formally in schools. Dealing with the pattern maintenance problem may also call for developing cultural patterns when necessary. For example, to maintain essential patterns of American culture during World War II it was necessary to develop new patterns of military service and of controls on the economy.

Integration. This problem involves the maintenance of the group's cohesion. The group would dissolve if internal conflicts of interest were not settled in a more or less orderly way and if individual tendencies to deviate from group norms were not checked. This fact can be illustrated by reference to almost any group—an office force, a church committee, a baseball team, a ship's crew, or a branch of government. Integration, as the term is used here, has to do with the relations of individuals and subgroups with one another. The first two functional problems, having to do with the environment, are called external problems. The second two are called internal.

The structure of every group that endures tends to be differentiated according to function. In other words, form tends to follow function. This tendency is never complete. But even in quite small groups roles often differ according to the nature, external or internal, of the problems to be faced. Informal conference groups, for example, usually develop a "task leader," who is a specialist in external problems, and a "best-liked" member, who usually has a talent for maintaining internal harmony. Similarly the so-called nuclear family, which consists of husband, wife, and children, has an essentially external specialist in the husband-father, who deals with the environment by going out to earn a living. The wife-mother, who is usually more concerned with the care and training of children, is essentially an internal specialist.

Relation of Sociology to Other Social Sciences. The division of labor among the social sciences is not clear-cut. On the whole, however, economics tends to deal with certain relationships involved in the production of goods and services, relationships called above the adaptive system of the society; and political science deals with the goal-attainment system of the society, in which the government plays a leading part. Sociology is largely concerned with the internal system of social groups, including, of course, societies. The relation between social, or cultural, anthropology and sociology is still being worked out and there is a great deal of overlapping. Social psychology is also very closely linked to sociology.

Sociology is also concerned with the processes (called "socialization") by which culture is transmitted to suc-

cessive generations of group members; the factors that make for conformity to social norms, in particular social systems or in social systems in general; the factors that tend to bring about alienation and deviation from norms, again in particular or in general; the forms of social deviation and the determinants of the different forms; the methods and processes of social control (that is, processes by which the motivation to deviant behavior is "corrected" or the deviant behavior itself is confined to narrow limits); and—a very important focus of scientific attention—the sources and processes of social change.

History of Sociology

Origins of Sociology. To pick a starting point for the history of sociology is an arbitrary decision. The reason is that only since about 1900 has the science clearly disentangled itself from religion, philosophy, and ideology, as well as from the other social sciences. Most medieval theorists of society were deeply influenced by religion. Many later writers simply shifted from religious emphasis to political and social emphasis. Thomas Hobbes (1588–1679), for example, wrote as a defender of monarchy. Jean Jacques Rousseau (1712–78) voiced new ideological aspirations as an advocate of democracy. In turn, Karl Marx (1818–83) won renown as a revolutionary socialist ideologist opposed to the capitalist system.

Many writers blended what is now called sociology with other social sciences. Among these were Hobbes and Rousseau, who might also be regarded as political theorists, and Marx, who was an economist as well as an ideologist and a sociologist. To cite another example, John Locke (1632–1704), the intellectual father of the Glorious Revolution of 1688 in England and the later American Revolution, was a philosopher whose work had an important influence on political science, economics, and sociology.

An understandable inclination in writing the history of sociological thought is to stress the forerunners of the most important modern theorists. Even with such a limiting emphasis, the list is necessarily long. Some men stand out for their contributions to the emancipation of social science from religious thinking. The Italian statesman and philosopher Niccolò Machiavelli (1469–1527) belongs in this category. He was also one of the first to understand clearly the vital part that moral norms play in human actions. Other thinkers are outstanding for having stated scientific problems, even if they could not solve them. Thus Hobbes stated clearly the problem of order. For him it was a matter of seeking to account scientifically for the sheer existence of any degree of order, or integration, in social life. Two centuries later Marx helped direct attention to two other problems: the functions, if any, of the division of society into social classes and the identification of the mechanisms of social change.

Modern Sociology. Modern sociology stems mainly from certain English, French, and German traditions of thought. The English utilitarians, who developed the science of economics, made great advances in the analysis of the rational elements in human action. They did nothing, however, to solve the problem of order. The German idealists, notably the philosopher G. W. F. Hegel (1770–

1831) and his followers, scored an advance in the recognition of the key significance of culture, including values and norms, in human societies. The shortcoming of the idealists was their inability to explain satisfactorily how ideals become involved in behavior and how they relate to the rational motives emphasized in particular by the English. The French rationalists also directed attention to the importance of culture. It was a contributor to the French rationalist tradition, Auguste Comte (1798–1857), who coined the word "sociology." Comte, nevertheless, was primarily a philosopher and mathematician. His chief renown in sociology was as a precursor of his fellow countryman, Émile Durkheim (1858–1917).

Durkheim ranks as one of the two great pioneers of modern scientific sociology and one of the major figures of his time. He fully appreciated the part played by normative factors in the integration of society. He also grasped the connection between *internalization* (the learning of culture, including norms, by the individual member of a society) and *institutionalization* (the process of incorporating norms into a culture as binding rules of behavior). This insight gave Durkheim an understanding of one of the most vital links between the *personality* and the *social system*. Another of Durkheim's achievements was his fundamental analysis of the close connection between religion and the normative integration of society (the idea, in a sense, that social institutions are "sacred"). Still another achievement was his contribution to the analysis of social differentiation. Durkheim's work had importance partly because of its functionalism. If that functionalism was not always explicit, the reason was that Durkheim took it for granted. He was well aware that society is a kind of system. Durkheim is also noted for his studies of deviant behavior, particularly suicide.

The other great pioneer of modern sociology was a German, Max Weber (1864–1920). He and Durkheim did not know each other's work, and they came out of somewhat different, although related, traditions. Weber, like Durkheim, appreciated the significance of values and norms in human action. He also clarified the role of ideas. In particular, he showed how religious ideas, by defining religious interests, play an important part in social change. He showed, too, how religious differences help explain other far-reaching differences among the great civilizations of the world. Weber's other major contributions included an analysis of types of social actions and groups and a description of the characteristics of bureaucratic organization. This description opened up a whole field of sociology and remains to this day a fundamental reference point for scientific work in the field. In addition, Weber wrote a brilliant study of types of political systems, which is important to sociology for its illumination of some aspects of social change.

The British anthropologists Bronislaw Malinowski (1884–1942) and Alfred Reginald Radcliffe-Brown (1881–1955) influenced sociology by helping to make the functional approach both explicit and systematic.

The pioneering American sociologist William Graham Sumner (1840–1910) clarified several concepts still basic to sociology in his monumental book *Folkways* (1906). According to Sumner, folkways, or customs, are evolved unconsciously through trial and error to meet material or imaginary needs. When folkways are regarded as morally good, or indispensable to social welfare, they are called *mores*. These exert coercion on the individual to conform, though they are not co-ordinated by any authority. The *laws* are those mores that, in addition to the unco-ordinated approval of public opinion, have the specific sanction of the political organization. Mores also develop into institutions (as the notion of religion or education) with accompanying structures (as the organization of the church or the school system). In any society the young are introduced to the folkways, thus guaranteeing the continuity of the particular culture. Sumner also established the concepts of *in-group—out-group* and *ethnocentrism*.

Among other early major American contributors to sociology were George Herbert Mead (1863–1931) and Charles Horton Cooley (1864–1929). They showed the social origin of personality and thus illuminated the process of socialization. Mead, whose work was especially notable, demonstrated the importance of symbolic communication (not simply confined to speech) to personalities and social systems. The demonstration was another step forward in the appreciation of culture's integrative function. Mead used the term "role" somewhat broadly, but his analysis remains vital to an understanding of the way in which roles are interrelated and become the centers of subsystems of the personality. The work of Mead and Cooley is linked to that of the founder of psychoanalysis, the Austrian Sigmund Freud (1856–1939). Freud's theory of identification and the formation of the ego and the superego is also vital to an understanding of socialization.

Since the 1930's Americans have probably been the most important contributors to sociology. Among contemporary American sociologists, Talcott Parsons is outstanding. Parsons has perhaps grasped most fully the theoretical contributions of Durkheim, Weber, and Freud, has clearly formulated the problems they did not entirely solve, and has carried forward their work. He has illuminated the relations between social systems and other types of "action systems," such as the personality, culture, and, in some ways, the organism. He has also clarified the relations of the social sciences to each other and to psychology and has contributed to the theory of social differentiation. One of his most striking and important contributions is an analysis showing that the processes of socialization, social control, and social change are very similar. His careful distinction, furthermore, between processes maintaining structure and those changing structure is in itself a valuable contribution.

Parsons' importance is also revealed in the achievements of his students. Robert King Merton has, among other things, clarified the nature of functional analysis, carried forward the analysis of social deviation (here building in part upon Durkheim), and contributed to the sociology of science (here building in part upon Weber). Robert F. Bales, in making carefully controlled experiments with small conference groups, isolated what now seem to be the basic functional problems of social systems. He also clarified their sequence, noting that in conferences there tends to occur a succession of phases with shifting emphasis on adaptation, goal achievement, and integration, in that order. Neil Joseph Smelser collaborated with Parsons on an important book dealing with the relation of the economy to the rest of society (one of Weber's chief interests). In this work Parsons and Smelser also made progress in the analysis of the process of social change. Smelser then used the theoretical framework thus developed for a detailed analysis of the industrial revolution.

Canadian sociology reflects a strong American influence. Léon Gérin (1863–1951), Canada's pioneer in sociology, may be cited as an exception, but most of his successors, as products of American graduate schools, have been basically American in their approach. Unlike some of the Americans, however, Canadian sociologists have shown no great interest in pure theory. Notable exceptions have been C. A. Dawson and C. W. M. Hart.

Sociology as a Profession

There is a well-established department of sociology in every major U.S. and Canadian university and in all but a few colleges. (Sometimes the departments of sociology and anthropology are combined.) The importance of sociology on the American scene is evident in the quick growth of the American Sociological Association (estab., 1905, as the American Sociological Society). In other countries sociology is not as well established, either academically or professionally, as in the United States and Canada, although interest is rising. The International Sociological Association (estab., 1950) embraces 7 sociological institutes, 35 national associations, and individual members from 15 countries without national associations.

Functions of Sociologists Today. The central function of sociologists is to develop sociology as a special social science. This function includes the training of the next generation of professional sociologists. Other functions lie in several fields of applied sociology. Some of the applications are direct: for example, in market research, other business activities, and the work of government bureaus and juvenile delinquency courts. The most important applications of sociology, however, are probably indirect. They involve the transmission to experts in other professions of the results of relevant sociological research. Transmission occurs naturally and habitually when, as is often the case, sociologists are attached to the staffs of schools of medicine, law, education, business, agriculture, and social work.

Sociologists have at least two other functions. The first is to help develop related fields, such as anthropology, social psychology, the psychology of personality, political science, and economics. Some of this help is given through direct collaboration with workers in these allied fields. Some of it stems from developments in sociology, developments that necessarily have meaning for the other social sciences, all of which, like sociology, are concerned with the phenomena of human behavior. Finally, sociologists have the function of teaching undergraduates who will not become professional sociologists. In performing this task, sociologists not only can broaden and deepen the layman's appreciation of the world he lives in, but also can help keep ideology from straying too far from verifiable fact.

See also CULTURE AND PERSONALITY; PSYCHOLOGY.

SOCIOMETRY [sō-sē-ŏm'ə-trē], a technique in social science research for measuring the social relations among members of a group. The term has been closely associated with the work of the psychotherapist J. L. Moreno, who used this technique in his study *Who Shall Survive?* (1934).

The data in sociometric analysis consist of information about the attractions and rejections among members of the group as indicated by their preferences for associates in some activity, real or hypothetical. The data are collected from interviews, questionnaires, and observations by researchers. In the analysis and presentation of sociometric data a wide variety of graphic, mathematical, and statistical methods are used, including the sociogram, a diagram depicting the pattern of choices and rejections within the group being studied.

To construct a sociogram, the researcher asks members of a group which persons in the group they would most prefer to have as leaders or partners in certain activities and which they would least prefer. From the replies the researcher draws a diagram on which positive choices or likes are indicated by solid lines and negative choices or dislikes are shown as broken lines. Sociometric techniques and sociograms have been applied in studies of such diverse topics as leadership, friendship formation, and power structure within groups.

Many early sociometric studies were published in *Sociometry: A Journal of Interpersonal Relations*, founded by Moreno in 1937. It was subsequently taken over by the American Sociological Association, which began publishing it in 1956 as *Sociometry: A Journal of Research in Social Psychology*, including reports covering a broad range of research in social psychology.

SOCIOPATHIC PERSONALITY, name of a group of personality disorders, formerly called psychopathic. The malfunction in conduct is expressed in inflexible and limited patterns of behavior, compatible at time with social success. It may be impossible to recognize the symptoms of personality disorder, especially when the particular features of the individual makeup are both accepted and rewarded by the culture.

According to psychoanalytic theory, neurosis and personality disorder may have the same background. A person with a character neurosis has conflicts which make it difficult for him to adapt to his own drives, his family, and job relationships. If such conflicts become incapacitating to others, rather than to himself, the person is said to have a personality disorder. Thus, neurosis and personality disorder differ only in their end product—the symptoms—but they have the same basic dynamics. Sociopathic behavior disorders are more common than psychoses but less crippling. The psychotic individual has lost contact with everyday reality and the neurotic suffers from his inappropriate attempts to reduce anxiety. The sociopathic personality, however, deals excellently with what *he* considers the world, and therefore he has no feelings of anxiety.

Characteristics. The sociopathic personality is characterized by emotional immaturity, with marked defects in judgment. He is prone to impulsive behavior without consideration of others and may come in constant conflict with his society's laws and behavioral standards. He often is quite intelligent and capable of mastering the most subtle occupational skills. In spite of these advantages the sociopath consistently fails·in all endeavors. He knows that his antisocial behavior will produce adverse consequences, but he lacks the emotional ties or the inner feelings of concern which would prevent him from committing those acts which, in his rational moments, he would condemn. Although he may simulate normal concern, he is callously indifferent to the welfare of others.

Sociopathic reactions against the social order are exemplified in the lawbreaker—the swindler, bigamist, or habitual thief. Sexual deviations include infidelity, prostitution, and perversion. Addiction most often appears as dependence on drugs or alcohol, but the sociopath may adhere to any type of irresponsible act. Certain general characteristics distinguish the sociopath from the neurotic. Sociopathy seems to depend more on the individual's constitution than his environment. The sociopath does not feel abnormal or ill, while the neurotic often looks for help. At present, therapy is generally unsuccessful, although the condition seems to improve with age.
See also NEUROSIS; PATHOLOGICAL LYING; PSYCHIATRY; PSYCHOANALYSIS.

SPEARMAN, CHARLES EDWARD (1863–1945), British research psychologist. He held the post of professor at the University of London from 1907 until his retirement. His work centered around the assessment of intelligence by means of intelligence tests and the statistical analysis of test scores. He developed a technique of "factor analysis," which led him to conclude that intellect was comprised of a central integrative factor, the "G" of general factor, with many specific ability factors contributing to distinct skills. This theory, that intelligence is the ability to discover relationships, as they exist in a mathematical problem, for example, is in opposition to the intelligence theories of the American psychologist Edward Lee Thorndike. Spearman's search for specific ability factors led to the development of useful statistical tools, such as the Spearman-Brown prophecy formula, used to estimate the reliability of psychological tests. Spearman's *Rho* statistic, a technique of correlation analysis, is in widespread use today.

SPEECH DISORDERS AND SPEECH THERAPY. It has been estimated that over 10% of children and roughly 5% of adults have speech deviations severe enough to warrant the attention of a speech therapist. Speech disorders are often divided into four categories: disorders of articulation, of voice, of language, and of fluency.

Speech Disorders

Disorders of articulation, consisting of the improper production of speech sounds, are by far the most common form of speech deviation, and are most frequently encountered in children. Articulatory errors usually take the form of omissions, substitutions, or distortions of sound. A child who omits a sound may say "at" for "hat" or "oo" for "you." Examples of the substitutions of one sound for another often heard in the speech of young children are "fumb" for "thumb," "yike" for "like," or "tate" for "cake." The distortion of a sound is heard in the "slurpy"

s or sh of children or adults who have a so-called "lateral" lisp.

Although a variety of psychological and physical factors may play a part in the causation of articulatory disorders, the majority of children who have such difficulties are emotionally stable and constitutionally sound. They also tend to be of normal or even superior intelligence. Most articulatory problems fall into a category which may be referred to as "infantile" or "immature" articulation. In such cases the child has persisted in articulatory habits which are commonly found in younger children. It is important to note that while some children appear to speak like adults almost from the moment they begin to talk, it is entirely normal for a child to use some "baby talk" until the age of six or seven. Before that age the important question is not whether a child has articulatory errors but which sounds he is failing to say properly, since some sounds are easier and are therefore learned earlier than others.

A child of four and a half who has not yet learned to say l, r, th, s, and sh merely has some normal baby talk. If he also has difficulty with sounds such as h, y, k, and g, however, his articulation is decidedly immature. At age three, few consonants are demanded of a child beyond the relatively simple m, p, b, w, and h. A useful rule of thumb is that a child should be understood outside the home on most occasions by the age of four and a half years. The child with immature articulation is not necessarily immature in his language development (that is, in his vocabulary and sentence structure) or social behavior, but it is likely that he has been somewhat slow at beginning to talk. In some cases there appears to be a family tendency toward late development of speech and infantile errors of articulation. It is not true that immature articulation is generally caused by talking baby talk to a child.

Not all articulatory defects involve persistent infantile habits. Some are caused by imitation of a parent's speech errors. Others result from malocclusion of the teeth ("bad bite") and require the help of an orthodontist. However, only the more severe degrees of abnormal bite will interfere appreciably with articulation, and then only with the production of the "sibilant," or hissing, sounds: s, z, sh, zh (as in "pleasure"), ch, and j. "Tongue-tie" is a condition in which the lingual frenum (the connective tissue beneath the tongue) is unusually short and attached close to the tip of the tongue. It was once thought to be an important cause of articulatory difficulties, but it probably interferes with speech in very few cases.

There are three major organic disorders which may result in very severe articulatory problems: (1) hearing impairment, (2) cerebral palsy, and (3) cleft palate.

Hard-of-hearing persons often have their greatest difficulty in the perception of high-pitched sounds. These persons may fail to hear sounds such as s, sh, and th and will therefore distort or omit them in their own speech. A sentence such as "He stuck in his thumb" will typically sound like "He tuck in hid tumb." A person who has a more severe hearing loss involving the low pitches as well may have difficulty articulating all or most of his sounds, and his voice may be harsh, monotonous, and unnatural.

Cerebral palsy is a disturbance of motor co-ordination caused by brain injury, usually at or near the time of birth. When the speech muscles are affected, articulation tends to be slow, clumsy, labored, and exceedingly indistinct.

Cleft palate is a congenital abnormality in which the roof of the mouth fails to close in prenatal life. This leaves a gap, or cleft, in the roof of the mouth through which air escapes into the nasal cavity during speech. The result is a nasal voice with extreme distortion of all those consonants for which it is necessary to build up air pressure inside the mouth cavity, as with *p*, *t*, *k*, *f*, *th*, *s*, and many others. A sentence such as "Peter is a tall boy" becomes something like, "Hmeener in a hnall moy." The speech of a person with cleft palate is sometimes virtually impossible to understand.

Disorders of voice may be divided for the most part into disorders of pitch, of loudness, and of quality. One of the most common disorders of pitch is "persistent falsetto" in the male. This is caused by unconscious resistance to voice change on the part of a pubescent boy and results in an unusual, high-pitched, falsetto voice which may persist into adulthood if not treated. Inadequate loudness for normal conversation may result from a variety of causes, but is most likely to be a personality problem. "Harshness," "hoarseness," or "huskiness" are disorders of voice quality. These terms do not have exact scientific meanings, but refer in a general way to a feeling of "roughness" or strain which is imparted by certain voices.

Such disturbances of voice quality may be produced by abnormal vibration of the vocal cords resulting from an excessive tension of the vocal cords, which is in turn associated with emotional pressures. Abnormal vibration of the cords may also be caused by paralysis, growths, or ulcerations of the cords, by moist deposits on the cords (seen in sinusitis), or by inflammation of the cords caused by disease. An especially common cause of husky voice quality is abuse of the voice. This leads to the formation of small growths on the cords, called vocal "nodes" or "nodules" which are in actuality tiny calluses produced by excessive friction between the cords. Vocal nodes are seen most often in persons who use their voices professionally, such as teachers, singers, or public speakers. Usually, however, the voice can withstand a remarkable amount of use if it is produced efficiently.

Nasality is a voice quality disorder caused by improper use of the nasal passages, where the voice is modified and reinforced, as resonators. In normal speech the nasal passages are employed only for the production of the "nasal" consonants *m*, *n*, and *ng*. An unpleasant "twangy" voice quality occurs if the nasal passages are used in the formation of other sounds as well, especially the vowels and vowel-like consonants. In most cases nasality is caused by the habit of keeping the soft palate in a relaxed (lowered) position, thus leaving the posterior entrance to the nasal passages open. This habit may be an imitation of home or community vocal patterns, or may be caused by removal of enlarged adenoids, or by other speech habits such as articulating with inadequate vigor.

Nasality is often confused with a distinctly different pattern of speech known as "denasality," which results from failure to nasalize the consonants *m*, *n*, and *ng* properly. Thus "Mister Miller" becomes "Bister Biller"; the person sounds as though he has a cold in his nose. Denasality is almost always caused by an organic obstruction of the nasal passages, for example, enlarged adenoids, deviated nasal septum (an abnormal position of the bone separating the nasal passages), or swelling of the walls of the nasal cavities as seen in cases of allergy or infection.

There are two major conditions in which the voice may be lost outright. In "hysterical aphonia" the person usually can speak only in a whisper. This is a neurotic symptom, unconsciously employed as a makeshift solution for acute emotional conflicts, and is similar to hysterical deafness or blindness. The other condition is the surgical removal of the larynx (laryngectomy) which is frequently performed in cases of laryngeal cancer. When the larynx, which houses the vocal cords, is removed the patient is in most cases unable even to whisper.

Disorders of language are disturbances in the use or interpretation of verbal symbols. They take two principal forms, the loss or impairment of language and the failure of language to develop.

Loss of language in whole or part is usually caused by brain damage: such cases are called "aphasia." The aphasic person may be unable to call forth familiar words (like the names for common objects) or may speak slowly, gropingly, and with errors in pronunciation and grammar. Some aphasics speak fluently, but in what may amount to an incomprehensible jargon. For example, in response to every question about his name, age, address, and so forth, a person with aphasia may consistently reply, "insofar as the girl is concerned," though he may be aware of the inappropriateness of his answer. On the receptive side, the aphasic may have difficulty understanding speech, though he may recognize that a familiar language is being spoken. Like the person who has not quite mastered a new language, he may feel that people are speaking too rapidly. In addition to having difficulties with spoken language, he may have similar problems in reading, writing, mathematics, and other activities involving symbols.

Delayed language development in children is one of the more common problems of speech therapy. The average child speaks his first word by about the age of one year and his first simple sentences by about age two. Children vary greatly in rate of speech development, however, and many normal children do not say their first words and sentences until considerably later. If a child does not speak any words at age two and a half years or sentences at three and a half years he should be examined carefully.

There are a number of factors which can seriously impede language development. One is mental deficiency. Many mentally deficient children never learn to speak at all. Another is deafness. The totally deaf child who is not carefully taught to speak by special techniques will not learn language. In such cases he is often referred to as a "deaf-mute." The deaf-mute ordinarily has perfectly normal speech organs. Still a third serious factor is cerebral palsy affecting the muscles of speech. In some cerebral palsied children these muscles are so severely paralyzed that no speech will ever be possible for them. A fourth factor is infantile psychosis, a very severe emotional disturbance in which contact with reality and normal relationships with others are impaired. Finally, some children with retarded speech probably have a congenital form of aphasia; that is, there has been injury or inadequate development in the "language areas" of the brain.

All of these factors are comparatively rare, and the ordinary child who is slow in learning to talk is not too likely to be suffering from any of them. There are many other reasons why children may be slow in talking. These probably include heredity, limited speech stimulation in the home, retarded physical development caused by illness or premature birth, and unwholesome parent-child relationships. Language development is never impeded by "something wrong with the child's throat."

Disorders of fluency are those in which the forward flow of speech is impeded—the chief example being stuttering, or stammering. The stutterer repeats sounds luh-luh-luh-luh-like this, or prolongs them lllllike this, or has complete stoppages like ------- this. These interruptions are usually accompanied by excessive tension in the muscles of speech and often by grimaces, gestures, bodily movements, breathing abnormalities, or extraneous words or sounds, as in the sentence, "John um Baker lives on well Tenth Street." The stutterer generally knows quite well what word he wants to say; he is simply unable for the moment to say it. He is likely to develop fears of inability to say particular words or sounds, to anticipate blocks on them beforehand, and to try to avoid them by such devices as saying, for example, "this evening" instead of "tonight," or "This is my mother's sister's son" instead of "This is my cousin."

Stuttering usually begins in early childhood and is more common in boys than girls by a ratio of about four to one. In many cases it disappears spontaneously during childhood. It appears chiefly in civilized societies and is not found at all among many "primitive" peoples. It frequently tends to "run" in families. It is a highly intermittent disorder; most stutterers are fluent when they sing, whisper, speak in unison with another person or talk to an infant or pet, when they are alone, and under many other conditions. They are most likely to have difficulty speaking when they expect to stutter and want very much not to. The stutterer exhibits no abnormality of bodily constitution or personality make-up which has been established to the satisfaction of most experts. He is not necessarily more "nervous" than anyone else or lacking in confidence, except about his speech. On the average, stutterers are as intelligent as other people.

Significance of Speech Impairment to the Individual

Impaired speech may gravely disable the individual in both his social and business life. A lisp may create a wholly unwarranted impression of immaturity on the listener. A person who distorts the *l* sound or has an unpleasant voice quality may feel chronically conspicuous and ill at ease in social situations. Children who stutter or have infantile speech are vulnerable to torment by their schoolmates. The sudden loss of speech in laryngectomy or aphasia is likely to be felt as a catastrophe and to be acutely demoralizing.

The lifelong communication problem of many persons with hearing loss, cleft palate, or cerebral palsy probably contributes considerably to the progressive attrition of personality sometimes associated with these disorders. The young child with severely delayed language development is frequently a behavior problem for want of adequate means of relating normally to others. Until he learns to speak he is also apt to appear intellectually retarded and

for all practical purposes to be functioning on a retarded level in an environment in which intelligence consists so largely of verbal ability.

The outstanding example of the social and emotional consequences of speech impairment is afforded by severe stuttering. There are few deviations from the normal which are so harshly penalized by society. The stutterer generally learns to dread the listener's look of amusement or shocked surprise, or his impatient "Hurry up, young man—I don't have all day." He may also bitterly resent the listener's attempts to help him with words, his expressions of pity, his tendency to look away, and his confident advice to "Take it easy."

To escape such penalties, many stutterers do everything in their power to pass as normal speakers. They may continually substitute synonyms or circumlocutions in order to avoid difficult words. In the classroom the stutterer may talk as little as possible and may tell the teacher that he does not know the answer or declare that he is unprepared in order to avoid stuttering. At great inconvenience he may avoid making phone calls, asking for directions, or going into stores. He may avoid dances, parties, and dates, sometimes convincing himself that he does not enjoy "small talk" anyway. Stutterers have been known to leave school because of their stuttering, to choose a vocation chiefly on the basis of how much speaking it requires, to hide their speech problem successfully from wives or husbands for many years, or to live in virtual seclusion because of their stuttering.

Aims and Prospects of Therapy

Generally speaking, improvement is easiest in cases of defective articulation based on habit. Here the therapist is often concerned simply with hastening the process of speech maturation. With the assistance of speech therapy, the great majority of these children can be expected to acquire normal speech in a reasonably short time.

When defective articulation is due to severe organic disorders, as a hearing impairment, cerebral palsy, or cleft palate, it is usually necessary to carry on an intensive program of therapy over a period of years and to aim for relatively intelligible rather than normal speech. This is particularly true in cerebral palsy. In the case of hearing impairment there are a few individuals who will show rapid improvement through the use of hearing aids which may enable them to perceive sounds which they were unable to hear before. In cleft palate, speech therapy is of little value until the cleft has been closed by means of oral surgery or an artificial palate known as an "obturator." The outcome of speech therapy then depends in part on how well this closure has been made. Sometimes normal speech can be achieved if it is possible to perform a successful operation on the palate early in the child's life, before speech habits have been fully formed.

In disorders of voice the prospects for improvement are excellent when the problem is one of improper habits of voice production. On the other hand, the presence of organic or emotional problems may create stubborn obstacles in some cases.

In serious language retardation in children the outcome

of therapy depends greatly on the cause of the problem. In cases of mental deficiency only limited improvement can be expected. The child may develop some language but will go no further than his restricted mental capacity will allow. In children diagnosed as having "congenital aphasia," on the other hand, the prospects for satisfactory language development through training aided by maturation may be very good. In loss of language in adulthood through a stroke or other brain injury (aphasia), there is nearly always a considerable amount of spontaneous recovery in the months immediately after the injury, but language is seldom restored to its former level, even with the aid of speech therapy.

Stuttering is often considered difficult to eliminate completely when it has been of long standing, but even in adulthood it can often be considerably reduced. It has been known to disappear with or without help at almost any age. In childhood the treatment of stuttering tends to be easier and is aided by a tendency toward spontaneous recovery. Brief episodes of stuttering are extremely common among young children, so that when it has been present for only a short time the outlook for spontaneous recovery is good.

Techniques of Therapy

Articulatory Disorders. When being treated for improper articulatory habits, the child is usually first taught the correct sound in isolation (as "ssss" rather than "soup" or "ess"). He must be trained to hear the sound accurately and vividly or, if necessary, instructed in the proper placement of his articulatory organs. He is then given practice in the use of the sound in progressively more complex contexts, as in syllables, words, sentences, and so on. Finally, he is taught to "carry over" his new articulatory habits to spontaneous speech.

The ordinary young child who has a few infantile errors can sometimes be helped by a parent or teacher. Usually it is not advisable to stop the child now and then in the midst of his conversation to demand that he repeat the word "soup" correctly. He should be taken aside regularly for a few minutes to work on the sound in isolation. The sound should be taught entirely by ear, that is, by imitation. The removal of tonsils and adenoids is of little benefit in cases of defective articulation unless the problem is chiefly one of "denasal" production of *m*, *n*, and *ng*.

When articulatory errors are complicated by organic abnormalities, the help of a trained speech therapist is always necessary. In the case of the child who is hard of hearing, therapy is usually made more effective by the use of hearing aids together with intensive training in the use of residual hearing. The cerebral palsied child usually requires intensive exercises in relaxation, control of speech rate, and accurate use of his speech organs. In cleft palate, special training needs to be given in directing the breath stream through the mouth instead of the nose.

Voice Disorders. The treatment of voice disorders makes use of such techniques as ear training, relaxation, and the habituation of more efficient pitch levels. In some voice cases psychotherapy or psychological guidance are necessary adjuncts to speech therapy. When the voice is lost through surgical removal of the larynx an effective substitute can usually be developed by teaching the patient to belch voluntarily while placing his speech organs in the usual positions for speech sounds. This is termed "esophageal speech."

Aphasia. Treatment of aphasia involves patient retraining in basic language skills which have been lost, as vocabulary, grammar and pronunciation. With children who have failed to develop language the essential procedure is to contrive situations in which verbal responses are made useful and meaningful. For example, the therapist may play ball with the child, continually repeating the word "ball" in the expectation that the child will be stimulated to say the word. It is not wise to withhold a desired object from such a child "until he says it," but whenever possible the name of the object should be spoken when giving it to him.

The Therapist

Speech and hearing therapy is one of the youngest professions. Although European physicians had been concerned with the treatment of speech disorders for many years, it was not until the 1920's that speech therapy began as an independent, nonmedical profession in the United States as a result of the awakening interest of teachers of speech and English, phoneticians, and psychologists. After World War II there was a particularly rapid increase both in the recognition of the importance of such services and in the size of the profession. At the same time audiology (hearing rehabilitation) came to be regarded as a major concern of the profession.

The fully qualified speech therapist has usually received graduate training in his field at an accredited university. This training ordinarily includes studies in hearing as well as speech rehabilitation (hearing testing, selection of hearing aids, teaching of lip reading, and so forth). The person generally regards himself as a member of the "speech and hearing" profession. The majority of speech and hearing therapists are employed in schools, hospitals, and in private practice. Persons with doctoral (Ph.D.) degrees in this area are generally employed in colleges and universities, where they may train therapists, conduct research, and direct speech and hearing clinics.

The professional organization of speech and hearing therapists in the United States is the American Speech and Hearing Association, which has offices in Washington, D.C. There are also many state speech and hearing associations which are affiliated with the national organization. The American Speech and Hearing Association disseminates information about speech and hearing services, publishes scientific journals, organizes annual professional conventions, and maintains relationships with organizations representing related professions.

Speech and hearing therapists are not licensed by state governments, as are physicians and teachers. The American Speech and Hearing Association, however, awards certificates of competency to those of its members who meet certain minimum standards of training and experience. In addition to fulfilling such requirements, certified speech and hearing therapists are bound by a code of ethics. It forbids them from promising "cures," advertising in a blatant manner, charging exorbitant fees, divulging confidential information about their cases, or behaving in any other way detrimental to the welfare of the speech and hearing handicapped.

STIMULANTS [stĭm′yə-lənts], a term applied in medicine principally to drugs which stimulate the central nervous system. These compounds have been used to increase mental alertness and efficiency, to counteract depression, and to stimulate breathing in certain cases of poisoning.

The amphetamines (Benzedrine and Dexedrine) have been widely used for some time to improve the mood of mildly depressed patients and those suffering from chronic illness. Newer drugs for this purpose, sometimes called "psychomotor stimulants," include piperidine derivatives (Pipradol and methylphenidate), the monamine oxidase inhibitors (Marsilid, Catron, Marplan, Niamid, and Nardil), and iminodibenzyl derivatives (Tofranil). While little is known about the nature of the action of these compounds, the monamine oxidase inhibitors are believed to prolong the action of certain hormones in the nervous system (serotinin, epinephrine, and norepinephrine). The psychomotor stimulants are also used to correct some behavior problems in children, to relieve despondency in the aged, and in chronically fatigued patients.

Stimulants used to counteract overdoses of barbiturates and similar depressant poisons are called "analeptics." These drugs, including Nikethamide, Picrotoxin, Metrazol, and Benzedrine are used in such cases to stimulate breathing and circulation and to combat drowsiness. At one time, Metrazol was also used in the treatment of schizophrenia and other mental disorders to produce convulsions.

SUBCONSCIOUS AND UNCONSCIOUS, terms used in medicine and psychology to describe mental activity outside of awareness. In medicine unconsciousness denotes a state of diminished awareness. An unconscious person is partially or completely unaware of his environment and usually has only partial possession of many of his normal body functions. The depth of unconsciousness is indicated by progressive loss of reflexes.

In psychology the usage of these two concepts cannot be sharply defined. Most often the unconscious is understood to be that part of the personality which shapes much of our behavior without the ego having immediate knowledge of it. The subconscious is a portion of the unconscious containing materials which may be recalled voluntarily to consciousness. The concept of unconscious determinants of behavior of which the individual is unaware is an ancient one. It stems from the observation that people may act irrationally, doing things which make no sense in relation to their nominal goals.

At present psychologists generally accept the existence of unconscious factors. The emphasis has now shifted to the conditions under which these factors operate and the degree of their influence.

Consciousness and unconsciousness as opposite concepts derive from subjective experience. They cannot be defined in terms of behavior but reveal their existence only through introspection. Nevertheless, the use of these terms is neither specious, as some schools of psychology

maintain, nor unscientific. Existence of the unconscious is a reasonable postulate that may clarify behavior in cases where other explanations are absent. However, schools of psychology which formulate their statements solely in such subjective terms cannot provide full insight into the causality of behavior. Even the most acute subjective observations make limited sense without correlated behavioral observations.

Some modern concepts regarding conscious and unconscious behavior arise from the evolutionary theory of central nervous system (CNS) functions. Hughlings Jackson, neurologist, postulated that the functions of the CNS are integrated at progressively more complex levels from simple reflexes to mental activity, the last being singular to man. Much of what our body needs to do for survival never comes into awareness. Much acquired knowledge becomes integrated and forgotten, and once we have learned an action, it becomes habitual and automatic.

Sigmund Freud was the first to outline specific techniques for the study of the unconscious. He theorized that each person is born with an unconscious, in which the life instincts are at work and which provides the energy for growth and development. Carl G. Jung proposed that the unconscious contains not only innate drives but also innate ideas, which bear upon our highest aspirations as well as upon our most primitive instincts. These ideas have arisen in the past of mankind and may relate to a collective unconscious shared by living beings.

It is possible to depict an arbitrary scheme of these concepts, starting with Freud's classical notion that the mind resembles an iceberg. Only one tenth of its contents can be seen above the surface—that is, are conscious—and nine tenths of the mind remains out of awareness. Some parts may be voluntarily recalled (subconscious), but most of the unconscious will remain hidden from awareness by the function of a censoring mechanism. It usually requires indirect methods, such as analysis of free associations, dreams, and involuntary errors, to reveal unconscious material. Uncensored unconscious processes show in daily life only in mental disorder.

This model is useful in the explanation of human behavior. The assumption that all actions are rational and can ultimately be analyzed in terms of reasonable causality only narrows the scope of many personality theories. It leads to an evasion of the question, rather than an explanation of man's actions.

In the treatment of mental disorder, the assumption that a patient is cognizant of his difficulties, only needing clarity in sorting out his problems, may not lead to assistance to the patient or understanding of his problems. Finally, it is impossible to account for fantasy, imagination, and creativity in an individual at present, without assuming that certain processes, thoughts, and feelings are outside awareness and cannot possibly be described subjectively. Insights or ideas may suddenly appear in the conscious mind, with little or no awareness of how they came into being. According to some authorities, such as Jean Piaget, the major portion of conscious thought is guided by unconscious patterns and is made conscious only in the formal expressions of logicians.

Nonpsychoanalytic psychology recognizes the unconscious as the repository of memory and as a major site of

MODEL OF THE MIND

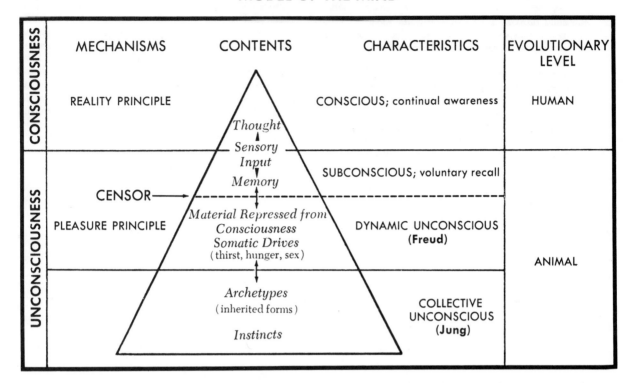

	MECHANISMS	CONTENTS	CHARACTERISTICS	EVOLUTIONARY LEVEL
CONSCIOUSNESS	REALITY PRINCIPLE	*Thought* ↑ *Sensory Input* ↓ *Memory*	CONSCIOUS; continual awareness	HUMAN
UNCONSCIOUSNESS			SUBCONSCIOUS; voluntary recall	
	CENSOR→ PLEASURE PRINCIPLE	*Material Repressed from Consciousness Somatic Drives* (thirst, hunger, sex)	DYNAMIC UNCONSCIOUS **(Freud)**	ANIMAL
		Archetypes (inherited forms) *Instincts*	COLLECTIVE UNCONSCIOUS **(Jung)**	

the activities associated with thought and perception. There is evidence that the mind unconsciously stores details of past experiences. Hypnotized subjects can remember minute details of childhood experiences, and electrical stimulation of certain parts of the brain may cause a patient to "relive" earlier experiences.

The importance of unconscious activity in perception has been demonstrated by experiments in which images, exposed too rapidly to be seen, left an impression on the mind. Some time ago there was a flurry of interest in such "subliminal" perception. It was feared that large groups of people could be "brainwashed" by high-speed suggestions flashed on television or movie screens. The viewer would be unaware of the image, but the message would nevertheless register on his unconscious mind.

Personality analysts point out that unconscious factors shape our perception of social facts, such as the impressions we form of people. We sometimes see a person for the first time and immediately like or dislike him but are unaware of why our reaction is so swift and certain. The answer may lie in the "subliminal" impression the person gives. There is a look in the eye, a curl of the lip, a tilt of the head, which coalesce in the unconscious mind and deliver to consciousness the fully formed impression of like or dislike.

Under certain circumstances portions of the unconscious may become detached from the main stream of personality (dissociation). This disorder may range from types of amnesia, in which unpleasant memories are segregated from consciousness, to the rare "multiple personality," in which consciousness is split into two or more distinct personalities.

See also CONSCIOUSNESS; DISSOCIATION; FREUD, SIGMUND; JUNG, CARL GUSTAVE; PSYCHOANALYSIS.

SUBLIMATION, a concept of Freudian psychoanalytic theory according to which primitive drives and desires are unconsciously transformed into socially acceptable goals. Freud conceived of sublimation as the basis of civilization. In his view the human infant is a small barbarian whose primitive desires must be curbed before he can live in civilized society. In Freudian terms, a classic example of sublimation would be the scholar or artist whose sexual energies are diverted (sublimated) into creative and intellectual activity.
See also PSYCHOANALYSIS.

SULLIVAN, HARRY STACK (1892–1949), American psychiatrist known for his clinical studies of schizophrenia and his stress on social factors in the development of the personality. Sullivan taught at the University of Maryland and was coeditor of the journal *Psychiatry*. His theories of human behavior, put forward in *Psychiatry: Introduction to the Study of Interpersonal Relations* (1948), have stimulated much psychiatric thought.

SUPEREGO. In psychoanalytic theory, the mind is comprised of three main parts—ego, id, and superego. Though in continual conflict, they remain balanced in the normal individual. The superego is that part which accounts for "the activities of self observation, conscience and the holding up of ideals" (Sigmund Freud). Although it has been popularly equated with "conscience," the superego covers a far greater area of behavior.

SUPEREGO

In the young child, two concurrent processes lead to the development of the superego. In the more important, the child takes as his own the parents' ideals, demands, and restrictions so that he becomes able to govern himself and establish standards for his own behavior. In the second, the child may decide that he deserves punishments more severe than his parents impose. This may explain why children with "mild" parents often develop harsh self-demands. Though the superego is built up gradually from the first year, it is not felt to be fully developed until the age of six or seven, when the child achieves a stable identification with the parent of the same sex.

In the adult, several aspects of behavior are connected with the superego, including perseverance at a task, sense of order and responsibility, attentiveness to the needs of others, and control of emotional expression. Depending upon the balance of these factors, the superego might be characterized as either harsh and uncompromising, inconsistent and corruptible, or, ideally, supportive and adequate. In some psychological illnesses there is felt to be a severe imbalance of these superego functions. The sociopathic personality may have a deficient superego, while those suffering from excessive feelings of guilt and worthlessness may labor under a too harsh and uncompromising superego.

See also CHILD DEVELOPMENT; PSYCHOANALYSIS.

T

TELEPATHY. *See* PARAPSYCHOLOGY.

TERRITORIALITY, a concept in animal behavior that refers to the tendency of individual animals or groups to occupy, mark, and defend a circumscribed region, and to return to that region after removal. In 1920 H. E. Howard's *Territory in Bird Life* established the concept of territory in behavioral terms. The male bird "isolates himself, makes himself conspicuous, becomes intolerant of other males (of his species) and confines his movements to a definite area." Knowledge of the function of territory is rapidly increasing. A summary at present can only be tentative, but there are several findings which seem significant for the study of behavior in general.

Territorial behavior is a complex pattern based on many simpler behavioral units. For example, territoriality in migrating animals is only visible at certain periods, notably in relation to procreation. Territorial behavior plays a part in mating, for instance, in the male challenge and his vocal display. It also plays a part in the defense of the nest by male and female after pairing. The male display has a double function. It is directed against other males, while simultaneously attracting the female. Thus a bird may, by its singing, indicate to his rival "this is my territory, stay way from it" and to his sweetheart "please come and look at my beautiful home."

Territoriality apparently serves several functions of great biological significance. The geographic spacing of animals probably plays a role in keeping the population at a level appropriate for the particular environment. Territorial behavior counters the influence of dominance and aggression by other animals which, if unchecked, would engage the animal constantly and cause needless stress. A territory provides security and motivates the animal to identify with "its space." This may well have been the origin of property in man, "possession" being that which one can sit on.
See also AGGRESSION.

TESTING, PSYCHOLOGICAL AND EDUCATIONAL, is now big business in America. It is used in the educational system from the kindergarten through the university; its techniques are used in the process of selecting students for important scholarships and honors, as well as for many routine applications in school administration, supervision, and guidance. Testing is used widely in industry for the selection of personnel, as a basis for promotion, and as a basis for allocating individuals to positions requiring special abilities. The majority of persons in the United States are affected by testing in one way or another, either directly in terms of measurement of their own characteristics or indirectly through the measurement of the characteristics of their children in school.

The Nature of Measurement in Psychology and Education

The word "testing" has been used in the title of this article, although test experts might prefer the more inclusive term "measurement" or the even more inclusive term "evaluation." A test implies an instrument made up of questions to which there are right and wrong answers. Many measurement devices used in education and industry are not scored in this way. Attempts to measure interests are examples of such instruments. There are still other evaluative devices involving rating scales and the like that do not yield a quantitative score of any kind. However, in the minds of most people outside the ranks of the test technicians, the word "testing" has a much broader meaning, being essentially equivalent to "evaluation."

Some kind of evaluation of ability and achievement has been going on as long as there have been schools, businesses, armies, and other institutions. Standardized testing, however, is a phenomenon of the 20th century. The scientific measurement of intelligence can be said to have begun with the work of the French psychologist Alfred Binet. In 1905 he issued, with the collaboration of Théodore Simon, the Binet-Simon Test of Intelligence. This test was prepared at the request of the French government for the practical purpose of identifying children whose mental ability was too low for regular schoolwork. The test consisted of a number of items graded from age 3 to age 12. A score, called mental age, was assigned on the basis of the number of items a child completed successfully.

Binet's test was designed for individual use. That is, one examiner could administer the test to but one child at a time. Work on a test that could be administered to groups was under way in the United States when that nation entered World War I. The Army, facing the problem of screening hundreds of thousands of recruits, used materials prepared by Arthur S. Otis, a psychologist at Stanford University, as the basis for the Army Alpha Examination. In the 1920's use of intelligence scales in the United States expanded rapidly, finding many applications in the schools (*see* INTELLIGENCE TEST).

Standardized testing of achievement in school also developed in the early 20th century, gaining impetus from the work of E. L. Thorndike at Teachers College, Columbia University. Statistical methods used in the psychology laboratory and in intelligence testing were applied to schoolwork. Studies of traditional grades showed the variability of teachers' judgments. For example, when copies of one mathematics examination paper were graded by a number of teachers, scores ranged from 28 to 92. Thirty-seven teachers marked the paper below 65; 47 marked it 75 or better; and 12 marked it 83 to 90.

TESTING

In an effort to provide more objective means of measuring progress, publishers began to issue standard tests for mathematics, reading, science, and other subjects.

Unlike measurement in the direct physical sense, measurement in education and psychology is indirect. The significance of the obtained score must be inferred by comparing the performance of an individual with other individuals, with whom he presumably has something in common. In the areas of achievement and of capacity to achieve (intelligence and aptitude), measurement is accomplished by providing standard tasks to be performed under standard conditions. The number of such tasks successfully performed under standard conditions (uniform directions, uniform timing, and the like) generally is the basis for determining the quality of the performance.

Varieties of Tests

Mental-Ability or Intelligence Tests. In the measurement of mental ability, general intelligence tests of the global type—that is, tests that measure many different aspects of mental ability without attempting to differentiate among them—still are in wide use. These probably will continue to be used extensively, especially at the younger age levels where differentiation among separate kinds of mental ability is of little import. Such tests of intelligence or mental ability began as paper and pencil copies of Binet-type individual tests of intelligence. Historically, the most important of these tests was the Otis Group Test of Mental Ability, developed while Otis was working as a student under Lewis M. Terman. Otis attempted to develop in paper and pencil form tests that would follow a pattern derived from the Binet individual examination. Subsequent group test developers experimented with different types of items, but in all cases responses were combined to yield a single score. This total score was then interpreted as a mental age and an IQ was computed by dividing mental age by chronological age (see INTELLIGENCE QUOTIENT).

Beginning in the 1920's much effort was made to differentiate among mental abilities that were more or less independent, and thus to discover those traits that were probably more nearly native or inborn. (The word "probably" is used advisedly since this problem of how much nature and nurture contribute to ability has never been solved.) The approach to the development of such tests was essentially statistical. It involved the study of the strength of the "going-togetherness" (correlation) between scores on many types of tests that were presumed to measure independent aspects of mental ability. This statistical procedure is called *factor analysis*. As a result of early developmental work by L. L. Thurstone and others, a number of factors were isolated that have tended to become generally accepted as real factors of mental ability, relatively independent of each other, and existing regardless of the pattern of training or experience to which an individual has been subjected. Extended experimentation in the study of such mental factors has tended to increase the number of so-called "factors" recognized by one experimenter or another, as those who have carried out these studies have come to accept substantially larger amounts of overlapping (higher intercorrelations) from one test to another. Among the factors often reported are the number factor, memory factor, space factor (ability to visualize objects in three dimensions), perceptual speed, and facility in understanding verbal meaning (see INTELLIGENCE). Studies made to date do *not* establish any single set of mental factors that can be generally agreed upon as being independent of each other. Within the

---

ACHIEVEMENT TEST ITEMS
Three excerpts from achievement test designed to measure each subject's competence in various academic fields are shown.

Below, a biology question. In such testing, the subject often marks his choice on a separate answer sheet.

Iron is needed by the body to form —

[a] nerve tissue   [b] red blood cells
[c] thyroxin   [d] strong bones and teeth

Below, an arithmetic question. The subject is usually provided with extra paper so that he may work out the problems if necessary.

What is the sum of 3 hr. 20 min., 4 hr. 15 min., 2 hr. 50 min., 1 hr. 5 min., and 5 hr. 10 min.?

[e] 17 hr. 25 min.   [f] 16 hr. 0 min.
[g] 16 hr. 40 min.   [h] 16 hr. 45 min.

DIRECTIONS: Read each group of words below. Decide if the words make *one complete sentence*, *more than one complete sentence*, or *no complete sentence*. Look at the answer spaces at the right or on your answer sheet (if you have one). If the group of words *can* be correctly punctuated as one sentence by merely putting a period or question mark at the end, fill in the space under the 1. If the group of words *could* be punctuated as two sentences (without changing or omitting any words), fill in the space under the 2. If the group of words is just part of a sentence, fill in the space under the N. ("N" stands for "not a complete sentence.")

SAMPLES

K In 1818 the flag had twenty stars . . .   K ● ○ ○

L In the right-hand corner of the flag . . .   L ○ ○ ○

A paragraph of directions prefaces an English grammar test. The supervisor often reads the directions aloud and discusses sample questions before permitting the subjects to begin the actual test.

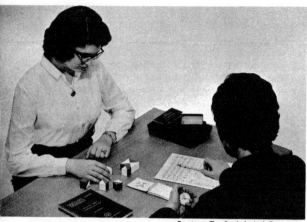

Courtesy, The Psychological Corporation

A subject takes the block design test, a subtest of the Wechsler Adult Intelligence Scale; a supervisor records the results.

whole area of factor analysis of mental ability there still are many contradictions, both in point of view and in techniques used.

Individual versus Group Intelligence Tests. Historically intelligence testing began with tests that were administered to a single individual one at a time, with the examiner exercising a substantial degree of control over the test situation. The first systematic intelligence test that followed the pattern typical of the present-day individual test was the Binet-Simon battery developed in France. In the United States the first individual intelligence test to become widely used was the Stanford Revision of the Binet-Simon scale, developed by Lewis M. Terman at Stanford University. First published in 1916, this battery of tests was in its third revision in the early 1960's.

The Wechsler test batteries by David Wechsler, a clinical psychologist at Bellevue Hospital, are another widely used set of measures of mental ability of the individual type. These tests differ substantially from the Stanford Revisions of the Binet-Simon tests. For one thing, these batteries yield both a verbal and performance IQ instead of a single measure of brightness.

It is generally assumed that an individual test is necessarily a better measure of mental ability than a group test, but this is not true. Giving and scoring individual tests are very time-consuming, and as a result such tests generally are less well standardized. They usually involve less precise statistical analysis, and are standardized (used experimentally so that scores can be established) on smaller and usually less representative groups of individuals.

Individual tests allow the examiner considerable latitude in encouraging the subject to do his best and in interpreting the performance of the individual being tested. If an examiner is properly trained, this individual attention can result in a more valid indication of a subject's level of mental ability; if he is not, his influence is a major source of error or variation from one test situation to another.

Group tests, on the other hand, are much more efficient in the sense that they permit an individual to solve many more problems per unit of time than individual tests do and, therefore, are generally more reliable as measures of

capacity. Because they can be administered to groups as large as several hundred at one sitting, many more individuals can be tested. Most group tests of mental ability in current use also permit very rapid processing, usually by means of a scoring machine.

Achievement Tests. In achievement testing the simplest types of tests are those that attempt to measure certain knowledges and skills specifically taught in school or in other special courses of instruction. A test in arithmetic computation is a good example of such an instrument within the school framework. Examples of achievement test items are shown on these pages. A test of ability to follow a wiring diagram in electronics might be an example of an achievement test in an industry training program.

In most achievement (and mental-ability) tests the trend is toward the objective type question, of which there is an almost infinite variety. The item type most frequently used is the multiple choice question. Several possible answers are given from which the individual chooses the one he thinks is right. A common variant of this is the multiple response question, in which there may be more than one right answer among the choices given. Another commonly used item type provides two lists of facts or other information that have to be compared or matched; hence the name "matching type" question.

All such objective type questions are in contrast to the free response type, in which the individual is allowed complete freedom of response to the stimulus. An example of the free response question would be, "How are you feeling today?" In this item the individual is allowed to respond just as he pleases. By contrast, one might say, "How are you feeling today?" and then give the following choices: (1) Energetic; (2) Lazy; (3) Tired; (4) Ill; (5) Strong. In such questions it sometimes is desirable to include "none of these" as an alternative. In the question above there could be two appropriate answers, in which case the individual would be justified in marking both of them. For example, he might mark "ill" and "lazy" or he might mark "energetic" and "strong." This question elicits an emotional response, thus illustrating the point that such objective type questions can be used in a wide variety of situations.

There is much discussion, especially among lay people, of the efficacy of the objective type question. Extensive research has shown that such items are more to be depended upon as valid and reliable measures than are the essay type or free response questions, which are very difficult if not impossible to score objectively.

Tests of Developed Abilities. Tests have been developed that purport to measure both mental ability and achievement simultaneously. These are sometimes called tests of "developed abilities." It is hypothesized that such instruments reflect not only the specific training an individual has had, but also the native mental abilities he brings to the task.

Aptitude and Prognostic Tests—Measures of Capacity or Potential. The Differential Aptitude Tests fall in this category to the extent that they are a mixture of measures involving skills little affected by specific in-school training, and measures of other skills definitely affected by school instruction. Such tests clearly serve a different purpose than the achievement measure intended to discover how much an individual has learned as a result of a specific course of instruction. They are intended to show to what extent the individual has profited by all of his learning experiences in an area, and how much this learning helps him in solving related problems. Such instruments generally are used for prediction purposes.

The so-called prognostic tests attempt to predict success in specific subject-matter areas. For example, there are prognostic tests for algebra and, more generally, for mathematics. There are prognostic tests for secretarial and stenographic courses. There are prognostic tests for science. All of these are generally similar in the sense that they attempt to predict what an individual will do in a subsequent course of instruction on the basis of knowledges and skills that he has inherited and developed up to the time the particular course of instruction is begun.

Historically, the term "aptitude" was thought of as applying to tests that measured capacities that were somewhat independent of general intelligence but were considered to exist as real dimensions of ability. The best examples are the art aptitude tests and musical aptitude tests developed in the 1930's or the mechanical aptitude tests developed even earlier. These tests are not now widely used in school, but find more use in industry.

Readiness Tests. The "kit bag" of tests available to a psychologist includes additional tests of capacity or potential that can be considered, in a sense, specialized intelligence tests. In this category would fall the so-called readiness tests used at the beginning of school to determine a child's ability to undertake formal instruction in reading and other subjects. Some readiness tests are much like group intelligence tests for use at this early age level; others are really simple achievement measures of knowledges likely to be developed by normal life experience. Their value in any particular situation depends on many local factors having to do with the organization of instruction and the type of curriculum in use.

Measures Requiring an Affective, Attitudinal, or Emotional Response. Within the broad category of measures of personality, interests, and aptitudes are a host of instruments that are not properly called tests, but that do record in systematic fashion the response of an individual to many situations found to suggest or "predict" in a loose sense certain psychological characteristics. For example, it is often helpful in school guidance or in industry to be able to characterize the individual as being generally an outgoing (extroverted) type of person or one who is comparatively withdrawn (introverted). Extroversion and introversion are at opposite ends of a kind of continuum, most individuals probably being somewhere in the middle and having some tendencies in each direction (see INTROVERSION-EXTROVERSION).

Similarly, other personality traits or characteristics have been described or defined. Attempts have been made to measure them by asking individuals to tell how they feel about certain related situations or activities and comparing their responses to those of many other individuals like them in age, sex, socioeconomic status, and other respects. Most of these instruments are not intended to identify or measure the extreme deviate, that is, the individual who is really mentally ill, but rather to describe the variations in personality found in normal persons. Following are some sample questions of the simpler type found in such personality tests:

> Do you let yourself go and have a gay time at a party?
> Do people consider you to be rather quiet?
> Do you like to be the chairman of a meeting?
> Are you sometimes considered to be cold and unsympathetic?

Other instruments in this category, on the other hand, are intended to probe more deeply and to provide the clinician with indications of deviations from the normal pattern that may demand professional treatment. Such instruments obviously are not for lay use any more than is a surgeon's scalpel.

A type of personality measure used to study both the normal and the mentally ill is the so-called projective test. The prototype of such tests is the Rorschach technique. For discussion of this and other projective tests, see PROJECTIVE TECHNIQUES.

Interest Inventories. Another type of measuring device widely used in schools, and to some extent in industry, is the interest inventory. While there are a substantial number of these on the market, the Strong Vocational Interest Blank and the Kuder Preference Record are predominant. The Strong inventory has been used with and standardized primarily on adults, while the Kuder Preference Record is commonly used in the junior and senior high schools. The primary purpose of such inventories is to find some evidence of the vocation in which an individual would be happy or contented, all other determiners of success being favorable. The results of the administration of such instruments do not predict success in any occupation except to the extent that job satisfaction is a contributor to success. These instruments are not aptitude measures.

The hypothesis underlying interest inventories is that when an individual makes a choice of his most preferred activity among several competing activities, he is revealing some generalizable information about himself, not just the obvious choice among three competing activities or preferences. By suitable statistical analysis, activities that cluster together can be identified and scored as a group to determine the strength of the individual's concern with that category of interest.

An example of an item in an interest inventory is given below:

> If your school took a poll to find out what kind of extracurricular activities students preferred, in which of the following would you be most interested? Which least?
>> c. Creative writing course
>> j. Competitive sports within school
>> g. Science Fair project

The statistical analysis required to construct an interest inventory is time-consuming and expensive. Judging the effectiveness of such instruments requires matching test results against subsequent success in a field. This is not only expensive but may require years of follow-up studies.

How Tests Are Constructed

A number of references have been made to the selection of test items and other steps in making a standardized test. A brief review of the process will further explain the nature of such measuring devices. When a publisher has decided to prepare a new test, items are usually drafted by subject-matter experts. An algebra achievement test, for example, would be drafted by mathematics teachers. Often the first draft is reviewed by other teachers as well as by the publisher's test editors. Then the preliminary form is tried out, perhaps by being given to several thousand students. Every effort is made to eliminate ambiguous or inappropriate items. The length of the test is adjusted to fit a desirable administration time. The revised form of the test is then administered to a large group so that standards for scoring can be established. In the standardization program for one widely used achievement battery, the tests were given to more than 500,000 students. As a result of extensive trials, the degree of validity and reliability of the test is determined and standards for interpretation are set up. These concepts are further discussed below.

The Nature of Test Validity. A valid test is one that measures the thing it is intended to measure. Some tests have what is called face validity; that is, they are obviously measures of what they are supposed to be. A test of arithmetic computation, which requires an individual to compute, would be such a test. In other tests ways to measure an ability, skill, or attribute are not nearly as obvious. Indirect evidence may be used to establish validity.

Validity depends on many factors, some of which are intrinsic, such as the quality of the items and the suitability of the instrument for the age and school grade of those taking it. Other factors vary with the individual or group being tested and the conditions under which the measure is used. An instrument used in a situation where there is considerable antagonism toward testing will not yield valid results in many instances. The validity of a test may be seriously weakened if a separate answer sheet is used without adequate preparation or if the answer sheet is carelessly marked so that the test scoring machine will not accurately score it.

The factors affecting validity are so complex that only a major treatise on this subject can properly deal with it. The most important single generalization is that every test given should yield a score that can be depended upon as being a reasonably good measure of what the test is desired to measure. Since a test that is not valid is no test at all, validity is perhaps the heart of the entire measurement problem.

Parents often misinterpret the results of standardized tests administered in the schools (and sometimes school people do also) in that they think of these tests as being measures of the specific outcomes of instruction within the local school. Actually such tests are measures of the extent to which the local group compares favorably or unfavorably with some other standard group, most commonly students across the nation. Thus a standardized test in spelling may include many words that do not appear in the local course of study, but do appear in many other courses of study used elsewhere over the country. The quality of performance is judged against the national performance on the particular measure. The local group may actually spell better or less well than average due to a difference in the amount of time given to the subject and the seriousness with which the subject is viewed by the local community. Such a spelling test may be a valid measure of spelling ability in terms of nationwide performance but not a valid measure of how well local spelling instruction meets local goals for spelling teaching.

Reliability. The reliability of a test generally is an estimate of the extent to which the test is stable. If another test just like it were given within a short period of time, would the individual rank about the same on the second test as he did on the first? Unless he does, the test is not very reliable. If the results for a group were exactly the same on two measures, the test could be said to have perfect reliability. Many factors affect reliability, and some of these factors also affect validity. The quality of the test items, the length of the test, and the extent to which the test is speeded or is a power test (an essentially untimed test) all affect reliability. Other factors include attitude toward the test (motivation), procedure in administration, adherence to time limits, and accuracy of scoring.

Interpreting the Results of Educational and Psychological Measures

The figure obtained by scoring an educational or psychological test often is not significant by itself. The initial result (usually called a raw score) must be interpreted before it can be used. This is done by comparing the performance of the individual with the performance of some representative group or persons who have taken the same test. This process is called standardization, or "norming." Generally speaking, the group on which a test is standardized, or normed, is supposed to be representative of some large geographic area or homogeneous group of individuals. For example, most school achievement tests purport to have national norms that are applicable to certain grades in any section of the country. Intelligence measures generally are standardized on very large unselected populations of individuals divided into age groups, regardless of grade and usually regardless of sex. The problem of providing norms for the interpretation of standardized tests is complex and difficult. It is perhaps the one area where the publisher of a standardized test is forced to compromise with what he knows to be the best practice, since he is not in a position to control the entire situation.

In order to establish norms for school-oriented tests, it is necessary to test many individual pupils, and the control over the schedule of individuals lies within the school systems where such individuals are to be found. School systems are reasonably co-operative in helping publishers standardize tests, but generally insist on receiving the materials, plus substantial amounts of service, either without charge or at a very nominal fee. This makes the process of large-scale norming very expensive, and really adequate norms can be established for a test or battery only when it is reasonable to expect a wide sale and consequently an adequate return on the investment involved.

Norms for Achievement and Related Types of Tests. Achievement test scores for tests administered in the public schools can be interpreted in a number of ways. Perhaps the most widely used basis for interpretation is the grade placement score or grade equivalent. This is the real or estimated average score of persons in the norm population at any stated grade level. For convenience in establishing such grade equivalents the school year is divided into 10 parts, called months of grade even though few school systems are actually in session for 10 full months. Such norms assume that no growth or development in the skills involved takes place during the course of the summer months, which is rarely, if ever, true. It is certainly less true for the more general or developmental types of tests, such as reading or spelling, than it is for other types where the instruction in a subject is largely confined to what goes on in the classroom.

Another type of norm widely used with achievement and similar types of tests at the high school level is the percentile rank. The percentile rank describes the pupil's position in a group by stating the percentage of pupils who fall below him. For example, if one hundred individuals representing a good cross section of the population to which the norms were to apply could be lined up along a wall in order of height from shortest to tallest, the percentile rank of an individual in such a group would be the number of pupils who were shorter than he. One advantage of percentile ranks is that they are comparatively easy to explain by simple illustrations such as the one given above. A major disadvantage, however, is that the units are not equal. Almost all of the measures to which such norms are applied yield score distributions that produce a bell-shaped curve when plotted on a graph. Many individuals are near the average score and fewer and fewer individuals earn scores at the extremes. Thus, it takes a fairly wide range of scores at the extremes to equal a certain percentage of the total number of individuals in the group, whereas a very small range of scores at the middle of the distribution will equal the same percent of cases.

Still another type of transformed score that is used widely is the standard score. This can be simply a straight line translation of the raw scores into a new set of numbers with a different mean and different (wider or narrower) range of scores or variability than the original scores. This is called a linear transformation. More and more, standard scores are becoming score scales, which means that the number of questions answered correctly, or its equivalent, is interpreted along a scale that has been adjusted so that the transformed scores follow generally the shape of the normal curve or some close approximation to it. (The normal curve is a special variety of the bell-shaped curve mentioned above. It has many cases piling up at the middle and a few cases at the extremes. It is a mathematically precise curve which can be expressed in equation form, and is very widely used in educational and psychological measurement.)

A simplified normalized standard score scale is the stanine. The word "stanine" stands for "*sta*ndard *nine*-step scale." Raw test scores are converted into scores that run from 1 (lowest) to 9 (highest). Stanines of 4, 5, and 6 indicate average performance. Stanines were first used extensively in the Air Force air crew selection program. They can be computed for any set of data with which it is possible to arrange individuals in rank order. Stanines are simple to compute and are sufficiently precise for almost all usual purposes. Their utility and simplicity have resulted in their increasingly wide use, especially as devices for interpreting achievement and mental-ability measures at the local level, although they are not limited to this use.

Norms for Mental-Ability and Similar Measures. Mental-ability measures can be interpreted in terms of percentile ranks, standard scores, including stanines, and age equivalents, which are comparable to the grade equivalents discussed previously. Most intelligence tests also make use of the intelligence quotient, or IQ.

Originally the intelligence quotient was defined as the mental age divided by the chronological age (see INTELLIGENCE QUOTIENT). The ratio IQ (MA/CA) has certain serious disadvantages related to the fact that growth in mental ability is most rapid in the very young, slowing up in the teen years and then stopping. This does not mean that an individual does not keep on learning; it simply means that his capacity to learn reaches its maximum. Under these conditions, if the chronological age divisor in the equation MA/CA was allowed to continue upward indefinitely as individuals got older, the result would be that everyone would appear to get duller as he got older. In practice this contingency has been met by carrying the chronological age divisor up to some maximum value. Usually this maximum value is 16-0, although this varies from one test to another.

The ratio IQ, because of its many disadvantages, has gradually been superseded by a different measure, which interprets the brightness of an individual in terms of his deviation from the average score of his own age group. This is called the deviation IQ and stems directly from the index of brightness first devised by Arthur S. Otis in the 1920's. Gradually, most intelligence measures of the omnibus type that are interpreted in terms of IQ's have swung over to the deviation rather than the ratio type of quotient. In many ways, the deviation IQ is akin to the standard score. It has a mean of 100 and a standard deviation or measure of variability of approximately 15 to 17 points, which is arbitrary. It generally is normally distributed and is free of any effect of increase in age, since this increase is taken care of by varying the reference point or norm from which the deviation is computed.

Norms for Inventory and Projective Type Measures. The problem of interpreting an inventory type measure or a projective measure is entirely different from that of interpreting achievement or ability measures. In the inventory or projective instruments, an expression of attitude is solicited or an emotional reaction is engendered and recorded. At best one can only compare the performance of an individual reacting to such a measure to what many other individuals do when they react to the same stimulus. Many times there is no way of determining the reasonably right answer, and a numerical score may not be possible.

All such measures need to be interpreted with a great deal of caution. The best use of the result is not so much to be found in the interpretation of the over-all score (if any score is given) as in the way the individual responds to the separate items, questions, or situations. Projective instruments can be evaluated only by experts. Whatever insights into personality such tests provide probably depend on the skill and understanding of the examiner.

The Proper Use of Test Results. The caution just expressed can be extended to the interpretation of all test results. No single test report can be taken as an exact measurement of capacity, achievement, interest, or personality. For example, an educational psychologist is healthily skeptical about any single measurement of a child's intelligence. He surveys the complete school record on the child. He regards an IQ as one useful part of the record and as a valuable predictor of success in school but not as a final verdict on ability.

See also:

INTELLIGENCE
INTELLIGENCE TEST
PSYCHOLOGY: *Educational Psychology*
SOCIOMETRY
VOCATIONAL GUIDANCE

THINKING. The nature of thinking has occupied man since he began to wonder about himself, and the studies of thinking by the great theorists of man make up a large part of the disciplines of philosophy, psychology, and education. The present article confines itself to certain leading approaches to thinking of modern experimental and genetic psychology.

Problem-Solving Behavior

The Puzzle Box. The U.S. psychologist Edward L. Thorndike (1874–1949) placed a cat in a box with an escape mechanism that could be operated by a lever or loop at one side of the box. Through the bars of the box the animal could see, but not reach, food. Thorndike observed that the cat would thrash about wildly, scratching and clawing the box until he inadvertently tripped the escape mechanism. In subsequent trials the thrashing gradually diminished as the animal learned to activate the lever smoothly whenever placed in the box. To Thorndike this was the model of problem-solving behavior, a blind groping, leading to accidental discovery of the solution, which was then "stamped in" by the reward of solving the problem.

The Maze. A more sophisticated concept of problem-solving activity was developed through experiments on maze-running problems in rats. The animals were "motivated" to solve the maze by rewards of food or water placed at the goal. From such experiments "behaviorist" psychologists constructed a scheme of thinking based on concepts such as "generalization" (if the rat is taught to run toward a short, wide rectangle, he will extend, or generalize, this response to a long, thin rectangle) and "goal gradient" (the closer to the goal the rat comes, the more intense is his response—that is, he runs faster as he nears the food box).

The concept of thinking derived from the behaviorists' experiments is essentially mechanical. A stimulus acts upon the organism, which responds in a certain manner according to simple laws of generalization, goal gradient, and so forth. Human thinking is held to be merely a series of stimulus-response sequences (S–R bonds), a richer combination of the principles by which the rat solves its maze problems.

Köhler and the Apes: a Gestalt View of Thinking. To the Gestalt psychologist the essence of thinking is the dramatic moment of insight when the solution of the problem is suddenly seen in terms of a total configuration or Gestalt. In a series of classic experiments performed on chimpanzees, the German-born psychologist Wolfgang Köhler (1887–) demonstrated the role of insight in problem solving. In one experiment Köhler placed a banana beyond the reach of a confined chimpanzee. Lying close by and well within reach was a long stick. At first the chimpanzee tried to reach the banana by direct groping. Failing in these attempts, he roamed about, angry and frustrated, until he suddenly seized the stick and used it to bring the banana within reach. Köhler stressed the suddenness of the act—the moment of rapid insight. Gestalt psychologists describe this solution as a sudden "restructuring" of the situation. The stick, which was clearly visible all the time, is suddenly seen as an instrument for obtaining the banana.

Thus to the Gestaltist the problem is solved suddenly by insight. The early attempts at solution are guided by intelligent searching, and problem-solving thought is essentially the change in the perception of a visual situation.

A Study of Concept Formation. In *A Study of Thinking* (1956) a group of U.S. psychologists led by Jerome Bruner (1915–) report researches in the problem of concept formation. Bruner discovered that his subjects preferred methods of approach, or "strategies," in problem solving that reduced mental strain. He also found that most people were better able to deal with "conjunctive" concepts, those based on the simultaneous presence of two attributes (a chair has legs *and* a surface on which to sit), as opposed to "disjunctive" concepts, those based on the presence of one or more of several properties (a man called "doctor" has an M.D. *or* a Ph.D. *or* a D.D.S. *or* other degrees). Although Bruner did not expand his studies into a general theory of thinking, his work is of interest in showing aspects of problem-solving behavior that do not fit into the traditional Gestalt and behaviorist schemes.

Computer Simulation of Human Thought. The "electronic brain" has been used to study human thought. The human subject is given a problem (such as one in symbolic logic) and instructions on how to manipulate the subject matter of the problem (such as the rules for changing one set of symbols to another). The subject is asked to think aloud and to write the phases of his solution as he proceeds. The machine is given the same problem and the same rules of manipulation. The machine is also given a method of approach, what in the language of the computer world is called a "program." The machine follows the program and produces a complete written record of all the stages preceding solution.

This record is compared with the spoken and written comments of the human subject. If the output of the machine and the human are reasonably close, it is presumed that the human is using the same program, or method of approach, as the machine. To the workers in this field, thinking is neither learning nor seeing, but is information processing. Information is given in the problem and is processed in the brain. The laws of thought constitute the program used by the brain.

Genetic or Historical Approach

Thinking in Children. In a series of studies extending over a 30-year period the Swiss psychologist Jean Piaget (1896–) has traced the growth of thought from infancy to adolescence. In infancy the development of thinking can be considered from two viewpoints: (1) learning how to act upon the world and (2) learning what the world is like.

Learning How to Act upon the World. At birth, the child is limited to reflexes involving grasping, sucking, looking, and hearing. Originally uncoordinated, these reflexes gradually mesh with each other—the child looks in the direction of sounds, grasps what he sees, and brings before his eyes that which he grasps. He learns to separate the components of acts. Thus grasping, first performed for its own sake, comes to be used as a means to an end, such as grasping to obtain a specific object. The highest point of this development, which signals the beginning of true thought, occurs when the child can perform "mental experiments." For example, when the child seizes a stick to bring an interesting object within reach, he has foreseen the entire action in his mind before actually grasping the stick. He is manipulating objects with his mind instead of his hands.

Learning What the World Is Like. The child at first is conscious only of sounds, images, and the pressure of objects against his skin. Persons do not exist, but are seen as faces that appear and disappear. Objects gradually emerge as the separate senses become coordinated, for example, as the sound and touch of a rattle become associated with its image. The crucial developments of this period occur when the infant searches for objects that disappear from sight (thus indicating that he knows they continue to exist) and when he anticipates the path of an object moving out of sight (as when an object passes behind a screen and the infant looks for it to emerge on the other side).

The Increasing Representation of the World in the Mind. The world moves "into" the mind, and consequently thought becomes less dependent on the world. This begins with the ability of the child to represent objects as images and thus to give them permanence. For example, he persists in searching for an object even if it is out of sight. A later profound development occurs when he learns the use of words. Initially the child regards the word as imbedded in the object. The word "sun" is considered almost as written into that heavenly body. Later the word is liberated from the object and the child recognizes that the sun could have been given any name.

A slightly different aspect of the inward movement of thought is revealed in a well-known experiment in which Piaget pours beads from a short, round container into a long, thin container. At one stage of development the child believes that the total number of beads has increased, although he has clearly observed that no beads were added or taken away during the passage from one container to another. Piaget attributes this to the inability of the child to take into consideration the fact that, although the column has become longer, it has also become thinner. The error results in part from the child's tendency to center his attention on the visually prominent length of the container.

Eventually his thought becomes liberated from direct perception and he becomes able to take into account both the width and height of the container. This progress from the concrete to the abstract can be observed again and again in mental growth and, interestingly, is often reversed in the case of brain injury when the victim may lose his capacity for abstract thinking.

The Increasing Complexity of Mental Processes. The earliest mental activities deal with images. More complex mental activities occur when the child can envision the use of a stick to reach a far object. A significant advance appears when symbols replace mental images in the course of the increasing abstractness of thought. This makes it possible for regularities of mental combination to emerge. Piaget refers to such regularities as "operation." To illustrate what is meant by this term we may return to the bead experiment. One of the difficulties the child faces, in addi-

tion to being rooted to the visual appearance of the long, thin column, is his inability to deal with situations in which changes in two dimensions compensate each other. Thus the child's mental experience up to this time enables him to consider that the object increases in height or decreases in thickness, but not that these changes occur simultaneously. Piaget calls this combining ability a multiplicative compensation. At the time the child learns this operation he will have reached the stage of mental development that will enable him to solve the bead problem.

Piaget further points out that operations do not exist independently in the mind, but combine into groups. The essence of the group and its importance as the principal instrument of thought is that eventually (at the level of "formal" thought) it permits the mind to move from the actual situation to envision all of the possibilities that could develop from that situation. Thus groups enable the chess player to construct possible moves, enable the scientist to construct experiments, and permit lawyers to examine the possible implications of new legislation. To Piaget problem solving becomes a question of which groups and operations are called into play to move from a problem to its solution.

Unity or Chaos: Do the Studies on Thinking Interrelate?

Both the casual reader and the student may properly ask if the studies on thinking described here relate to each other in any way at all, or if they are, as they seem, completely without connection.

Some understanding may be gained from considering the hypothetical situation of a group of social scientists who set out to study a newly discovered country. Each is determined to understand the society and each proceeds in a different way. One examines the economy and describes the country in terms of the flow of goods, the distribution of wealth, and the gross national product. Another studies the religious structure and considers the relation between church and state, the concept of parent-child relationships as structured by the church, and the religious legends and myths which flavor the arts. A third scholar concerns himself with the political structure—the legislative bodies, the distribution of power, and the selection of leaders. The fourth takes a historical approach and studies the growth of the society, including the evolution of its religion, its politics, and its economy.

The experimenters who based their work on rats in mazes, on perception, or on concept formation and computer studies may be compared to the scholars who study religion, politics, and economy. Each develops a view based upon the area he chooses to study and encounters difficulty when he attempts to expand his theory to describe thinking as a whole. In the same way the student of politics, religion, or economy would distort the picture of the entire culture if he attempted to describe it solely in terms of one of these areas. At the same time the theories may adequately describe the facts in their limited areas and are perfectly acceptable for that purpose alone.

Piaget's approach resembles that of the historical scholar, and for this reason may surpass the others in its ability to deal with a broad range of phenomena in the area of thinking. The interpretive power of Piaget's concepts has gradually become appreciated in the interna-

tional psychological community, and the extension of his ideas into the field of adult thought may eventually make possible the unification of thought on "thinking."
See also ASSOCIATION OF IDEAS; MEMORY.

THORAZINE [*thôr'ə-zēn*], trade name for chlorpromazine, a major tranquilizing drug used to reduce anxiety and agitation in mental illness, in alcoholic delirium tremens, and in certain cases of neurosis. Thorazine, in common with other tranquilizing drugs, produces sedation without causing extreme drowsiness or unconsciousness. It is also valuable as a pain reliever in combination with narcotics, as an antiemetic (to prevent vomiting), and as a treatment for hiccups. Side effects such as headache, lowering blood pressure and body temperature, and dizziness, palpitations, and jaundice may be seen. Thorazine enhances the effects of alcohol and consequently should not be given to persons under its influence.
See also TRANQUILIZERS.

THORNDIKE, EDWARD LEE (1874–1949), American psychologist known for his studies in animal learning and educational psychology. Thorndike tried to demonstrate the evolutionary hypothesis that the mind as well as the body has developed in the transition from lower to higher animals. His general method was to observe the amount of ability animals have in solving problems, specifically whether they could find their way out of puzzle boxes. He discovered that many animals learn by trial and error, initially finding the answer by accident. If the animal responds more quickly to the situation and the answer is repeated in the next trial, it has learned. From these findings Thorndike evolved the theory of connectionism, in which the animal makes a bond between a situation and a response. Reward is the factor that maintains and strengthens this bond.

Thorndike was connected with the Teachers College of Columbia University from 1899 to 1940. In the field of education he introduced intelligence tests which distinguished between the ability to learn and previously acquired knowledge. He demonstrated that the study of a particular subject, such as Latin, does not result in a general increase of learning ability. Rather, he found that transfer of knowledge occurred only in areas sharing common elements. Thus, knowledge of Latin roots can increase English vocabulary. This compartmentalized effect of training was in agreement with Thorndike's theory of intelligence, that mental abilities are independent of one another, so that someone with mathematical aptitude might lack verbal skill. This theory is in opposition to the general factor theory of the English psychologist, C. E. Spearman, which holds that a global intelligence factor ("G") underlies all mental capabilities.

TITCHENER [*tĭch'nər*], **EDWARD BRADFORD** (1867–1927), English psychologist who promulgated in America the psychological doctrine of structuralism, that is, that the mind is composed of elements, such as images, thoughts, and feelings. Titchener was trained at Oxford and in Leipzig, Germany. In 1893 he went to Cornell University in New York State, where he established a psychological laboratory. Although Titchener was a prominent figure in his time, his psychology did not exert any important influ-

ence after his death. His textbooks, though now outdated, testify to his thorough experimental approach and encyclopedic command of the field. Among the best known of his works are *Experimental Psychology* (2 vols., 1901, 1905) and *Elementary Psychology of Feeling and Attention* (1908).

TRANQUILIZERS [*trang'kwəl-īz-ərs*], group of drugs widely used in psychiatric practice to calm excited patients and to control anxiety. These compounds are distinguished from sedatives, such as the barbiturates, by their ability to calm the patient without producing extreme drowsiness or unconsciousness. They have been used to control psychotic patients, to combat alcoholic hallucinations and delirium tremens, and to relieve anxiety in some forms of neurosis. Since their introduction in the 1950's the tranquilizers have done much to quiet the previously tumultuous wards of mental hospitals. An important advantage of the drugs is their ability to make otherwise intractable patients suitable for psychotherapy.

The earliest and best known of the tranquilizers are the Rauwolfia alkaloids, which include reserpine, rescinnamine, and deserpidine. These are obtained from the roots of plants of the genus *Rauwolfia*, found in parts of the tropics. Less than one-thousandth of an ounce of reserpine can reduce excited or violent behavior and relax anxious or fearful subjects. A disadvantage of the drug is its tendency to produce serious depression. A medically important action of reserpine is its ability to lower high blood pressure.

Chlorpromazine, the best known of the phenothiazines, has the same general quieting effects as reserpine but is preferred because it is less likely to produce depression. It is also an excellent antiemetic (an agent used to reduce nausea and vomiting) and is widely used for this purpose. Both the Rauwolfia and the phenothiazine compounds are capable of causing undesirable side effects, particularly when given for prolonged periods. These effects include nervous disorders (Parkinsonism), attacks of low blood pressure, skin rashes, and jaundice.

A number of newer tranquilizers have been introduced, which, although differing in their properties, also produce sedation and quieting without marked drowsiness. These include meprobamate, phenaglycodol, and benactyzine. The manner in which tranquilizers produce their effects is still not understood. According to one theory, they alter the quantities of certain potent substances (for example, serotonin or acetylcholine) which are normally present in the brain.
See also PSYCHOPHARMACOLOGY.

TRANSFERENCE [*trăns-fûr'əns*], psychoanalytic concept describing the transfer to the analyst of attitudes and feelings which the patient once directed toward his parents, brothers, or sisters. This is considered an important part of the therapeutic process since it enables the patient to re-experience important past feelings and thus to gain greater understanding of his emotional difficulties and their origins.
See also PSYCHOTHERAPY.

TWINS, PSYCHOLOGICAL STUDIES OF. These have been largely concerned with exploring a long-standing controversy in psychology: the relative contributions of inheritance and environment to the development of the individual. Identical twins are particularly useful in this respect since they receive an identical inheritance. Fraternal twins are no more similar than nontwin brothers and sisters. Studies of identical twins, fraternal twins, and nontwins thus offer the possibility of assaying the importance of heredity and environment in determining intelligence, character traits, and other psychological characteristics. Conclusions from such studies rest on the assumptions that:

(1) Both heredity and environment are highly similar for identical twins (they are usually dressed in the same way and spend most of their time together).

(2) The environment for fraternal twins is also highly similar (they are also dressed alike, and so forth), but, as noted, their biological inheritance is not the same as in the case of identical twins.

(3) Nontwins differ in both heredity and environment (one child will be older than the other, may attend different schools, may have different friends, and so forth).

Thus in the three cases identical twins have identical heredity and environment, fraternal twins have different heredity and similar environment, and nontwins differ in both heredity and environment. Therefore differences between fraternal twins and nontwins can be attributed to the similar environment of the fraternal twins, and differences between fraternal twins and identical twins can be attributed to the similar inheritance of the latter.

Among the major findings of these studies are:

(1) In intelligence test scores, using a measure of similarity called a correlation (a correlation of 1.0 means both groups score the same), identical twins show correlations of about .90, fraternal twins about .65, and nontwins about .50. These correlations are similar, but smaller, for specific aptitudes.

(2) Certain mental abnormalities, such as schizophrenia, seem to be greatly influenced by heredity, as they are more likely to occur in identical twins than in fraternal twins or nontwins.

(3) For many psychological characteristics extreme differences are more likely to occur in cases of fraternal rather than identical twins.

V

VOCATIONAL GUIDANCE as a formal procedure is largely a 20th-century development. In the past, guidance in planning a career was often provided by parents or friends. A boy often chose his father's career or went to work for a relative or acquaintance in his town. For girls the expected career was as housewife and mother. In the present-day world there are thousands of jobs that were completely unknown a generation or so earlier. The U.S. Department of Labor *Dictionary of Occupational Titles* lists and describes more than 22,000. One effect of automation is to accelerate a trend toward reduction in the proportion of unskilled jobs and increase in the proportion of jobs that require special skills. More and more professional and technical jobs require four or more years of college training. Such preparation is so expensive in money as well as time that few people can afford to train for one field and then shift to an unrelated field. Choosing a vocation is one of the most serious decisions a man or woman makes—important to the country as well as to the individual. In American society economic and social status is to a great extent dependent upon occupation. Moreover, a suitable occupation can provide lifelong satisfaction to emotional as well as economic needs. Vocational guidance services are offered to help with these decisions. One of the major tasks of school guidance services is helping students plan appropriate and satisfying careers. Some tentative career choices have to be made in junior high school, so that the student can enroll in a suitable course of study.

Principles of Vocational Guidance

Vocational guidance involves studying the requirements of occupations and the qualifications of individuals and trying to match individuals with jobs or related groups of jobs. It also seeks to discover how people arrive at occupational choices. Many studies have been made of the characteristics of men and women employed in various occupations. One large-scale investigation (R. L. Thorndike and Elizabeth Hagen, *Ten Thousand Careers*, 1959) produced findings that were not on the whole surprising. College professors as a group ranked well above average on measures of general intellectual ability, reading comprehension, and visual perception and below average on measures of mechanical ability. Engineers ranked high on all factors, including mechanical ability. Architects stood high in visual perception—higher than artists and designers—and well above average in general intellectual ability. Accountants, auditors, treasurers, and comptrollers ranked high on measures of numerical fluency.

Such results must be considered with due caution. There are differences between job families—groups of related occupations—but there is also a wide range of abilities within an occupational group. Engineers as a group rank higher than machinists. The highest-ranking machinists,

however, score higher than the lowest-ranking engineers. Unusual ability is not by itself a guarantee of success in a field, nor does average ability necessarily doom a person to failure. Sustained interest, initiative, good health, stamina—such factors contribute to getting ahead in any vocation. The qualities that make some people so outstanding that they are called geniuses are not well understood. The fact remains, however, that people in related professional groups tend to have similar abilities.

The same generalization holds true for personality traits other than the abilities mentioned above. Salesmen, for example, tend to like social and athletic events. These findings match the stereotype of the salesman as outgoing, talkative, extroverted, a "good mixer" rather than a scholar. Again, a note of caution is in order because of the great variety of jobs and of individuals. Selling professional textbooks may require the attributes of a professor. Selling industrial machinery may require the background and interests of a mechanical engineer.

Studies of how people select jobs indicate that vocational choice is a developmental process rather than a single incident or act. Once the process has reached the point of decision, drastic change is difficult. The approach to the choice must be careful and realistic.

All vocational choices are determined by a combination of various forces. To differing degrees, in each individual, choice is influenced by the economic and social situation in which he has been reared. The amount and quality of education a man gets doubtless play a significant role as a vocational determinant. Vocational choice is highly influenced by emotional forces and personal needs. The ultimate choice, unconscious as it often is, is an achievement of self-fulfillment. The vocational role, especially in men, represents a life style of work which hopefully will provide maximum satisfaction. In making a vocational choice, the individual must balance limitations against opportunities. It is important for him to remember that any choice is inevitably a compromise.

Guidance Procedures

There is no certain and simple way to assess an individual and tell what vocation he is suited for. There is likewise no such thing as a sure predictor of success in a given career. One reason why success is difficult to predict is that the word means different things to different people. To a writer it may mean praise from the critics, or making money, or both. To an administrator, enlarged responsibility may mean success. Income is often used as a criterion of success, but incomes may vary greatly from field to field. Despite such variables, however, it is possible to assist an individual to review his strengths, weaknesses, interests, and preferences and match them against the requirements and rewards of varied professions. The counselor provides information and guidance, but the decision remains a personal responsibility. Professional procedures involve the following steps.

Studying the Individual. To make a realistic career plan for any individual it is necessary to have information about his physical health, level of intellectual ability, special abilities (as in art, music, or shop work), aptitudes, interests, and other personality traits (for example, does he like to work alone or as one of a group? Can he work long hours under pressure? Can he postpone immediate satisfactions in favor of efforts for long-range goals?). By the time a boy or girl reaches high school, much valuable information is already in school records.

Psychological testing is extensively used in schools, colleges, and guidance centers to provide one source for assessing the probability of success or failure in a vocation. Such tests are valuable in furnishing a personal picture of the individual not otherwise obtainable. Even when tests are interpreted by highly competent counselors or psychologists, however, they cannot indicate what single career an individual should pursue. They are actually measures of interest, intelligence, aptitude, and other traits. These measures alone cannot become *predictors;* that is, they cannot tell which occupation a person will be successful in. Combined with other information, such as individual likes and dislikes, test results can help rule out occupations that are most likely to be unsuitable and to suggest which ones will be most suitable for exploration prior to final choice.

The interests and preferences of high school students are likely to change. They show increasing stability with each additional year.

Analyzing Occupations. Vocational counselors divide jobs into categories such as "white collar," manual, service, and farming. These fields are subdivided. White collar occupations, for example, include professional and technical, managerial, clerical, and sales jobs. Career fields can also be grouped according to the level of ability required, the major interests involved, or the school subjects related to them. Counseling an individual means helping him to decide which broad field of work matches his qualifications and aspirations. Within the field he can narrow his choice to a specific occupation.

The Characteristics of the Field: What specific work is done? Who are the employers—industry, government, or universities? What special skills have priority (speaking, writing, designing, or organizing, for example)? Do many people work as individuals (as doctors do)? Are jobs clustered in some parts of the country or widely distributed?

Qualifications: Are physical strain and risks involved (as in forestry and mining engineering)? Are there health hazards (as in some branches of atomic physics)? Are certain personality traits necessary (interest in working with people is vital in teaching and social work, for example)? Is a license required (as for architects, physicians, pharmacists, psychologists, and civil engineers, to cite a few examples)? How many institutions give training courses accepted by the licensing body? What are the requirements of professional associations and labor unions in the field?

Education and Training: What is the minimum education required—technical school certificate, bachelor's degree, or master's degree? Is a doctor's degree essential for advancement? Is on-the-job training required after graduation from college? How much will education cost? Are fellowships, scholarships, loans, and government training programs available?

Income: What is the normal range of salaries for men in the field? For women? Do salaries vary markedly from employer to employer or from region to region?

Prospects for Employment: How many men and women are now employed in this field? Is it difficult for women to enter this vocation? Is the field growing? What factors affect the rate of growth (population growth, consumer demand for products, and government spending for research, to give a few examples)? What is the relation of supply of and demand for trained personnel in this field?

Matching the Individual to a Field. The third step in vocational guidance is to help the individual review his qualifications and preferences and match them against the requirements and attractions of a career field. The final choice, as already noted, is a compromise. After a young man or woman has sufficiently explored the realities of the world of work, it usually becomes evident that no one occupation can provide all the satisfactions desired or utilize all the interests and skills he or she possesses. On the other hand, certain careers demand more time and money for preparation than some people can afford. Frank consideration of the motivation, perseverance, and energy required to become successful may impose other realistic limitations on the final choice.

Counselors advise young people to think in terms of job families rather than of fixing all their hopes on one and only one occupation. Some young people, for example, want to be doctors but either cannot afford the lengthy training or fail to complete the course. An interest in medicine can still be put to good use in such related careers as pharmacy, nursing, occupational therapy, and medical technology. Some people make the mistake of pursuing their interests (or their parents' wishes) too far, striving to get into a vocation in which they cannot be successful. There is no value in spoiling a good technician to make a poor engineer. A white collar job is not necessarily preferable to a blue collar job. Moreover, scientists and engineers in all fields depend on the help of large numbers of technicians.

A general guide is that men and women should get as much training as they can benefit by. More and more professionals and technicians are needed, and the better positions tend to go to those who are ambitious and highly trained. Since training requires time, and basic courses must be taken as prerequisites to advanced courses, vocational planning should be done early and with all possible care. The degree of success of career planning affects both personal happiness and the efficiency of industrialized society.

See also GUIDANCE AND COUNSELING, EDUCATIONAL; TESTING, PSYCHOLOGICAL AND EDUCATIONAL.

W

WATSON, JOHN BROADUS (1878–1958), American psychologist known as the champion of behaviorism. Watson received his doctorate in 1903 and taught at Johns Hopkins from 1908 to 1920. His views were widely quoted in the press, helping to establish him as the leading American exponent of behaviorism. Watson held that complex feelings and emotions, such as love, are compounded out of simple habits built upon physiological needs of sex, hunger, and so forth. He also felt that thinking is based upon faint muscular contractions (internalized speech) and that the capacities of the individual depend almost exclusively on his upbringing. The latter view led him to declare that he could make any child entrusted to his care into a genius or a criminal by modifying the child's upbringing. His influence in American psychology later declined considerably, following the sustained assault of Gestalt psychology on behaviorist thinking.
See also LEARNING; PSYCHOLOGY; THINKING.

WEBER, ERNST HEINRICH (1795–1878), German physiologist known for his work on "Weber's law," the principle that noticeable differences in sensation occur when the stimulus is increased by a constant fraction of the original. For example, 1 lb. added to a 10-lb. weight might be perceived, but 5 lb. would have to be added to a 50-lb. weight in order for the change to be noted. This principle became a pillar of "psychophysics," the earliest branch of systematic psychology. He is also remembered for his investigation of the sense of touch and his description of the bones of the labyrinth of fishes.

WERTHEIMER [vĕrt′hī-mər], **MAX** (1880–1943), German psychologist known as the founder of the school of Gestalt (Ger., "pattern," "configuration") psychology. It stresses the existence of independent, unlearned, enduring patterns in thought and perception. Wertheimer received his doctorate at Würzburg in 1904 and taught at Berlin and Frankfurt. He fled the Nazis in 1933, joining the faculty of the New School for Social Research in New York City, where he remained until his death.
See also LEARNING; PSYCHOLOGY; THINKING.

WORLD FEDERATION FOR MENTAL HEALTH, organization which originated in 1920 as the International Committee for Mental Hygiene. The founders were Clifford Whittingham Beers, a leader in U.S. mental health programs, and Clarence Meredith Hincks, pioneer in Canadian programs. The present name was adopted in 1948. The federation co-operates with the World Health Organization on problems of mental health. Headquarters are in London.

WUNDT [vŏŏnt], **WILHELM MAX** (1832–1920), German philosopher and psychologist who founded the world's first psychological laboratory at the University of Leipzig in 1879. Wundt was a prodigious worker who contributed over 50,000 pages to the literature, ranging from works on logic and ethics to studies in physiological psychology and the massive 10-volume *Völkerpsychologie*, which treated the psychology of religion, language, and art. Wundt was by far the most influential psychologist of his day, and his laboratory attracted many students from abroad, among them future psychologists of great repute, including William James and E. B. Titchener. In 1881 Wundt founded the *Philosophische Studien*, the first journal devoted exclusively to psychology.

INDEX